NUTRITIONISM

ARTS AND TRADITIONS OF THE TABLE
Perspectives on Culinary History

NUTRITIONISM

THE SCIENCE AND POLITICS

OF DIETARY ADVICE

Gyorgy Scrinis

COLUMBIA UNIVERSITY PRESS   NEW YORK

COLUMBIA UNIVERSITY PRESS
Publishers Since 1893
NEW YORK   CHICHESTER, WEST SUSSEX
cup.columbia.edu

Library of Congress Cataloging-in-Publication Data

Scrinis, Gyorgy.
Nutritionism : the science and politics of dietary advice / Gyorgy Scrinis.
pages cm — (Arts and traditions of the table : perspectives on culinary history)
Includes bibliographical references and index.
ISBN 978-0-231-15656-1 (cloth : alk. paper) — ISBN 978-0-231-52714-9 (e-book)
1. Nutrition—Public opinion.   2. Food—Composition.   3. Functional foods.
4. Public health—Political aspects.   I. Title.

RA784.S435   2013
613.2—dc23   2012050819

Columbia University Press books are printed on permanent
    and durable acid-free paper.
This book is printed on paper with recycled content.

Printed in the United States of America

c 10 9 8 7 6 5 4 3 2 1

Cover design: Mary Ann Smith
Cover images: Food pyramid by Brian Hagiwara/Getty Images
    Laboratory bottle by Buena Vista Images/Getty Images

References to websites (URLs) were accurate at the time of writing.
    Neither the author nor Columbia University Press is responsible for URLs
    that may have expired or changed since the manuscript was prepared.

CONTENTS

ABBREVIATIONS

AHA   American Heart Association

ALA   alpha-linolenic acid

AMA   American Medical Association

AND   Association for Nutrition and Dietetics (formerly the American Dietetic Association)

BMI   body mass index

CSPI   Center for Science in the Public Interest

DASH   Dietary Approaches to Stop Hypertension

DHA   docosahexaenoic acid

DHHS U.S. Department of Health and Human Services

EPA   eicosapentaenoic acid

FDA   U.S. Food and Drug Administration

GI   glycemic index

GL   glycemic load

HDL   high-density lipoprotein

LDL   low-density lipoprotein

NAS   National Academy of Science

RDA   Recommended Dietary Allowance

USDA   U.S. Department of Agriculture

NUTRITIONISM

CHAPTER ONE

A Clash of Nutritional Ideologies

In appearance, colour, luster, and plasticity, margarine is superior to butter; in taste and flavor the recent improvements show excellent results. . . . The nutritional qualities of margarine, too, can be modified with comparative ease, either by action on the constituents of the fat phase, or by the inclusion of useful additives.

—ROBERT FERON, *MARGARINE,* 1969

Margarine has been the chameleon of manufactured food products, able to transform its nutritional appearance, adapt to changing nutritional fads, and charm unwitting nutrition experts and nutrition-conscious consumers.[1] While research published by nutrition scientists in the early 1990s on the harmfulness of the *trans*-fats in margarine temporarily unveiled its highly processed and degraded character, margarine has subsequently been reinvented as a *trans*-fat-free, cholesterol-lowering "functional food."

The history of margarine reflects some of the broader shifts in nutritional paradigms across three distinct eras of nutrition science and dietary advice over the past century and a half. From its invention by a French chemist in the late nineteenth century and up until the 1960s, the public generally regarded margarine as a cheap imitation of butter, and margarine was largely consumed by those who could not afford the real thing. The manufacturing of this highly processed spread involved hardening the vegetable oil by chemically reconstituting the polyunsaturated fats in the oil, a process that produces both saturated fats and novel forms of *trans*-fatty acids. A number of other ingredients were added to help simulate the appearance, taste, texture, and nutrient profile of butter, including yellow coloring agents and vitamins A and D.

In the early 1960s, American nutrition scientist Ancel Keys and others found evidence of an indirect relationship between saturated fats and the increased risk of heart disease. Saturated fats raised blood cholesterol levels, which in turn was associated with the increased risk of heart disease, while polyunsaturated fats decreased blood cholesterol levels. So began the idea of distinguishing between "good" and "bad" nutrients, and between "good fats" and "bad fats" in particular—signaling the emergence of a new nutritional era. Despite the preliminary nature of this new nutritional theory regarding saturated and polyunsaturated fats, such was the conviction of Keys and other advisors of the American Heart Association (AHA) that this discourse of good and bad fats eventually came to dominate not only dietary guidelines for heart disease but also the broader nutriscape.[2]

It was entirely on the basis of the emerging hypothesis regarding good and bad fats that many nutrition scientists came to promote those margarines manufactured from polyunsaturated-rich vegetable oils as "healthier" than saturated fat–rich butter. These experts considered the beneficial effects of polyunsaturated oils, and the detrimental effects of saturated fats, to be more important than the types of processing and additives used in the manufacture of margarine.

The promotion of margarine over butter by nutrition experts and manufacturers has exemplified a number of the features and limitations of what I call the ideology of nutritionism.[3] This ideology has framed and shaped nutrition science research since the late nineteenth century and has increasingly informed dietary advice, food labeling regulations, food engineering and marketing practices, and the public understanding of food. Nutritionism—or nutritional reductionism—is characterized by a reductive *focus* on the nutrient composition of foods as the means for understanding their healthfulness, as well as by a reductive *interpretation* of the role of these nutrients in bodily health. A key feature of this reductive interpretation of nutrients is that in some instances—and especially in the case of margarine—it conceals or overrides concerns with the production and processing quality of a food and its ingredients.

In the early 1960s, Keys himself had briefly raised concerns about the healthfulness of *trans*-fats and chemically hardened vegetable oils, having conducted studies showing that they seemed to raise cholesterol levels in much the same way as saturated fats did. But neither Keys nor many other scientists pursued this research into *trans*-fats and instead focused on stigmatizing the saturated fats that naturally occurred in many foods, particularly animal products.

The wheels only started to fall off the margarine bandwagon in 1990 when two Dutch scientists published a study claiming that *trans*-fats were in fact more harmful than saturated fats, since they raised so-called bad cholesterol in the blood (low-density lipoprotein, or LDL, cholesterol), while also lowering "good cholesterol" (high-density lipoprotein, or HDL, cholesterol).[4] In the following years, further studies were published by other researchers, including Walter Willett of the Harvard School of Public Health, that demonstrated an association between *trans*-fat consumption and the increased incidence of heart disease, as well as the role of *trans*-fats in promoting inflammation in the body and other detrimental health effects.[5] These studies directly contradicted the earlier advice of most nutrition experts that margarine was a healthier alternative to butter. In the name of improving the heart health of citizens, nutrition experts—by their own admissions—may have in fact been sending them to an early grave.[6] A new scientific consensus eventually coalesced around the idea that "*trans*-fats are bad fats" and are the worst fats of all, even more harmful than the supposedly "artery-clogging" saturated fats.

The history of margarine and *trans*-fats described thus far—and the reportedly harmful properties of *trans*-fats—should be fairly familiar to most readers. But what happened next illustrates how little has been learned from this *trans*-fat fiasco. Rather than opening up for questioning or challenging the reductive interpretation of foods in terms of their fat or nutrient composition, the *trans*-fat controversy has become an opportunity for nutrition experts to reinforce the nutritionism paradigm. The reference to *trans*-fats as bad fats, for example, has been used to reinforce and extend the language and assumptions regarding good and bad fats, as well as of good and bad cholesterol. Public health institutions such as the AHA have also used the *trans*-fat issue to reinforce their long-running campaign against saturated fats, even characterizing saturated fats as the more dangerous of the two fats because people consume more of it.

Importantly, the focus on types of fats has maintained the attention of nutrition experts and the public on the presence or absence of *trans*-fats in margarine, rather than on the processing techniques and ingredients used in its production. Since the mid-1990s margarine producers and other food manufacturers have reformulated their products, and fast-food restaurants have changed the oils they use for deep-frying, in order to reduce or remove the *trans*-fats. Yet few experts have questioned or alerted the public to the new techniques that margarine manufacturers are now using to solidify vegetable oils, or examined what the health implications of these alternative techniques and ingredients might be. In this "virtually *trans*-fat-free" era, food manufacturers now use a combination of techniques, including interesterification, fractionation, and full hydrogenation, to reconstitute and solidify the fats in vegetable oils. The hydrogenation process that produces industrial *trans*-fats is in many cases still being used, but in such a way as to avoid or minimize the creation of *trans*-fats. While the end product may have fewer *trans*-fats, it is not necessarily any less processed or chemically transformed: the fats have simply been reconstituted in another form. Interesterified fats—or *i*-fats for short—have come to replace some of the *trans*-fats in margarine and other products.

While the *trans*-fat controversy was unfolding throughout the 1990s, some margarine producers, such as Unilever, quietly began reducing the *trans*-fats in their products. But around this time they also simultaneously developed a premium line of "cholesterol-lowering" margarine products fortified with plant sterols. The production of these margarines involves adding highly processed plant components—sometimes derived from wood pulp—to an already heavily processed food product. These margarines and spreads are now permitted to carry the health claim, approved by the U.S. Food and Drug Administration (FDA), that they "may reduce the risk of heart disease."[7] These health claims are based on the same hypothesis linking blood cholesterol levels and heart disease risk that has informed dietary guidelines since the 1960s, rather than on any direct evidence that consuming these varieties of margarine leads to a reduction in the incidence of heart disease.

The idea that you can actively reduce your risk of heart disease if you consume these fortified products is characteristic of the present era of *functional nutritionism*. Rather than just avoiding the bad nutrients, the dominant nutritional discourse has now shifted to the goal of optimizing your consumption of beneficial nutrients. Rather than just aiming to be healthy, some of the imperatives of functional nutritionism are that you enhance your health and target particular bodily functions and processes. To achieve this enhanced and optimized state of health and bodily functioning, we must keep up with the latest nutrition research and expert advice if we are to identify the whole foods or processed "functional foods" that deliver the desired health benefits. The food industry is ideally placed to respond to and cultivate consumer demand for these health-enhancing functional foods.

NUTRITIONALLY REDUCTIVE SCIENCE
AND DIETARY ADVICE

The *trans*-fat fiasco is one of a number of cases of revisions and back-flips in scientific knowledge and dietary advice that have contributed to the common public perception that nutritional advice is constantly changing.

These revisions include advice regarding dietary cholesterol, eggs, low-fat diets, and beta-carotene supplements.[8] However, my critique of nutritionism is not based on a concern that nutrition scientists sometimes get it "wrong"—indeed, the claim that there is a clear-cut "right" answer or scientific truth regarding the health effects of nutrients is one of the features of nutritionism itself. The point is not that nutrition science has not yielded valuable insights into the relationships among nutrients, foods, and the body, but that these insights have often been interpreted in a reductive manner and then translated into nutritionally reductive dietary guidelines. This reductive interpretation includes the decontextualization, simplification, and exaggeration of the role of nutrients in determining bodily health.

It is also important to make clear that nutritionism and nutritional reductionism—as I define these concepts here—do not simply refer to the study or understanding of foods in terms of their nutrient parts. If that were the case, then all scientific research into nutrients, and all nutrient-specific dietary advice, would necessarily be reductive. Rather, it is the *ways* in which nutrients have often been studied and interpreted, and then applied to the development of dietary guidelines, nutrition labeling, food engineering, and food marketing, that are being described as reductive. This suggests that there are other (less reductive) ways in which nutritional knowledge could be developed and applied.

The past century and a half of scientific research has highlighted the immense complexity of relationships between food and bodily health. Foods are combinations of many nutrients and food components in various quantities and combinations. These nutrients may interact with other nutrients and other components within the body, and the health effects of a food may also depend on the other foods they are combined with in a meal. At the same time, various food processing techniques and additives may significantly transform—and in some cases reduce or degrade—the nutritional quality of whole foods. Understanding the health effects of this range of foods, additives, and processing techniques is also challenging because most bodily functions, diseases, and health conditions are likely to be affected by multiple dietary and nondietary factors. Single-nutrient deficiency diseases, for example—such as vitamin C deficiency causing scurvy—are now the exception rather than the rule in highly industrialized countries.

Despite the complexities of these food-body interactions, nutrition experts have consistently elevated their limited and often quite preliminary understanding of nutrients to the status of nutritional certainties or truths. From the nineteenth-century attempts by scientists to calculate the precise quantity of macronutrients and calories required for normal growth and to prevent deficiency diseases, this nutritional hubris has been extended to issuing definitive dietary advice for reducing the risk of chronic diseases, such as heart disease, cancer, and diabetes. More recently, nutrition experts claim to be able to identify the nutrients and foods capable of not only maintaining good health but also optimizing our health and enhancing specific bodily functions. This *myth of nutritional precision* involves an exaggerated representation of scientists' understanding of the relationships among nutrients, foods, and the body. At the same time, the disagreements and uncertainties that exist within the scientific community tend to be concealed from, or misrepresented to, the lay public.

A key characteristic of nutritional reductionism has been that nutrition scientists' understanding of nutrients has been systematically decontextualized. The role of nutrients has often been interpreted outside the context of the foods, dietary patterns, and broader social contexts in which they are embedded. Nutrition experts have, for example, made definitive statements about the role of single nutrients, such as the role of fat or fiber, in isolation from the foods in which we find them. This single-nutrient reductionism often ignores or simplifies the interactions among nutrients within foods and within the body. It has also involved the premature translation of an observed statistical association between single nutrients and diseases into a deterministic or causal relationship, according to which single nutrients are claimed to directly cause, or at least increase the risk of, particular diseases. Nutrition scientists have also tended to exaggerate any beneficial or detrimental health effects of single nutrients. For example, the detrimental effects of total fat, saturated fat, and dietary cholesterol—and the benefits of polyunsaturated fats, omega-3 fats, and vitamin D—have all, arguably, been exaggerated, if not in some cases seriously misrepresented, over the years.

Nutrition science has for much of its history been preoccupied with studying the naturally occurring nutrients found in whole foods, rather than the highly processed and novel foods and food components that have proliferated over the past century. At the same time, nutrition experts have promoted or vilified particular whole foods on the basis of their underlying nutrient profile, and according to the quantities of good and bad nutrients they contain. Eggs and butter, for example, have been stigmatized for their cholesterol or saturated fat content.

Yet the major changes in eating patterns since the early twentieth century have been toward an increase in the consumption of heavily processed foods containing highly refined, extracted, chemically transformed, and reconstituted ingredients. It is only during the past decade that some of these processed ingredients and foods have begun to be studied in a more systematic manner. It was not until the early 1990s, for example, that researchers began to pay serious attention to chemically reconstituted *trans*-fats. Until recently, the study of the precise metabolic consequences of high sugar consumption—beyond its caloric value—has similarly been neglected. There are also few studies that examine specific highly processed food products. Instead, nutrition scientists have primarily evaluated highly processed foods on the basis of the relative quantities of the so-called good or bad nutrients they contain, such as their vitamin content or lack of fiber. But this ignores the way processing techniques may also substantially transform and damage the original "food matrix"—that is, the unique combination of food components and the way they are all held together in a whole food.[9]

Since the 1970s, nutrition and public health experts have increasingly translated nutritionally reductive scientific knowledge into nutricentric dietary guidelines for the lay public. They have framed dietary guidelines and mainstream nutritional advice in terms of the need to consume more or less of particular nutrients and food components, telling us, for example, to eat more of the good nutrients (unsaturated fats, fiber, vitamins, calcium, and antioxidants) and less of the bad nutrients (saturated fats, *trans*-fats, cholesterol, refined carbs, and calories). This nutrient-level dietary advice inevitably involves a deliberate and pragmatic simplification of any more complex, detailed, nuanced, or multinutrient scientific knowledge.

The low-fat recommendation that dominated dietary guidelines in the 1980s and 1990s represents the pinnacle of this oversimplified, decontextualized, and exaggerated interpretation of single-nutrient advice. Most nutrition experts and institutions such as the FDA were unequivocal when telling the public that eating too much fat was a cause of obesity and a range of chronic diseases, regardless of the other nutrients, foods, or dietary patterns that the fat came packaged in. Many experts and the public alike assumed that eating reduced-fat foods of any kind was a healthier option than eating their full-fat equivalents, such as the replacement of full-fat with reduced-fat milk. The quality of the foods in which these fats were contained, and whether these fats were naturally occurring in whole foods or were added, transformed, or degraded during processing, were subordinated to concerns about the quantity or percentage of fat in these foods. The low-fat discourse has for many years also been challenged by its mirror image, the low-carb diet. However, many low-carb proponents have similarly decontextualized, simplified, and exaggerated the health effects of carbs.

Dietary advice and the everyday language we use to talk about food and dietary health has also been steadily colonized by a proliferation of nutritional categories and concepts. This nutri-speak has systematically replaced references to actual foods or to food quality. Nutrition experts typically use nutrient-level terms such as *empty calories, refined carbs, energy-dense,* and *high-GI* to refer to the nutritional character of refined and highly processed foods of poor nutritional quality, while the terms *nutrient-dense* and *low-GI* are often used as nutritional euphemisms for good-quality, whole foods.

THE COMMODIFICATION AND CORPORATIZATION OF NUTRITIONISM

Nutritionism has provided a powerful conceptual framework for transforming nutrients and nutritional knowledge into marketable food products and for further commodifying food production and consumption practices. Food manufacturers construct a *nutritional facade* around a food product, a facade for advertising some of the nutrients in the food product. (For definitions of this and other terms and concepts relating to nutritionism, see the appendix.) This nutritional facade distracts the attention of consumers from the ingredients, additives, and processing techniques employed in the production of the food. For example, highly refined breakfast cereals with 38 percent sugar content, such as Cocoa Krispies, are advertised as a "good source of vitamin D," a promotion of nutritional benefits common among cereal manufacturers.[10] Since the mid-1990s, in the United States and in other countries, government regulators have also allowed various types of direct health claims to appear on food labels and in food advertisements. This includes functional claims such as "calcium helps build strong bones" and disease prevention claims such as that the soluble fiber in oats reduces the risk of heart disease. These health claims further exaggerate the role of single nutrients, or of single foods, in the cause or prevention of diseases and other health outcomes.

The introduction of reduced-fat, low-calorie, and vitamin-fortified food products during the 1970s and 1980s has since diversified into the production of a broader range of nutritionally engineered foods with added food components that target a wider range of health conditions. This includes plant sterol–enriched cholesterol-lowering margarine and probiotic yogurt that improves gut health. Nutrition experts and the food industry often refer to these nutritionally engineered and marketed foods as "functional foods," since they supposedly enhance specific bodily functions or health conditions.

There is a deep complicity between nutritionism and the commercial interests of food manufacturers in the present era—a complicity that nutrition experts have been relatively slow to recognize. The food industry has certainly exploited nutrition science in various ways, such as selectively appropriating nutritional research, funding its own nutrition studies, and using government-endorsed health claims to market their products. However, the food industry has now also appropriated and taken control of the nutritionism paradigm itself and has become central to its maintenance, dominance, and public dissemination. Food corporations have colonized the nutriscape, flooding the food supply with nutritionally engineered products and nutritional marketing claims and accentuating the nutritional anxieties and nutritional needs of consumers—needs that these corporations are well placed to commodify and exploit. Yet many nutrition experts seem to ignore or be oblivious to this corporate capture of nutritionism, or corporate nutritionism.

A CLASH OF IDEOLOGIES

Back in the 1980s, it was nutrition experts' promotion of margarine over butter that led me to question this reductive interpretation of nutrients. At the time I was eating a mostly vegetarian diet, motivated by concerns for animal welfare and the environmental impacts of meat production. But I had also unquestioningly accepted the standard arguments of nutrition experts—and of the countercultural whole foods movement—that too much meat is essentially bad for your health due to its fat and saturated fat content, and so the less eaten the better.[11] My diet then (and still today) largely consisted of minimally processed, plant-based foods, including staples such as lentils, my home-baked sourdough bread, and eggs from our own free-ranging chickens.

However, my standard breakfast of a fried egg on buttered, white, sourdough toast seemed to break a number of the nutritional rules of the day, steeped as this meal is in saturated fats, cholesterol, and even so-called refined carbohydrates. Being told to spread margarine on my toast instead of butter did not sit well with the whole foods ideology I had embraced. I came to view this as a contradiction between my whole foods ideology and the ideology of nutritionism—a clash of nutritional ideologies. The focus on nutrients in scientific research and in dietary guidelines was producing what seemed to me to be some distorted dietary recommendations, and to be undermining obvious dietary choices. At the same time, food manufacturers were promoting their highly processed foods using nutrient content claims, and the meat and dairy industry had worked around the stigmatizing of saturated fats by focusing the public's attention on the protein, iron, and calcium in their products.

What surprised me more, however, was the lack of recognition or reflection on this ideology of nutritionism within the scholarly or popular literature on food and nutrition. Over the past fifty years, few nutrition experts have seriously questioned—or even raised as a topic for a sustained discussion—the reductive focus on nutrients per se within nutrition science and dietary guidelines.[12] Nutrition scientists have debated the merits of particular nutritional theories. Dieticians have focused on communicating this nutritional knowledge through nutrition education programs and dietary advice. Public health nutritionists have translated this taken-for-granted scientific knowledge into public health policies and strategies for changing food consumption patterns and the food supply itself. Many nutrition experts, as well as some food activist and consumer movements, have drawn on the dominant nutritional theories to highlight the poor quality of highly processed foods, such as their high fat content or lack of fiber. They have also criticized the food industry's manipulation and misuse of this nutritional knowledge to market their food products. Counternutritional movements, such as the low-carb diet and paleo diet communities, have arisen to challenge the nutritional orthodoxy of the anti-saturated fat and anti-meat hypotheses, though they have often merely put forward their own alternative nutrient-level advice. Occasionally, the reductive focus on nutrients has been commented on in passing in nutrition journals and commentaries, especially in the context of justifying the benefits of studying individual foods or dietary patterns directly. But apart from a few notable exceptions discussed later, food and nutrition experts have not closely examined the limitations and implications of nutritional reductionism.

The critique of nutritionism presented here is a product of my research into the philosophy and sociology of science and technology, social theory, and the sociology and politics of food. It draws on a framework I have developed for understanding scientific knowledge and technological relations in terms of how they are manifestations of distinct levels of engagement with nature.[13] Technologies of agricultural production and breeding, for example, can be distinguished in terms of whether they engage with and transform nature at the organic, chemical, or genetic levels. Applied to nutrition science, this framework highlights the way the nutrient level has been prioritized over the level of food and dietary patterns. It also focuses attention on the relationship *between* these levels of engagement with food, for example, the way that the comparison of foods at the more abstract level of nutrients may undermine or blur the qualitative distinctions we make at the level of foods, such as between minimally and highly processed foods, or between animal and plant foods. In this sense, the framework highlights and enables the examination of the ways in which the nutricentric approach to food has "effects," quite aside from the particular nutritional theories or advice being promoted.[14]

NUTRITIONISM AS PARADIGM AND IDEOLOGY

I have referred to nutritionism as an ideology as well as a paradigm in order to focus attention on how it represents a distinct, coherent, and systematic way of thinking about food and nutrition. The concepts of paradigm and ideology can each be used to highlight various features of this way of understanding and engaging with food and nutrients.

Scientific paradigms are the overarching worldviews, explicit theories, and implicit assumptions that frame a particular scientific discipline or body of ideas.[15] All scientific knowledge is generated within particular paradigms—or frameworks of understanding—that organize the study and interpretation of the world. There can be no purely objective, paradigm-free—or, for that matter, ideology-free—scientific knowledge and practices, since all scientific knowledge is necessarily an interpretation of the "facts" or the evidence. A scientific paradigm can also include the technologies, practices, and social structures and institutions associated with a body of ideas. Alongside the dominant paradigm within a particular scientific discipline, there are often other coexisting and competing paradigms, and every so often there can be major changes or revolutions from one dominant paradigm to another.

Nutritionism has, I argue, been the dominant paradigm of nutrition science since the mid-nineteenth century and has framed scientific research over the past century and a half. By the early twentieth century, nutritionism was beginning to infiltrate the public understanding of food and dietary health. By the 1970s, nutritionism had colonized and transformed dietary guidelines in its own image. By the 1980s, nutritionism had become a dominant strategy guiding the food industry's marketing practices. I divide this long history of nutrition science and nutritionism into three historical periods: the era of quantifying nutritionism, the era of good-and-bad nutritionism, and the era of functional nutritionism. Within these three eras, nutritionism has taken a distinct form, or paradigm. Each of these specific paradigms carries the same name as the eras in which they have been dominant—that is, the paradigms of quantifying nutritionism, good-and-bad nutritionism, and functional nutritionism. These particular forms or paradigms of nutritionism have defined how nutritional knowledge has been produced, interpreted, and disseminated within each of these eras.

In the era of quantifying nutritionism, running from the mid-nineteenth to the mid-twentieth century, the focus of nutrition scientists was on discovering and quantifying the nutrients in foods and the nutritional requirements of bodies. The aim of quantifying nutritionism was to identify the "protective" nutrients required for normal body functioning and growth, and particularly to prevent nutrient deficiency diseases. The era of good-and-bad nutritionism beginning in the 1960s was notable for the emergence of the novel idea of "good" and "bad" nutrients and for the emphasis on the need to avoid or reduce bad nutrients in particular. Negative dietary messages dominated this era, such as the low-fat campaign urging everyone to eat less fat. Dietary advice also shifted from the aim of preventing nutrient deficiencies to that of reducing the risk of chronic diseases, particularly heart disease. The present era of functional nutritionism began in the mid-1990s. Its distinctive feature is the rise of a more positive and targeted view of nutrients and foods as "functional" in relation to bodily health. Functional nutritionism also carries the expectation that particular nutrients, foods, and dietary patterns can enhance and optimize our state of health or particular bodily functions.

The key drivers and promoters of nutritionism have shifted across these three historical eras. The quantifying era was a time of prominent individual scientists who dominated scientific research and controlled the nutritional agendas, such as the German scientist Justus von Liebig and American scientists Wilbur Atwater and Elmer McCollum, and who established and promoted the reductive nutritionism paradigm. In the good-and-bad era of nutritionism, it was government and public health institutions, such as the U.S. Department of Agriculture, the FDA, and the AHA, that were instrumental in the establishment and promotion of nutricentric—and often simplified—dietary guidelines and food labeling regulations aimed at promoting dietary recommendations for reducing the risk of chronic diseases.

In the functional era, it is the food industry that has taken the lead in promoting nutritionism, through the nutritional marketing and nutritional engineering of their food products, their funding of nutrition research and of expert organizations, and their promises of health-enhancing and targeted foods. The power to define, shape, and promote the nutritional agenda has now decisively shifted from state institutions to food corporations. Many features of functional nutritionism enable food companies both to market their products and to cultivate consumer demand for these products. Food corporations' appropriation and control of nutritionism—or corporate nutritionism—also reflects the more widespread dominance of corporations across every sector of the global food system.

While nutritionism can be described as the dominant paradigm of nutrition science, I initially referred to nutritionism as an ideology because it reflects a number of characteristics of other political, social, or economic ideologies. For example, nutritionism constructs and preserves the scientific authority and material interests of nutrition experts, on the basis that only they are able to produce and interpret this scientific knowledge of nutrients. The authority of traditional and cultural knowledge of food, or of people's own sensual and practical experience with food, has been correspondingly devalued. The ideology of nutritionism also ultimately serves the financial interests of the food, dietary supplement, and weight-loss diet industries, by creating an extremely effective framework for commodifying and creating a new market for nutrients, nutritional knowledge, and nutritionally engineered products.

Nutritionism also functions as an ideology in the way it profoundly shapes how the lay public understands and experiences food. Nutritionism has produced *nutricentric persons*—the subjects of nutritionism—who identify with and respond to this ideology in various ways and who have come to see their own understanding and experience with food and their bodies mirrored in this approach to food. Nutricentric consumers are also more open and responsive to the nutritional marketing practices of the food, dietary supplement, and weight-loss diet industries.

The reductive focus on nutrients that characterizes this ideology is also embodied in the *nutritional gaze* of both the nutrition expert and the lay public. The nutritional gaze is a way of seeing and encountering food primarily as a collection of nutrients, and in terms of a set of standardized nutritional concepts and categories, such that it overwhelms other ways of seeing and encountering food.[16] Butter is encountered as full of artery-clogging saturated fats, milk as bone-building calcium, and broccoli as rich in protective antioxidants. Nutrition experts have focused their nutritional gaze on the food consumption practices of individuals and populations. They have also directed the nutritional gaze at—and increasingly within—the body, which is encountered and measured in terms of a number of internal and external biomarkers, such as blood cholesterol levels, blood pressure, blood sugar, insulin, and body mass index (BMI). However, nutricentric individuals have also increasingly adopted the nutritional gaze, often employing this gaze when wandering down the aisles of a supermarket, scanning the nutrient-contents claims on food labels.

Most of us are now nutricentric individuals to a certain degree. This is not to suggest that we uncritically believe and accept mainstream nutritional guidelines or nutritional marketing claims. Indeed, there has been a proliferation of counternutritional movements that challenge the status quo and that have been enabled and fueled by the growth of the Internet and the availability of diverse sources of information. Nor has the nutricentric view of food totally overwhelmed other ways in which we understand and choose healthy foods, such as on the basis of how it has been processed, or of the food knowledge embedded in our own cultures and traditions. Nevertheless, this nutricentric orientation has framed, and sometimes undermined, these other ways of knowing and engaging with food.

STRONG AND WEAK CRITIQUES OF NUTRITIONISM

A distinction can be drawn between strong and weak critiques of nutritionism among food and nutrition experts and commentators. The strong critique I develop in this book involves questioning how the scientific knowledge of nutrients and foods is generated and interpreted, how this knowledge is translated into dietary guidelines and food labeling regulations by government institutions and nutrition experts, and how this knowledge is utilized by food companies or weight-loss diet promoters to market their products. While some experts and commentators adopt such a strong critique of nutritionism, others adopt a softer or weak critique, focusing instead on the way scientific knowledge is mistranslated into dietary guidelines and thereby confuses the public, or is misused or exploited by food companies to market their products. While acknowledging some of the limitations of nutricentric or single-nutrient research, such weak critiques of nutritionism tend to exonerate or defend mainstream nutrition science and expert advice.[17]

An early and strong critic of some features of nutrition science was the late Canadian nutritional biochemist Ross Hume Hall. In his 1974 book *Food for Nought: The Decline in Nutrition*, Hall put forward an original analysis of what he called the "chemically biased nutrition paradigm." He focused on the way modern agricultural and processing technologies were degrading the nutritional quality of foods, such as by removing or chemically transforming foods and food components. But he argued that nutrition science had obscured, rather than shed light upon, this decline in food quality in the twentieth century.[18] Hall was not concerned with scientists' focus on nutrients per se, or with their biochemical level of engagement with food. Rather, he was critical of the way they had remained constrained within a narrow set of "outdated" chemically classified nutrient categories, such as polyunsaturated fats and protein. For Hall, this narrow focus on chemically defined nutrients had hindered the development of a deeper and more rigorous biochemical analysis of food:[19] "[This] concept of nutrition stems from nineteenth century studies that classify foodstuffs as proteins, fats, carbohydrates, and accessory factors. To nutritionists, protein is protein, whether in the form of a piece of beef steak or in the highly processed form of a synthetic bacon bit."[20]

Hall instead advocated a more detailed biochemical analysis of how modern food technologies and production methods were transforming and degrading these nutrients and food components. Unfortunately, his critique of nutrition science was not taken up and developed by other experts at the time. When Hall came to write his next and final book on food, a popular nutrition guide called *The Unofficial Guide to Smart Nutrition* published in 2000, he seemed satisfied that nutrition science had progressed to the point that it is now supposedly able to offer a more comprehensive and adequate biochemical analysis of food and its effects on bodily health. In this book, Hall explained his dietary recommendations from the perspective of what he called the "cell's eye view" of food and nourishment, including recommending dietary supplements for a range of claimed health benefits.[21] Nevertheless, his focus remained on the quality of foods, and he developed a classification system for differentiating foods based on the level and type of processing they are subjected to, which will be discussed in chapter 9.

The nutrition educator and advocate of sustainable food production systems Joan Dye Gussow has long been a critic of the nutricentric focus of nutrition education and dietary guidelines. In occasional articles and lectures since the 1980s, Gussow has emphasized some of the limitations of nutricentric research and the nutrition confusion that may result from the attempt to convey dietary information in nutritional terms.[22] She has noted, for example, the futility of trying to educate the public to understand the dizzying array of novel food products on the supermarket shelf by urging them to study the nutrition facts panel. Gussow has also been a strong and early advocate for broadening the scope of nutrition and dietary guidelines to integrate ecological issues.[23]

Nutritional epidemiologist David Jacobs has emerged as the most consistent scientific critic of nutritional reductionism in recent years. In a series of coauthored academic papers, Jacobs and his colleagues have highlighted the limitations of the reductive focus on single nutrients within scientific research for explaining diet-disease relationships. He argues that one of the problems with this focus on single nutrients is that it tends to "oversimplify a complex system and even does harm."[24] He instead emphasizes the synergies that occur among nutrients within foods, and the need to study foods simultaneously at the level of nutrients, foods, and dietary patterns. Nevertheless, Jacobs otherwise relies on standard epidemiological and metabolic research in support of these food-level and dietary-level studies.

Some nutrition experts have been more inconsistent in their criticisms of aspects of nutritional reductionism. Nutritional epidemiologist Colin Campbell, for example, has been critical of "scientific reductionism" within nutrition research, and particularly of the attempts to explain chronic diseases by studying single nutrients in isolation. He instead emphasizes the importance of studying foods and dietary patterns in a way that takes into account interactions between nutrients. Now retired, Campbell's own research involved using broad epidemiological data on large populations to identify causal relationships among foods, nutrients, and health. Despite Campbell's criticisms of scientific reductionism, his characterization of all animal foods as detrimental to health leads him to interpret any piece of nutrient-level, food-level, or dietary-level data as definitive evidence for the harmfulness of animal foods. For example, in his recent popular book *The China Study*, Campbell has no hesitation indicting cholesterol and all animal proteins as dangerous to human health and arguing that "eating foods that contain any cholesterol above 0 mg is unhealthy."[25]

The best-known and most influential American public health nutritionist, Marion Nestle, has criticized the food industry's manipulation of dietary guidelines and nutrition information to promote its products. In her seminal book *Food Politics: How the Food Industry Influences Nutrition and Health*, Nestle gives a compelling account of the way the food industry has shaped the form and content of national dietary guidelines and food labeling regulations. For example, she documents how the "eat less" messages of the government's dietary guidelines usually make reference to nutrients (e.g., eat less saturated fat) rather than to actual foods (e.g., eat less meat) so as not to offend the food industry.[26] She is particularly critical of the food industry's use of nutritional marketing and health claims to promote highly processed foods. Nestle has also noted the limitations of single-nutrient research: "Nutrition arguments are almost invariably about single nutrients taken out of their food context, single foods taken out of their dietary context, or single risk factors and diseases taken out of their lifestyle context."[27] However, Nestle also defends many aspects of the dominant nutritional paradigm and its prevailing single-nutrient theories, such as the low-fat and low–saturated fat dietary guidelines.[28] In recent years Nestle has focused on the calorie and the energy-balance equation—that is, calories in minus calories out—as the nutritional certainty that explains weight gain and loss. At the same time she downplays the uncertainties, inconsistencies, and changes in the scientific evidence and dietary advice over the past fifty years. Nestle instead presents any limitations in dietary guidelines—and the nutrition confusion that the lay public seems to experience—as primarily the result of the food industry's distortion of otherwise sound scientific knowledge, and of governments' eagerness to appease the food industry.[29]

Each of these critics mentioned so far has tended to focus on particular aspects or manifestations of nutritional reductionism, rather than on the broader nutritionism paradigm as I define it. Their critical interventions have also remained largely isolated, rather than referencing and building upon one another's work. It is also worth noting that most of the critics of reductionism within nutrition science that I have referred to—and who directly engage with the limitations of the science itself—are themselves either nutrition scientists or public health nutritionists rather than social scientists. Other food experts and academics who have examined the nutricentric focus of nutrition science include historian Harvey Levenstein's two volumes on the history of food and eating in America, *Revolution at the Table* and *Paradox of Plenty*, and Warren Belasco's *Appetite for Change* on the food and the counterculture in America in the 1960s and 1970s. In the United Kingdom, journalist turned public health nutrition expert Geoffrey Cannon has also been a consistent critic of the "chemical principle" in nutrition science and food labeling.[30]

It is journalist Michael Pollan's number one best-selling 2008 book *In Defense of Food* that has by far had the greatest impact in bringing the critique of nutritional reductionism, as well as my nutritionism concept, to a wide American and international audience.[31] His book has also brought this critique to the attention of many nutrition and food experts and has sparked and focused debate in academic as well as popular forums.[32] Pollan's book has been effective in highlighting the nutricentric focus of nutrition research and dietary advice and the exploitation of nutritional knowledge by the food industry. He emphasizes how difficult it can be to conduct nutrition research and to isolate the role of particular nutrients. Pollan draws on some of the characteristics of nutritionism I have identified in earlier work, such as the way it forms a coherent ideology or overarching framework, the blurring of qualitative differences among foods, and the framing of nutrients into good and bad types. He also draws on the work of Joan Dye Gussow, Marion Nestle, and others to identify some of the consequences of this reductive focus on nutrients. Yet for all his success in popularizing some of the general limitations of a reductive focus on nutrients, Pollan's understanding of my nutritionism concept is somewhat limited and misconstrued. The analysis of nutritionism he presents is at times deeply inconsistent and contradictory. He often repeats and reinforces, rather than questions, a number of conventional nutritional arguments and characteristics of the nutritionism paradigm.

Pollan often uses the terms *nutritionism* and *reductionist* to refer to all scientific research and knowledge relating to nutrients, rather than to a particular way in which nutrients and foods have been studied and interpreted.[33] Indeed, because he defines reductionism so broadly and loosely, he even sees reductionism as a necessary, and perhaps the only, means by which scientists can gain nutritional knowledge.[34] For Pollan, the problem with nutrition science is not so much the *way* it studies and interprets nutrients, but that the nutritional advice it generates has so often been "spectacularly wrong."[35] He suggests that "it has seldom been the case" that nutrition science and the policy recommendations based on that science have been "sound."[36] Pollan thereby adheres to a view of scientific knowledge as essentially "right" or "wrong" rather than understanding that scientific knowledge is always an interpretation of the world that is based on particular paradigms or ideologies.[37] His characterization of nutrition science as a rather primitive and inaccurate science is reinforced by his quip that this science "is today approximately where surgery was in the year 1650—very promising, and very interesting to watch, but are you ready to let them operate on you?"[38]

Yet having spent the first part of *In Defense of Food* largely dismissing nutrition science as being hopelessly inaccurate and misleading, Pollan inexplicably spends the rest of the book drawing fairly uncritically on the very same body of nutrient-level science in order to support his criticisms of the so-called Western diet and to explain the health benefits of whole foods, such as that some whole foods contain more omega-3 fats. Nor does he provide another way of interpreting this nutrient-level knowledge, instead continuing to draw on mainstream scientific research—including nutrient-level, food-level, and dietary-level studies—that has been generated with the same experimental protocols and assumptions that he otherwise derides.

Pollan not only questions the accuracy and usefulness of most nutrient-level scientific knowledge and dietary advice but also puts forward the surprising claim that this advice has been seriously detrimental to public health, arguing that "most of the nutritional advice we have received over the last half century (and in particular the advice to replace the fats in our diets with carbohydrates) has actually made us less healthy and considerably fatter."[39] Yet Pollan's own specific dietary advice—eat food (i.e., minimally processed foods), mostly plants (i.e., eat less animal foods), not too much (i.e., eat fewer calories)—merely repeats most nutrition experts' standard dietary advice over the past 50 years.[40] His mantra borrows from and combines Joan Gussow's suggestion to "eat food" with Marion Nestle's advice to "eat less; move more; eat fruits, vegetables and whole grains; and avoid too much junk food."[41]

In these respects and others, Pollan tends to repeat and reproduce both the form (the nutricentric justification) and the content (the specific advice) of mainstream nutritional discourses. For example, Pollan suggests people are getting "fatter" and "sicker" because they are eating a so-called Western diet—which he defines as a diet high in meat and processed foods. Yet his description and explanation of diet-related health problems are thoroughly conventional, repeating the standard explanations of nutrition experts since the 1970s, including their conflation of animal foods and processed foods as the twin causes of ill health. Even his conflation of being "fat" with being "sick" uncritically accepts and repeats the dominant "obesity epidemic" discourse promoted by many nutrition and public health experts. Pollan also suggests that mainstream nutritional advice, such as the low-fat campaign, can somehow carry much of the blame for these dietary patterns, as if such advice were a primary driver of the increase in consumption of highly processed foods since the 1980s. He thereby exaggerates the influence that dietary guidelines have over people's consumption practices. Pollan even seems to endorse the arguments of low-carb proponents such as Gary Taubes that it is the carbs, rather than the fats or calories, that make us fat, thereby simply buying into an alternative nutrient-level explanation for obesity.

Due to its popularity, *In Defense of Food* has been an important intervention in nutrition discourses and dietary debates in the United States, particularly for bringing some of the limitations of nutritional reductionism to a broad lay and expert audience. However, it also illustrates the need to go beyond just the focus on nutrients in scientific research and dietary advice, and whether the experts get it "right" or "wrong," and instead to identify and critically examine the various characteristics and assumptions of the nutritionism paradigm and the various forms of reductionism it promotes.

From Nutritionism to the Food Quality Paradigm

There are many reasons beyond a concern for personal health why we eat the foods we do, such as pleasure, convenience, cost, and cultural tradition. Even in terms of health, nutritional knowledge is by no means the only way in which nutrition experts and the public identify healthful foods. Another common approach is food production and food processing quality—that is, in terms of how a food has been grown and raised, or processed and prepared. Many laypeople—and nutrition experts—trust in the healthfulness of whole and minimally processed foods, as well as of fresh, organically grown, and free-range produce, and are fully aware of the disvalue of many types of fast foods and highly processed foods.

Over the past couple of decades there has been a growing emphasis within popular and expert food discourses on the need to eat what is now often simply referred to as "real food," and which typically means whole, "natural," or traditional foods. This demand for real food has in fact become a movement—and an ideology—in its own right. People's ability to regularly eat these types of foods is often limited by their relatively high cost, limited availability and accessibility, the demand for convenience, or inadequate time for preparation, rather than a lack of understanding or appreciation of their healthfulness. Food manufacturers have also responded to this widespread demand for whole foods by redesigning and marketing their products with a focus on the presence of "whole" and "natural" ingredients.

While the nutricentric and real food approaches have sat alongside each other, and are in many respects compatible, there has also been considerable tension between them. Nutrition experts and mainstream dietary guidelines have long promoted whole and minimally processed foods as the most healthful foods, though primarily on the basis of the quantities of the beneficial nutrients they contain. However, the reductive focus on nutrients at times displaces and contradicts a more straightforward appreciation of food production and processing quality. The food industry's ability to appropriate and manipulate this reductive understanding of food for their own ends has accentuated and intensified this contradiction at the heart of the nutritionism paradigm.

These limitations and contradictions—in particular, the contradiction between nutritionism on the one hand, and food production and processing quality on the other—have created a crisis of legitimacy for nutritionism. It is out of this ideological contradiction that opposition and alternatives to nutritionism may arise, even if this contradiction has not yet been clearly identified or articulated by food or nutrition experts or the various food movements.[42] One manifestation and response to this contradiction has come from nutrition experts' belated interest in studying foods and dietary patterns in their own right. Public health experts and institutions are also increasingly challenging the food industry's exploitation of nutritional labeling and marketing to sell junk foods, particularly to children. The loss of legitimacy of conventional nutritional theories and mainstream dietary advice manifests in the growth of counternutritional or counterdietary movements since the 1990s, such as the low-carb and paleo diet movements.

At the same time, many nutrition experts have attempted to address some of the limitations of nutritionism—and to defend and reassert the dominant paradigm—through the development of new, more sophisticated, and nuanced nutritional theories and concepts, such as the concept of nutrient density, nutrigenomics, nutrient profiling systems, and claims to ever greater scientific precision at the molecular level of food and the body. This has in fact precipitated the shift to the present era of functional nutritionism and to the claim of experts and food manufacturers to be able to deliver enhanced and targeted health benefits and personalized dietary advice. In some respects, functional nutritionism, on the one hand, and the real food or food quality movements, on the other, represent two divergent responses to the limitations of nutritionism since the 1990s.

If the nutritionism paradigm now stands in contradiction to a proper appreciation of food quality, then the alternative paradigm outlined in this book places food production and processing quality at the center of our understanding of the relationship between food and bodily health, and subordinates and reinterprets—rather than rejects—the scientific understanding of nutrients. I define the *food quality paradigm* as such a framework for integrating four distinct approaches to food and the body: food production and processing quality, traditional-cultural knowledge, sensible-practical experience, and nutritional-scientific analysis. Traditional dietary patterns and cultural knowledge, for example, can act as a guide for preparing and choosing tasty and healthful foods, for combining foods and food groups, and for giving a sense of the proportion and quantity of foods to consume. The selection of foods on the basis of sensual experience and the practical experience of growing and preparing foods are other ways of coming to know and appreciate healthful foods and diets.

In terms of evaluating food processing quality, beyond generic terms such as *whole foods*, *highly processed foods*, and *junk foods*, we lack a set of more precise terms and categories to distinguish between levels of food processing. I will identify three categories of foods in terms of the types of processing they have been subjected to, with each representing a shift to more refined, extracted, concentrated, reconstituted, and degraded food products. The first category is whole, minimally processed, and beneficially processed foods and ingredients, such as fermented whole grain bread, whole milk, and eggs. The second category is refined and processed foods that contain relatively concentrated quantities of refined or extracted ingredients, such as cane sugar, vegetable oils, white flour, and poorer-quality minced meat. The third category is processed-reconstituted foods, which are foods that have little if any direct relation to whole foods but have instead been reconstructed—from the ground up—out of the deconstituted components of whole foods, refined or extracted ingredients, and other reconstituted or degraded ingredients and additives. Such detrimentally processed ingredients and foods include *trans*-fats, artificial flavors, deep-frying oils that have been repeatedly used, and reconstituted meat products such as chicken nuggets.

The food quality paradigm does not deny the usefulness of nutrition science or nutritional knowledge but instead offers a framework within which to contextualize the scientific knowledge of nutrients, foods, and dietary patterns. For example, dietary studies can be designed to compare foods and dietary patterns in terms of the level and types of processing they are subjected to. We ultimately require different ways to conduct and interpret nutrition science and to translate that scientific knowledge into dietary guidelines. In part, this involves a reorientation of scientific research to the study of food and dietary patterns, a shift that has already started to occur over the past decade. But it also means conducting and interpreting nutrient-level, food-level, and dietary-level knowledge in a less reductive manner and addressing a number of limitations of nutritionism, such as the tendency toward the decontextualization, simplification, exaggeration, and determinism of these scientific insights. The food quality paradigm is a framework within which to interpret nutritional and scientific research and to translate this research into dietary guidance, food labeling regulations, and food and nutrition policies. However, given the power of food corporations within the contemporary food and nutrition system, any challenges to nutritionism will require not only very different understandings of food and the body but also strategies to combat the power of such corporations to exploit this nutritional knowledge and to shape government policies.

The aim of this book is to present a distinct philosophy and social theory of nutrition, one that interrogates forms of nutritional knowledge and their manifestations in scientific research, dietary guidance, food industry practices, and personal identities. I identify the various characteristics of nutritionism through a critical examination of the history and debates in nutrition science, dietary advice, and nutritional marketing in the United States over the past century and a half. I review the scientific literature, expert debates, government-issued dietary guidelines and reports, popular books, and public discourses on food and nutrition in the United States. This includes an examination of the diet-heart hypothesis, weight-loss diets, the reduction of food to calories, the low-fat campaign, the counternutritional low-carb and paleo diet approaches, the history of margarine and *trans*-fats, the mania over vitamins, the *Dietary Guidelines for Americans*, the *Food Guide Pyramid*, the celebration of the Mediterranean diet, nutrition and health claims and nutrition labeling on food packaging, functional foods, and the new science of nutrigenomics. I also examine the various forms that nutritionism has taken within the three eras of nutrition science I have identified. In the final two chapters, I consider alternative approaches to food and nutrition and outline the features of the food quality paradigm. In the course of the book I introduce and define a number of concepts, terms, and categories I have developed to help identify the characteristics of nutritionism and of other approaches to food quality. These are gathered together in the Nutritionism and Food Quality Lexicon in the appendix.

Throughout the book the term *nutrition experts* is used to refer to nutrition scientists, trained dieticians, and public health experts and institutions that conduct largely independent research or translate this research into dietary advice, nutrition education programs, or nutrition policies.

Nutrition experts are the recognized experts in the nutrition field who enjoy the trust of governments and the lay public and are perceived to be relatively independent from commercial interests. They include university-employed nutrition scientists, registered dieticians, public health nutritionists, and public health institutions such as the AHA and the federal committees that put together national dietary guidelines and food labeling and marketing regulations. These experts can be distinguished from the scientists and dieticians in the direct employ of food companies, the promoters of popular weight-loss diet books, and other parties that either lack the requisite qualifications or have direct financial interests in promoting food products or dietary supplements.

While nutritionism has been the dominant paradigm framing expert research and dietary discourses since the nineteenth century, nutrition experts do not equally adopt or embrace all aspects of this paradigm. Some public health nutritionists have been more critical of the narrower biochemical focus of nutrition science than have others. The New Nutrition Science project, for example, was launched in 2005 by an international network of nutrition experts who advocate that nutrition science needs to better integrate the biochemical, environmental, and socioeconomic dimensions of nutrition.[43]

Nutritionism has framed nutrition science and dietary discourses in many countries, particularly in the United States, Canada, Europe, the United Kingdom, Japan, and my own country of Australia. I have chosen to explore nutritionism through the history of nutrition and food in the United States for a number of reasons. American scientists and institutions have been at the forefront of nutrition research internationally since the late nineteenth century and have therefore shaped nutrition science and dietary guidelines worldwide. America has a rich and well-documented history of nutrition and dietary debates and controversies over dietary guidelines and weight-loss diets. The American public itself has led the way in embracing and incorporating nutritional knowledge and scientific eating practices, from the early twentieth-century obsessions with calorie counting and vitamania to the low-fat and low-carb diet fads of today. Yet perhaps for this reason, it is also the country in which an explicit challenge to nutritionism is beginning to emerge.

CHAPTER TWO

The Nutritionism Paradigm

Reductive Approaches to Nutrients, Food, and the Body

High protein levels can be bad for the kidneys. High fat bad for your heart.
Now Reaven is saying not to eat high carbohydrates. We have to eat something.
—ROBERT SILVERMAN, 1986

For Robert Silverman of the National Institute of Diabetes and Digestive and Kidney Diseases, the question of what we should eat had come down to a choice between proteins, fats, and carbohydrates. Silverman was responding to a presentation by Stanford University nutrition scientist Gerard Reaven at a 1986 diabetes conference, at a time when nutrition experts were promoting a low-fat/high-carb diet as a means of addressing diabetes, heart disease, cancer, and obesity.[1] But far from helping people with diabetes, Reaven argued that a high-carb diet could pose further risks to their health. Silverman's frustration was that the scientific research into fats, carbohydrates, and proteins was progressively ruling out all of the three main courses available on the nutritional menu.

Silverman's comment that "we have to eat something" is tongue-in-cheek, but it still articulates a key assumption of the dominant nutritional paradigm—that the health effects of foods and dietary patterns can adequately be understood in terms of their nutrient composition, independently of the specific types of foods or dietary patterns in which they are found. The macronutrient profile of foods in particular—that is, the ratio of fats, carbohydrates, and proteins—remains one of the touchstones of nutrition research and dietary advice and is assumed to reveal important truths about foods and their implications for bodily health.

The way nutrition experts have understood and ranked fat, protein, and carbs has changed significantly during the three eras of nutrition science.

In the era of quantifying nutritionism—running from the mid-nineteenth to the mid-twentieth century—nutrition scientists celebrated protein for its role in promoting and accelerating growth. In the era of good-and-bad nutritionism, beginning in the 1960s, scientists turned their attention to the role of different types of fats and carbohydrates in foods and their roles in heart disease and other chronic diseases. Ancel Keys, in particular, led the vilification of saturated fats as the "bad fats" that promoted heart disease, while polyunsaturated fats assumed the role of the "good fats." National dietary guidelines also promoted "complex" carbohydrate foods over "refined" or "simple" carbohydrates such as white flour and sugar. By the 1980s, the more simplified idea that "all fats are bad" and "all carbs are good" had overshadowed this distinction between good and bad fats and carbs. The 1980 *Dietary Guidelines for Americans* and the 1992 *Food Guide Pyramid* presented the low-fat/high-carb diet as the best means for reducing the risk of heart disease, cancer, and diabetes.[2] Low-carb, high-fat diets such as those promoted by Robert Atkins also formed a countermacronutrient strategy throughout that era.

In the present era of functional nutritionism that began around the mid-1990s, many nutrition experts have quietly acknowledged that the low-fat/high-carb advice was oversimplified, confusing, and potentially harmful to public health, particularly if it led people to eat more foods high in refined grains and sugars. Instead, mainstream dietary guidelines have shifted back to the "good and bad fats" and "good and bad carbs" discourse, though these good and bad nutrients are no longer framed exactly as they were in the 1960s and 1970s. *Trans*-fats have joined saturated fats in the "bad fats" category, while nutrition experts now celebrate one family of polyunsaturated fats—the omega-3 fats—for their supposed ability to reduce the risk of heart disease and other chronic conditions while also enhancing the health of the brain and other bodily functions. The good and bad carbs discourse has also come to the fore, with some nutrition experts now defining bad carbs as either the "refined carbs" or those with a high glycemic index (GI). Meanwhile, for its claimed ability to satisfy our appetites, protein has reemerged as a prized nutrient in a number of weight-loss diet plans.

The common assumption running through these dietary recommendations and weight-loss plans is that we can adequately explain the health implications not only of individual foods but also of dietary patterns simply by looking at their macronutrient profiles. Subscribers to this view consider that once the ideal macronutrient ratio has been established, the actual foods we choose to eat to achieve the optimum macronutrient profile are more or less irrelevant. From this perspective, foods are primarily viewed as interchangeable vehicles for the delivery of isolated nutrients.

In this chapter I introduce and examine some of the general characteristics and limitations of the nutritionism paradigm. This examination includes an analysis of the various forms of nutritional reductionism with respect to nutrients and the body (summarized in appendix table A.1), as well as how they have transformed the way scientists and the public think about food and dietary health. Nutricentric terms, for example, now dominate scientific and popular dietary discourses and blur, undermine, or even replace food-level terms and distinctions. These nutritionally reductive ways of understanding food have been translated into reductive food production practices, such as nutrient-fortified food products and nutritional supplements. Here I also outline the different forms nutritionism has taken in three historical eras.

Nutritional Reductionism

Nutrition scientists have given us great insights into the nature and health effects of foods and food components. They have helped us to better understand many nutrient deficiency diseases, such as scurvy, rickets, and anemia, as well as the nutrients and foods required for growth and bone health, such as protein, calcium, and vitamin D. But scientists have a necessarily incomplete understanding of the nutrient composition of foods, the complex interactions among nutrients and other components within foods, and the ways in which the body—and, indeed, different bodies—metabolizes these nutrients and foods.

Some of the inherent limitations in conducting nutrition research make it difficult for scientists to understand these relationships and interactions. These limitations include the challenges of monitoring and precisely measuring the dietary intake of individuals and populations and of isolating from confounding factors the health effects of particular nutrients, foods, or dietary patterns. In dietary intervention studies, for example, any attempt to modify the intake of one nutrient or food invariably alters the intake of other nutrients and foods. For instance, given that foods are combinations of proteins, fats, and carbohydrates, adopting a reduced-fat diet usually leads to an increase in the proportion of carbohydrate intake.[3]

One way to frame the various ways of understanding food and bodily health is to identify them in terms of distinct *levels of engagement with food and the body.*[4] I distinguish three levels of engagement with food: the nutrient level, which refers not only to nutrients but also to food components and to the biochemical composition of foods; the food level, which corresponds to the level of single foods, food groups, and food combinations; and the dietary level, which refers to the level of the overall dietary pattern or cuisine.[5] This framework for distinguishing among levels can be used to highlight the characteristics of each of these levels, as well as the relationships between levels.

Engaging with food at the level of nutrients can be described as a more abstract way of encountering food since it involves a less embodied level of engagement.[6] We generally do not directly engage with nutrients through our unaided senses. Instead, scientists bring to bear technoscientific instruments that mediate their understanding of food and its effects on the body. Nutritional categories, such as protein and carbs, are themselves abstract concepts—they abstract from the characteristics of particular types of foods as they present themselves to our unaided senses. These abstract nutritional categories also cut across the distinctions among types of foods and food groups, such as between plant and animal foods, and between whole and highly processed foods, in the sense that all of these foods are encountered as just different combinations of nutrients. While this more abstract nutrient level of engagement with food gives us new insights into food composition and quality, at the same time it potentially conceals other (more concrete) perspectives or levels of understanding and engaging with food.

There are a number of ways in which nutrition science—and modern science more generally—has been described as reductionist, although this term is often employed loosely, and without precise definition.[7] Reductionism is typically used to refer to any attempt to study the role of single nutrients or other components of food. Some nutrition scientists consider the study of foods in terms of their component parts as a strength of nutrition science and a feature of the scientific method.[8] By contrast, others highlight some of the limitations of this focus on single nutrients, such as that it may obscure the complexity of the composition of foods and diets and "fails to adequately describe the multiplicity of metabolic effects on the entire organism."[9] In short, "the whole is more than the sum of its parts" is the refrain of these critics of reductionism.[10]

I define nutritional reductionism as referring to both the reductive focus on the nutrient level and the reductive interpretation of the role of nutrients in bodily health. I also distinguish between two forms, or orders, of nutritional reductionism, which otherwise tend to be conflated or confused in discussions of reductionism in nutrition science: a first-order reduction to the nutrient level, or *nutrient-level reductionism*, which refers to the reduction from the levels of food and dietary patterns to a dominant and often exclusive focus on this nutrient level; and a second-order reduction within the nutrient level, which typically takes the form of *single-nutrient reductionism*.[11] Some of the characteristics of the reductive interpretation of nutrients are the decontextualization, simplification, fragmentation, and exaggeration of the role of nutrients and a deterministic understanding of nutrient-health interactions.

Nutrient-level reductionism—and the nutritionism paradigm in general—is where the nutrient level becomes the dominant level of understanding food, such that this level does not merely inform and complement but instead tends to undermine, displace, and even contradict other levels and other ways of understanding and contextualizing the relationship between food and the body. It carries the assumption that the healthfulness of foods can be adequately studied—and translated into dietary advice—on the basis of the quantities of some of its nutrient components. However, this reductive focus on nutrients does not give due attention to the quality of foods and what kinds of processing they might have undergone, or to the broader cultural contexts within which food is consumed (including traditional and culturally specific understandings of the healthfulness of foods), or to what we learn about food and nutritional quality through our senses and practical experiences of eating, preparing, or growing food.

This nutrient-level reductionism has often taken the more simplified form of single-nutrient reductionism, whereby individual nutrients are analyzed in isolation from other nutrients and food components, as well as from foods and dietary patterns. This single-nutrient reductionism also commonly carries the assumption that single nutrients can be extracted or synthesized and then consumed in isolation from particular foods, such as in the form of nutritional supplements or nutritionally fortified foods.

Nutrients are decontextualized in the sense that they have typically been studied and interpreted by scientists out of the context of the foods and dietary patterns in which they are consumed. Single nutrients are studied in a fragmented manner and assumed to exert specific health effects regardless of the other nutrients or foods they are combined with or embedded within. One expression of this nutritional decontextualization is the macronutrient reductionism referred to earlier, whereby nutrition experts and weight-loss diet book authors search for a diet with the optimal macronutrient ratio, as if the actual foods consumed to achieve this macronutrient profile are more or less irrelevant. Similarly, the reductive understanding of food and the body in terms of calories—or caloric reductionism—assumes that eating 100 calories of sugar has the same impact on a person's body weight as eating 100 calories of carrots. This is captured by the *everyday nutritionism*—that is, the oft repeated nutricentric expression—that "a calorie is a calorie."

The quantitative logic that pervades the nutritionism paradigm also tends to focus on even small differences in the quantity or proportion of desirable or undesirable nutrients found in foods and to exaggerate the health implications of these quantitative differences. An example of such ostensibly precise evaluations is the interpretation of the glycemic index (GI) of foods—a quantitative measurement that predicts how a food will increase a person's blood glucose levels. For instance, leading Australian GI researcher Jennie Brand-Miller encourages people to switch from jasmine rice (GI = 87) to basmati rice (GI = 57) purely on the basis of their respective GI scores—and regardless of what other foods these rice varieties are consumed with—as if such a substitution between varieties of white rice will make a meaningful difference to their blood sugar levels or overall health.[12]

The tendency to prematurely interpret an association between nutrients, foods, or biomarkers and health conditions as a one-to-one, cause-and-effect, deterministic relationship can be referred to as *nutritional determinism*. While this cause-and-effect model was useful and effective in identifying single-nutrient deficiency diseases in the early twentieth century, our understanding of the diet-related causes of chronic diseases, such as heart disease and cancer, has proven to be less amenable to this nutritionally deterministic model.[13] For example, nutrition scientists have interpreted the "diet-heart hypothesis," which links saturated fats to elevated blood cholesterol levels and, in turn, to atherosclerosis and increased risk of cardiovascular disease—as a series of cause-and-effect relations.[14] Yet arguably, we still do not know how (or even whether) saturated fats directly cause heart disease.[15] As discussed in chapter 4, nutrition and medical researchers have more recently shown that the association between fats and cholesterol levels, and between blood cholesterol levels and heart disease risk, is more complex than the original diet-heart hypothesis suggested.[16] At the same time, they have identified a number of other dietary influences on blood cholesterol levels, such as *trans*-fats, refined grains and sugar, and an insufficient intake of omega-3 fats. They have also suggested other biochemical pathways linking dietary components and heart disease, such as oxidative stress and chronic inflammation, thereby downplaying the importance and focus on blood cholesterol levels as a causal factor.[17]

The saturated fats and blood cholesterol story highlights how early scientific evidence on the health effects of particular nutrients can lead to an overemphasis or exaggeration of the role of these nutrients, particularly in the absence of evidence on other food components, known or unknown. These initial hypotheses have often been interpreted and presented as nutritional certainties, as if they are based on a precise understanding of the role of nutrients and foods in the body—what I have referred to as the myth of nutritional precision—and without acknowledging the limitations, uncertainties, and debates over this knowledge. As more nutrient-health interactions have been uncovered, a more complex understanding of food, nutrients, and the body has been constructed. Yet definitive pronouncements of the precise role of single nutrients or food components continue to be a feature of scientific publications and dietary guidelines for the public. The U.S. Food and Drug Administration's (FDA) approval of health claims for these single food components—such as that soy protein or soluble fiber reduce heart disease risk—illustrates this form of nutritional exaggeration.

Scientists' study of single nutrients is not in itself necessarily reductive. Indeed, the identification of single-vitamin deficiency diseases demonstrates the value of studying foods at the level of nutrients. Nevertheless, single nutrients can—and often have—been studied and interpreted in a fragmented and nutritionally reductive manner. For example, while in the early twentieth century scientists discovered that certain single vitamins were essential for preventing particular diseases, they did not necessarily understand the various interactions among vitamins and other food components, interactions that scientists to this day are still coming to appreciate.

The limitations and possible dangers of taking single nutrients out of the context of the foods in which they are contained are illustrated by the beta-carotene supplement controversy. In the early 1980s, carotenoid-rich colored plant foods, such as carrots, had been associated with the reduced risk of some cancers. Some scientists suspected that beta-carotene—one of many carotenoids in these foods—was the active nutrient that may have inhibited cancer growth.[18] In the absence of specific studies on the cancer effects of beta-carotene, the U.S. National Research Council's 1982 report *Diet, Nutrition and Cancer* attributed the apparent benefits of carotenoid rich foods to their beta-carotene content. This knowledge of the claimed benefits of beta-carotene was then translated into the nutrient-level practice of consuming beta-carotene supplements. However, subsequent clinical trials in the early 1990s involving people given high doses of beta-carotene supplements failed to support this hypothesis and even found that they were associated with an increased risk of lung cancer.[19]

Dietary advice at the nutrient level also tends to be delivered one nutrient at a time, since any more complicated advice regarding multiple nutrients and their interactions would be harder to convey, and might not be readily understood by members of the lay public. For example, the low-fat advice that dominated dietary guidelines in the 1980s and 1990s was in part intended by nutrition experts to be a simplification of the more nuanced advice to reduce the consumption of saturated fats, as well as calories. These experts considered the distinction between types of fats to be too complex for the public to digest.[20]

The distinction between nutrient-level and single-nutrient reductionism can be illustrated with the types of nutrition labeling commonly found on the front and back of food packaging. The Nutrition Facts label on the back of packaged foods is a product and a symbol of nutrient-level reductionism. The panel lists the quantities of a range of nutrients contained in foods, and this nutrient information typically appears much more prominently and in larger type than the ingredients list below it. This labeling presents nutrient-level information as the true indicator of the healthfulness of the food product and tends to deflect attention from the types of ingredients, additives, or processing techniques used in its production.[21] Despite the level of detail the Nutrition Facts label presents, its nutrient-level information is also limited and incomplete. For instance, it fails to distinguish between nutrients intrinsic to the ingredients in the food and those added during processing.[22]

Single-nutrient reductionism, on the other hand, is represented by the often-inflated nutrient-content claims on the front of packaged foods that focus on the presence or absence of single nutrients, such as "low fat" or "high in calcium." These front-of-pack nutrient claims implicitly promote both forms of nutritional reductionism: first, they shift attention from the ingredients list to the nutrient composition; and second, they shift the focus from the overall nutrient profile of the food to the presence or absence of particular nutrients. The food and diet industries have been the most enthusiastic proponents of this single-nutrient reductionism as a strategy to market their products.

Surprisingly few scientific studies have focused on foods or dietary patterns in their own right, although such studies have become more common over the past decade. When foods and dietary patterns have been examined, scientists have often reduced their claimed health effects to the action of particular nutrients. Nutrition researchers have tended to look for the active nutrients in foods and dietary patterns that explain their health effects, such as the presence of saturated fat or cholesterol in animal foods, the antioxidants in fruits and vegetables, or the monounsaturated fats in the olive oil–rich Mediterranean diet.

In recent years, nutrition scientists' criticisms of single-nutrient reductionism have become more common, as have their calls for more complex and integrated models for understanding food and the body. These models include studying the interactions among nutrients in foods, as well as studying foods, food combinations, dietary patterns, and cuisines.[23] Nutritional epidemiologist David Jacobs from the University of Minnesota has coauthored a number of papers critical of reductionism within nutrition research, particularly in terms of its focus on single nutrients: "Nutrition science has favored a reductionist approach," writes Jacobs, "that emphasizes the role of single nutrients in diet-disease (or diet-health) relations."[24] He argues that the single-nutrient focus of much scientific research tends to "oversimplify a complex system," since single nutrients interact "synergistically" with other nutrients and food components within a "food matrix."[25] Particular phytonutrients in plant foods, for example, may produce their beneficial effects only in synergy with other phytonutrients and food components in these foods. The results of long-term clinical trials on beta-carotene and vitamin C supplements have also shown the potential for detrimental health outcomes when single nutrients are isolated from the food matrix in which they belong and when they have been consumed in concentrated forms.

For Jacobs, the evidence thus demonstrates that "food synergies are important: the compounds in question are parts of foods that appear to be healthy, but do not work outside their food matrix."[26] His main concern with this form of reductionism is that it impedes the development of more accurate scientific knowledge. A more fruitful approach, he suggests, is to study the interactions among nutrients in the context of the natural food matrix in which they are found, as well as the synergies found in combinations of single foods and in broader dietary patterns.[27] This more integrated research into nutrients, foods, and the body is likely to yield new, more detailed—and perhaps more robust—scientific knowledge. Such attempts to integrate these levels of understanding food are examined further in chapter 10. However, food-level and dietary-level studies can also potentially reproduce some of the limitations and problems associated with nutrient-level reductionism and with the nutritionism paradigm more generally, as I will discuss in chapter 7.

NUTRIENT MARKERS AND CONFOUNDERS OF FOOD QUALITY

A significant problem for nutrition researchers analyzing epidemiological data is addressing the so-called confounding of results. This confounding occurs when the nutrient, food, or dietary pattern under investigation is strongly associated with other dietary and nondietary factors. When two variables are strongly correlated, their individual effects are difficult to untangle. Despite the sophistication of scientists' statistical models, it is a challenge to adjust for these confounding factors, especially when a nutrient is strongly correlated not only with other food components but also with overall dietary patterns.[28] In these situations, the health benefits or detrimental effects of one food component may be mistakenly attributed to another food component, or the positive or negative impacts of a food component may be greatly exaggerated.

A number of types of confounding occur in nutrition studies. Some nutrients or food components may commonly be packaged together within particular foods, such as beta-carotene, vitamin C, and other antioxidants that are contained in many fruits.[29] Similarly, two nutrients or foods may be strongly correlated within particular dietary patterns.[30] For example, in the 1950s and 1960s when epidemiologist Ancel Keys found an association between saturated fat consumption and heart disease in a number of countries he studied, he argued for a causal association between them. At about the same time, the British physiologist John Yudkin found that sugar, too, was correlated with heart disease in a number of countries and put forward the rival hypothesis that high sugar consumption was a key cause of heart disease. Yudkin also observed that in the countries he studied, saturated fat consumption was strongly correlated with sugar consumption, and therefore fat and sugar may be mutually confounding variables.[31] So, was heart disease caused by fat, by sugar, by the synergistic combination of fat and sugar, or by neither?

Many nutrients and food components are closely correlated within either good- or poor-quality diets, and this may exaggerate or otherwise distort the apparent health effects of a nutrient or food. Some nutrients can therefore act as reliable *nutrient markers of food quality*. For example, a good-quality diet might include whole or minimally processed foods such as fish, free-range eggs, whole meat, richly colored vegetables, and whole grain bread, and tends to be high in vitamins, fiber, omega-3 fats, anti-inflammatory agents, and antioxidants. In this case, a high omega-3 intake is likely to be associated with—and is in this sense a nutrient marker of—a good-quality diet. The health benefits that have been attributed to a high omega-3 fat intake in many studies may therefore be due to, or amplified by, its association with other beneficial nutrients and foods. Similarly, some stigmatized nutrients or foods—such as saturated fat or red meat—may be associated with an overall poor-quality (highly processed) diet, with such confounding leading to a kind of "guilt by association."[32]

NUTRITIONAL LEVELING AND THE BLURRING OF QUALITATIVE FOOD DISTINCTIONS

The nutrient level of engagement with food abstracts from the qualitative distinctions between types of foods, such as between minimally processed and highly processed foods, between fresh and preserved foods, or between animal- and plant-based foods. At this more abstract nutrient level, these qualitative distinctions between types of foods are flattened out and blurred, or *nutritionally leveled*. Within the nutritionism paradigm, foods are instead ranked and compared on a one-dimensional scale, based on the relative quantities of beneficial or harmful nutrients they contain. Within this nutritionally leveled playing field, highly processed or fabricated foods can—on the basis of the presence or absence of particular nutrients—be considered "nutritionally equivalent" to, or even healthier than, whole foods.[33]

In his 1974 book *Food for Nought*, Ross Hume Hall argued that nutrition science had failed to shed light on the way modern agricultural practices, and food processing techniques and additives, had degraded the nutritional quality of foods. Instead, he argued, scientists had remained focused on a narrow set of chemically classified nutrient categories that were developed in the nineteenth century, particularly fats, carbohydrates, and proteins. In doing so, they had largely ignored the way these nutrients and other food components were being technologically transformed. Hall also noted the interrelated developments in food labeling in the early 1970s. The U.S. Food and Drug Administration (FDA) had passed new regulations that mandated a Nutrition Facts label on many food products. At the same time, the FDA also deemed that the long-standing requirement that "imitation foods" be explicitly labeled as imitations would no longer apply in cases where the imitation was deemed to be "nutritionally equivalent" to the original.[34] This new ruling allowed food manufacturers to manipulate the nutrient composition of foods in order to achieve nutritional equivalence and to thereby "balance the numbers," as Hall put it.[35]

While blurring the qualitative distinctions between types of foods, nutritionism also creates a quantitative hierarchy of foods *within* particular food categories and can thereby accentuate and exaggerate the differences between foods within the same category. Within the category of plant-based whole foods, for example, some vegetables and fruits, such as broccoli, are celebrated as "superfoods" for their relatively high concentrations of antioxidants. Within the category of animal-based whole foods, dietary guidelines have valued chicken meat and fish for their high polyunsaturated and omega-3 fat content and have devalued red meat, full-fat milk, and cheese because of their saturated fat content. Within the category of processed foods, nutritionism encourages the consumption of nutritionally engineered or nutritionally "improved" products—such as low-fat, low-calorie, or *trans*-fat-free varieties—rather than simply eating less of these foods.

NUTRIENT-DENSE LANGUAGE AND NUTRI-SPEAK

The pattern of nutrient inadequacy in the face of caloric excess is the result of nutrient-poor food choices, too many energy-dense foods, and sedentary lifestyles.
—ACADEMY OF NUTRITION AND DIETETICS, "NUTRIENT DENSITY: MEETING NUTRIENT GOALS WITHIN CALORIE NEEDS," 2007

Nutrition experts' reductive focus on nutrients is also evident in the nutricentric language and terminology they have developed to describe foods and dietary patterns. The above statement from the Academy of Nutrition and Dietetics (AND, formerly the American Dietetic Association) is an attempt to describe the nature of the standard American diet entirely using nutrient-level terms—that is, in nutri-speak—without actually referring to foods or food groups. They describe foods as "nutrient-poor" and "energy-dense," while dietary patterns are described in terms of their "nutrient inadequacy" and "caloric excess."[36]

Nutrition experts have introduced a range of terms to refer to the nutritional quality of foods, such as nutrient density, energy density, high or low glycemic index, empty calories, discretionary calories, refined carbs, and, more recently, solid fats and SoFAS (solid fats and added sugars).

Their language for talking about foods has itself become nutrient dense, even if many of the foods Americans consume are not. This suggests that nutrition experts are more confident and comfortable speaking of nutrients, while seemingly avoiding wherever possible having to refer to foods. This is perhaps understandable, given that much of the scientific research they draw upon is indeed focused on the nutrient level.

The nutricentric focus of dietary guidelines has often favored the food industry. Marion Nestle argues that since the late 1970s the American agencies responsible for publishing dietary guidelines have avoided referring by name to the foods they recommend the public eat less of, largely in order to appease food companies who sell these products.[37] Instead, some of these nutrient-level recommendations act as euphemisms for particular foods. Whereas "eat less beef" called the meat industry to arms, "eat less saturated fat" did not. "Eat less sugar" sent sugar producers right to Congress, but that industry could live with "choose a diet moderate in sugar."[38] Dietary guidelines still urge the public to eat less sugar, salt, saturated fat, and refined grain yet rarely mention the highly processed foods and beverages in which these food components tend to be concentrated.

Since the 1990s, the AND and other nutrition experts have promoted the idea that there is "no such thing as good and bad foods, only good and bad diets."[39] The food industry, too, is particularly fond of this expression, because it suggests that no single food should be vilified in terms of its health impacts, and that even the poorest-quality foods can form a part of an overall healthy diet.[40] However, despite their reluctance to make clear statements and definitive judgments about the quality of foods in good/bad terms, the AND and most other nutrition experts are willing to describe nutrients as definitively good or bad. Food quality is thereby reduced to the "quality" of the nutrients contained, by which nutrition experts typically mean the ratio and quantity of so-called good and bad nutrients in a food, rather than the way the foods have been produced or processed.

One of the latest nutricentric terms introduced by the U.S. Department of Agriculture (USDA) is *solid fats*, which refers to animal fats and hydrogenated vegetable oils that are high in saturated fats and *trans*-fats and are therefore solid at room temperature. The term *solid fats* was used extensively for the first time in the 2010 *Dietary Guidelines for Americans*, which urged people to drastically reduce their consumption of these fats. For the USDA, the term *solid fats* performs two functions. In providing a single category to refer to the two "bad fats," the term collapses the distinction between naturally occurring saturated fats and chemically reconstituted *trans*-fats.[41] The term also acts as a nutritional euphemism for the foods that contain saturated or *trans*-fats and thus avoids reference to animal foods or to the types of processed foods that may contain these fats.

A number of calorie-centric terms are currently in use by nutrition experts, such as *empty calories*, *discretionary calories*, and *energy density*. The term *empty calories* is used to refer to foods and beverages that lack many beneficial nutrients yet provide ample calories. The term was originally coined in 1970 to refer to sugary and highly processed breakfast cereals that had been stripped of beneficial nutrients.[42] It is now more commonly used to describe sugary sodas that contain mostly sugar and water. However, in recent years some nutrition experts, and the 2010 *Dietary Guidelines for Americans Committee Report*, have also started to define empty calories so as to include not only foods high in added sugars but also foods high in "solid fats" (i.e., saturated fats and *trans*-fats).[43] Some whole foods high in saturated fats, such as whole milk, cheese, and fatty cuts of meat, are thereby stigmatized as empty calories, despite being rich in a range of beneficial nutrients.[44]

Another nutricentric term that deserves close examination is *refined carbohydrates*, which is commonly used by nutrition experts to refer to two types of high-carb foods that have been through a refining process: refined grains and extracted/refined sugars. Within the discourse of good and bad carbs, refined carbs are designated the bad carbs or poor-quality carbs. Experts began to use the term *refined carbohydrate foods* in the 1950s and 1960s, but by the early 1970s they had shortened it to *refined carbohydrates*.[45] British surgeon Thomas Cleave was one of the first to use this shortened phrase in his 1975 book *The Saccharine Disease*, in which he argued that the steep rise in consumption of refined flour and sugar throughout the twentieth century was responsible for an increased incidence of many chronic diseases. Low-carb diet pioneer Robert Atkins also used the term *refined carbs* in his 1972 book *Dr. Atkins' Diet Revolution*.[46]

The term *refined carbohydrate foods* correctly refers to the way the carbohydrate-rich foods themselves have been passed through a refining process, and is a way of distinguishing between, say, whole wheat and refined wheat. At the level of nutrients, however, a distinction between whole carbs and refined carbs is not so clear-cut. Refined grain and whole grain both contain fiber and other classes of carbohydrates found in the outer shell, although in refined grains the amount of many types of these fibrous carbohydrates is greatly reduced. While refined grains are stripped of many—though not all—of their vitamins and minerals, they retain much of their protein. This overlap in the nutrient composition of whole and refined grains makes distinguishing between them at the nutrient level less clear-cut.

By grouping together refined grains and refined sugars, the term *refined carbs* also suggests that these two types of foods have similar nutritional characteristics and effects on the body. But while there may be some similarities in terms of their health effects, the term conceals important differences between them. Refined grains, such as white rice and white wheat flour, largely consist of starch (quickly broken down to glucose in the body) but still contain other beneficial nutrients such as protein and some fiber and vitamins. But sugar (sucrose) is little more than pure, concentrated fructose and glucose and has no other nutritional benefits.[47] In the 1970s British nutrition scientist John Yudkin refused to use the term *refined carbohydrates* precisely because it gives "the impression that white flour has the same ill effects as sugar."[48] Unlike Cleave, Yudkin considered sugar to be far more harmful to health than refined grains.

NUTRITIONALLY ENGINEERED AND TRANS-NUTRIC FOODS

So far I have been describing the various reductive ways of understanding nutrients and foods. But it is not only how we think about and describe food, but also the practical ways in which we engage with and produce food, that can be nutritionally reductive. Over the past forty years, the food, pharmaceutical, and alternative health industries have increasingly translated nutricentric scientific knowledge into nutritionally reductive technological products, in the form of nutritionally engineered foods or dietary supplements. Dietary supplements are the purest expression of a nutritionally reductive technological practice, since the nutrients or other food components they contain not only have been technologically isolated but also are then consumed in isolation from any particular foods. In this sense, supplements represent the materialization of a more simplified, single-nutrient reductionism. In the case of vitamin supplements, for example, a particular fraction of a complex of vitamins may have been extracted or synthetically produced, thereby representing the further simplification, isolation, and reduction of the vitamin in comparison with the form in which it is contained and consumed in foods. Many nutrition experts continue to recommend a multinutrient supplement as a nutritional insurance policy for individuals perceived to be consuming inadequate diets.[49]

Foods that have been nutritionally engineered differ to some extent from supplements in that the added nutrients are consumed along with other nutrients and food components contained within the foods. In some cases, food manufacturers enhance or reduce a nutrient already present in the food, such as in the case of low-fat milk or vitamin C–fortified orange juice. In other cases, however, they introduce nutrients not otherwise found in that particular food (or only in very small quantities), such as adding plant sterols to augment dairy products and margarine, calcium to orange juice, and vitamins to water.[50] I refer to these food products as trans-nutritionally engineered foods—or simply *trans-nutric foods*—as they involve the transfer of nutrients across recognized food categories or boundaries.[51]

The nutritional engineering of foods is a *nutritional techno-fix* for the perceived nutritional inadequacies of foods and diets and for the health problems associated with them. However, there is good reason to question the health benefits and effectiveness of these nutrient-fortified foods. The claimed benefits of the added or subtracted nutrients may be exaggerated and taken out of the context of the role they play within broader dietary patterns. To the extent that these nutritionally engineered products "work," in many cases they may work in a nutritionally reductive manner. While these foods will deliver to the body a substantial dose of extracted or synthesized nutrients and food components, the way the body metabolizes these nutrients may be compromised if they are not consumed with the other nutrients and food components we get when we eat the whole foods in which they are otherwise contained.[52]

The nutritional modification of foods in order to "improve" their nutrient profile can, in some cases, lead to the further degradation of the quality of the food, such as the replacement of whole food ingredients with refined-extracted and processed-reconstituted ingredients. For example, the incentive to produce reduced-fat foods in the 1980s and 1990s often led manufacturers to replace naturally occurring fats with chemically modified starches, refined and artificial sugars, or artificial fats such as Olestra, in order to mimic the taste and texture of fat. Similarly, manufacturers have used calorie-free artificial fats and artificial sweeteners to produce reduced-calorie foods.

BIOMARKER REDUCTIONISM AND REDUCTIVE APPROACHES TO THE BODY

Nutrition science's reductive approach to food and nutrients has also been accompanied by an equally reductive approach to understanding the body and bodily health. Just as nutritionism breaks foods down into their component parts, so too does it represent the body in terms of its component parts and biochemical and genetic processes. Since the 1960s, nutrition experts have focused on a relatively small number of internal biomarkers (biological markers) of disease risk. They include the measurement of LDL and HDL blood cholesterol levels, blood sugar levels (hemoglobin A1c, and the glycemic index), hormones such as insulin and leptin, the energy requirements of the body measured in calories, and the body mass index (BMI).[53]

The reductive approach to the body often takes the form of what I call *biomarker reductionism*, in which bodily health is reduced to a number of these quantifiable biomarkers and biochemical and genetic processes. Biomarker reductionism shares a number of characteristics of nutritional reductionism, such as its reductive focus on single biomarkers, the claims to a precise understanding of the way foods and nutrients affect biochemical processes, the decontextualization and simplification of the understanding of these biomarkers and their relationship to bodily health, and the differentiation of biomarkers into "good" and "bad" types. Within the nutritionism paradigm, these biomarkers are often interpreted by nutrition experts not just as risk factors or indicators of possible problems with one's diet or state of health, but are instead taken as definitive representations of one's health, and even as determining one's health (i.e., biomarker determinism).

A key example of this biomarker reductionism has been the focus on blood cholesterol levels. In the 1950s and 1960s medical scientists interpreted the correlation between blood cholesterol levels and heart disease incidence as a causal or deterministic relationship, even though the precise causal pathways remained unknown. In the 1970s, this "lipid hypothesis" shifted from total blood cholesterol levels to measuring levels of cholesterol carried in LDL and HDL particles in the bloodstream. However, as I discuss in chapter 4, the characterization of LDL as bad and HDL as good is an oversimplification and exaggeration of scientists' understanding of the role of these cholesterol carriers in the body and in the development of cardiovascular disease. Nutrition scientists have in turn formulated their dietary fat recommendations primarily on the basis of this deterministic understanding of blood cholesterol.

BMI is another type of biomarker, one that refers not to internal biochemical processes but to an external measure of body size. Within the dominant obesity discourse promoted by obesity experts and public health institutions, BMI is treated not simply as a marker or indicator of possible inadequacies or problems with a person's diet, exercise patterns, or bodily health. Rather, it is interpreted as directly representing, and even determining, a person's state of health and risk of diseases, regardless of what they eat and how they exercise. The claimed statistical correlation between above "normal" BMI (i.e., BMI > 25) and ill health has thereby been translated into a deterministic or causal relationship. This reductive interpretation of BMI can be referred to as a form of BMI reductionism or BMI determinism. Like other forms of biomarker reductionism, BMI reductionism involves taking the BMI out of the context of whole bodies and exaggerating its role and significance.

Critics of the dominant "obesity epidemic" discourse have highlighted the limitations of BMI as a marker of bodily health and have questioned the evidence of a direct association between BMI scores and health outcomes, as well as the claimed causal relationship between them.[54] For example, a study by researchers at the U.S. Centers for Disease Control and Prevention estimated that people in the "overweight" category (with a BMI between 25 and 30) had a risk of mortality from some diseases the same as, if not lower than, those in the "normal weight" category (BMI between 18.5 and 25).[55] This is not necessarily to deny that being very large (i.e., having a very high BMI) is not sometimes associated with increased risks of various diseases or health conditions, and it may be an indication of poor dietary habits. Rather, it is to argue that many obesity experts have reductively interpreted and represented the BMI. This reductive and deterministic interpretation of BMI has also led to a focus on weight loss as an end in itself, based on the assumption that this will improve health outcomes, rather than to a focus on healthful eating and exercise patterns. Alternative approaches to body size and weight will be discussed in chapter 9.

THE NUTRICENTRIC PERSON

These nutritionally reductive ways of representing and manipulating food and the body have profoundly shaped how the lay public understands and engages with food and the body. Nutritionism has in many respects come to dominate the lay public's understanding of the relationship between food and bodily health and has given rise to what I call the nutricentric person—a type of person that to a certain extent accepts, embraces, and internalizes this nutricentric understanding of food and the body.

Nutritionism shapes individuals' approaches to nutrients, foods, and their own bodies in ambiguous and contradictory ways, producing disempowered, confused, and dependent individuals, on the one hand, and active, empowered, and critically informed individuals, on the other. First, nutritionism creates the conditions for nutrition confusion, a dependence on nutrition experts, a susceptibility to food marketing claims, and a general sense of anxiety about "what to eat." It contributes to the creation of new needs and to the idea that people are "in need"—in need of nutrition information, dietary advice, and nutritionally engineered foods.[56] The nutricentric person may perceive that nutrients are scarce and be anxious about the nutritional adequacy of modern foods and of their own dietary habits. Caught on the *nutrient treadmill*, they are compelled to keep up with the latest scientific studies reported in the media, to understand and incorporate the proliferation of nutrient categories and biomarkers, to accept nutrition experts' celebration or condemnation of particular nutrients and foods, and to purchase nutritionally engineered foods containing the latest wonder nutrients.[57]

The nutricentric person may equally, however, feel empowered and critically informed, rather than disempowered and confused, by this stream of expert advice and is able to follow the dietary debates in the media, to see beyond the more inflated nutritional marketing hype, and to make informed decisions in putting together a "healthy" diet. Nutricentric individuals may be nutritionally savvy, in the sense that they are able to selectively accept and integrate the nutrient-level knowledge they consider relevant to their own personal circumstances. These individuals thrive on having some familiarity with the basic categories of nutrition science and a capacity to explain and rationalize the connections among foods, nutrients, and their own functional bodies. The popularity of the concept of the glycemic index, for example, may in part be due to the way it offers a simple and accessible explanation of the relationship between foods and biomarkers, for example, that low-GI foods convert carbohydrates into blood sugar more slowly. By grasping and articulating such simplified scientific explanations, the nutricentric person can feel empowered to take ownership of these nutritional concepts.

Many nutrition experts and food writers have responded to these nutritional needs and anxieties by offering an endless stream of advice on "what to eat," thereby adding to what French sociologist Claude Fischler has referred to as the "nutritional cacophony" of conflicting dietary messages and voices.[58] Harvard University historian of science Steven Shapin has observed the lay public's unfailing demand for and trust in expert advice, whether it be from nutrition scientists or popular diet book authors such as those by Dr. Atkins:

> In our society, it is just not possible for food to be bought, prepared, and ingested unaccompanied by thoughts flowing from bodies of technical expertise. . . . If one strand of dietetic expertise is treated with scepticism, then residual faith in the existence of expertise seems to be transferred to another claimant. The laity assert their freedom to pick and choose which expertise is credible, while giving few signs that they find the whole domain of dietary expertise wanting.[59]

The Internet has made readily available to the lay public a much wider range of nutritional perspectives, with countless websites and blogs dedicated to promoting alternative dietary approaches, such as the low-carb and paleo diets. However, rather than uncritically accept this expert advice, follow conventional nutritional guidelines to the letter, or believe the nutritional and health claims on food labels, nutricentric individuals are increasingly compelled to actively construct their own diets and nutritional worldviews. They have little choice but to do so in the face of competing nutritional claims and the erosion of traditional ways of understanding food. Nutricentric individuals may also be motivated to put together their own personalized package of foods—and their own nutritional menus—in order to meet their perceived nutrient needs and to optimize the nutrient profile of their diets and the functional performance of their bodies.

The heightened form of health consciousness that has emerged since the 1970s—or the ideology of *healthism*, as medical sociologists have referred to it—has also fueled the rise of this nutricentric person. Healthism has elevated the pursuit of personal health and well-being to a supreme goal or super-value.[60] This ideology often takes a highly individualized form, characterized by an emphasis on the need to take personal responsibility for one's own health, rather than address the socioeconomic and environmental conditions that affect public health. This pursuit of good health goes beyond just being free of disease and illness, but involves a more active engagement in health-affirming practices, with the ultimate goal of attaining an optimal or enhanced level of health. As sociologist Julie Guthman characterizes this ideology, "Since health can never be achieved once and for all, it requires constant vigilance in monitoring and constant effort in enhancing."[61] Dietary healthism can be defined more specifically as where an obsession with healthy food overwhelms and subsumes other ways of engaging with food.[62] Food and nutrients may also be imbued with an exaggerated sense of their ability to cure or prevent a range of health issues, or to enhance the health and performance of the body and mind.

The nutricentric person is, of course, an ideal type and simply refers to one aspect of contemporary identities. We are all to some extent nutricentric, though in different ways and to varying degrees. To refer to the nutricentric person is not to suggest that nutritionism now totally overwhelms or dominates our understanding of food in relation to our health. Other approaches to food continue to coexist with this nutricentric approach. An appreciation of food production, and processing quality in particular, continues to inform people's understanding of food, and over the past decade this appreciation has been accentuated, such as in the form of the "real food" movement. There are also signs of disillusionment with nutritionism and a growing cynicism among many consumers with respect to the reductive and misleading nutritional marketing practices. These counter-dietary movements will be discussed further in chapter 9.

THREE PARADIGMS AND ERAS OF NUTRITIONISM

While nutritionism has been the dominant paradigm of nutrition science since the mid-nineteenth century, it has taken three distinct forms over this period.[63] These three specific forms or paradigms of nutritionism—quantifying nutritionism, good-and-bad nutritionism, and functional nutritionism—have framed scientific research, dietary guidelines, and food engineering and marketing practices and have defined how nutritional knowledge has been produced, interpreted, and applied. These paradigms are not necessarily defined by any particular nutritional theories or dietary recommendations (such as specific theories regarding fats, vitamins, or calories). Rather, these paradigms encompass the more fundamental assumptions that determine what counts as good science and common sense, and they incorporate the broader aims and motivations that frame the nutritional and health imperatives of the producers and disseminators of this knowledge. Each of these three paradigms of nutritionism has also been dominant within three distinct historical eras and bears the same names: the eras of quantifying nutritionism, the era of good-and-bad nutritionism, and the era of functional nutritionism (summarized in appendix table A.4). These three nutritionism paradigms essentially define the nutritional zeitgeist of each era.

Quantifying nutritionism was the dominant paradigm of nutrition science from the late nineteenth century until the mid-twentieth century in the United States. It is characterized by the logic of nutri-quantification—a calculating and quantifying approach to food, nutrients, and the body—whereby only information about those nutrients that are identified and measurable and whose function can be explained is accepted as legitimate knowledge about food and bodily health. In this era, nutrition scientists considered nutrients to be essentially good, "protective," growth promoting, and literally nutritious. The focus of nutrition experts was on the need to consume an *adequate* quantity of nutrients, particularly to avoid nutrient deficiency diseases and to promote normal bodily growth and general good health.[64] The quantification of calories and the importance of consuming enough protein and vitamins were at the center of much nutrition research and dietary advice. The discovery of vitamins also led to a public perception that modern foods and dietary patterns are nutrient scarce—a perception that persists, and indeed has been accentuated in recent years.

The good-and-bad form of nutritionism first emerged in the early 1960s and framed nutritional discourses up until the mid-1990s. Good-and-bad nutritionism is primarily characterized by the differentiation of nutrients, as well as biomarkers, into good and bad types. It is particularly distinguished by the emergence of a view of many scientists that some nutrients are bad or harmful and are thought to contribute to the incidence of chronic diseases.[65] The focus of research and dietary advice had shifted from nutrient deficiencies to reducing and preventing chronic diseases. The other important development in this period was the shift to nutricentric dietary guidelines, dominated by an obsession with reducing fat.

From the mid-1990s there was a further shift from good-and-bad nutritionism to functional nutritionism, which is characterized by a heightened sense of the relationship between foods and nutrients, on the one hand, and specific bodily functions, health conditions, and biomarkers, on the other. There has been a further proliferation of "good" and "bad" categories of nutrients, with each nutrient more precisely targeted to particular bodily functions and health outcomes. However, dietary guidelines and food advertising now place a greater emphasis on the positive and beneficial attributes of nutrients, combined with the need to "optimize" the quantities consumed and to personalize diets for individual bodies. The food industry has also developed a new range of "functional foods" that they claim can deliver these nutritional and health benefits.

The nutritional fate of the egg illustrates some of these changes in the understanding of foods and nutrients across the three eras of nutritionism. In the first half of the twentieth century, the egg was promoted as a cheap, compact, and convenient source of many desirable and protective nutrients, such as protein. Following the stigmatizing of dietary cholesterol in the good-and-bad era of nutritionism, eggs were condemned by the American Heart Association (AHA) in the early 1970s on the basis of their cholesterol content, and the AHA recommended that consumption be limited to a maximum of three eggs per week in order to minimize heart disease risk.[66] However, by the late 1990s nutrition experts had largely exonerated eggs following the release of new egg studies and due to a waning of scientists' concerns over dietary cholesterol. The AHA and the 2010 *Dietary Guidelines for Americans* now concede that about one egg a day is acceptable, but not much more than that, based on their recommended maximum cholesterol intake of 300 milligrams per day.[67] Over the past decade the egg has also been reinvented by nutrition experts and the poultry industry as a nutrient-dense, functional food and celebrated for its various nutritional benefits, such as its high-quality protein, omega-3 fats, and choline content. The industry has also developed designer eggs with enhanced omega-3 fat content that are usually produced through the nutritional engineering of chicken feed.[68]

These shifts from one nutritional era to another have to a certain extent involved responding to a "crisis" or a perceived contradiction within the previous nutritional paradigm. For example, the shift from the quantifying era to the good-and-bad era was in part a response to the "epidemic" of heart disease and other chronic diseases in the mid-twentieth century. The dietary recommendations of the quantifying era promoting animal products rich in fat, saturated fat, and cholesterol—that aimed to prevent nutrient deficiencies and promote growth—were suspected of contributing to these new disease patterns. The shift from the good-and-bad era to the functional era has in part been driven by the new imperative to move away from the negative nutritional messages of the good-and-bad era and to embrace new nutritional components and foods that claim to enhance and optimize health and wellness. Each of these three forms of nutritionism has not so much come to replace but instead has overlayed and reframed the previously dominant forms of nutritionism, so that aspects of each of these forms now coexist in the present era.

The way in which the body has been understood, represented, and experienced by nutrition experts and the lay public has also changed significantly across the three eras of nutritionism. In the quantifying era, scientists conceived of the body in quantitative and mechanical terms. This *quantified-mechanical body* was most evident in the representation of the body as a machine, the characterization of food as "fuel," and the measurement of food intake and energy expenditure in terms of calories. With widespread concerns over the scarcity of vitamins and other nutrients in modern-industrial foods, and concerns over nutrient-deficiency diseases, this quantified-mechanical body was also represented and perceived as being nutrient-deficient. In the good-and-bad era, the body came to be understood and experienced as being "at risk" of chronic diseases, particularly due to the overconsumption of bad nutrients and calories. This *at-risk body* has thereby been represented as being overnourished, in stark contrast with the nutrient-deficient body of the previous era. In the functional era, bodies are now encountered as "functional," because there is a greater focus on the links among nutrients, foods, and internal bodily functions. The *functional body* is also characterized as being nutritionally enhanced, since functional nutrients and foods are understood to target and optimize the functioning and performance of the body.

While the specific form and characteristics of nutritionism in each era have been defined by nutrition experts, nutritionism has been shaped, disseminated, and promoted by different social actors and institutions in each era. In the quantifying era nutrition scientists themselves formulated and promoted this reductive understanding of food and nutrients, drawing upon and reproducing the chemically reductive paradigms that characterized other scientific disciplines in this period. A number of pioneering scientists drove the nutritional agenda in the United States and Europe. In the late nineteenth century, for example, Wilbur Atwater was the dominant figure in American nutrition science who developed and promoted a reductive focus and interpretation of foods in terms of calories.

In the good-and-bad era, government agencies such as the USDA took a more active role in translating nutrition science into simplified and decontextualized dietary guidelines that they promoted to the wider public. While earlier government-endorsed dietary advice was largely in the form of food-based guides, the first *Dietary Guidelines for Americans*, released in 1980 and jointly published by the U.S. Department of Health and Human Services and the USDA, was largely framed in terms of nutrients, reflecting the focus of much scientific research. The concern of government agencies and public health experts with the rise of chronic diseases also hastened the translation of the highly contested hypotheses on fat and saturated fat into definitive dietary advice. Public health and consumer advocacy institutions such as the AHA and the Center for Science in the Public Interest also actively promoted the form and content of these nutricentric dietary recommendations.

In the functional era, the food industry—enabled by government policies and regulations—has been able to set the nutritional agenda and to promote the most reductive forms of nutritional knowledge and food products to the wider public. With the power to advertise not only nutrient content claims but also direct health claims since the mid-1990s, the enormous marketing budgets of food corporations have allowed them to dominate the dietary messages circulating in the nutriscape and to overwhelm any more nuanced, qualified, or integrated dietary advice from nutrition and public health experts and government institutions. Food corporations now set the nutritional agenda in many other ways, such as through their funding of scientific research, their funding of nutrition and public health institutions, and their lobbying of politicians for more favorable government policies.

This corporate capture of nutritionism—or corporate nutritionism—has also followed the rise to dominance of transnational food corporations along the entire food chain, particularly since the 1980s. Sociologists Philip McMichael and Harriet Friedmann refer to the contemporary global food system as characterized by a "corporate food regime" in which these powerful corporations control the production, processing, trade, and retailing of food within and across borders. This control has in part been enabled by the reduction in barriers to international trade.[69] This corporate food regime superseded the industrial food regime of the early and mid-twentieth century, when national governments had a more prominent role in controlling, supporting, and regulating both food production and trade. The shift from government-led to corporate-led nutritionism thus parallels this broader shift in global food regimes.[70]

The three nutritional paradigms have also mirrored and been shaped by the broader paradigms of medicine and health care. Sociologist Adele Clarke and her colleagues have recently identified three historical eras in the organization of medicine, health, and illness.[71] The first era (1890–1945) they call the "rise of medicine," a second era (1940–1990) that of "medicalization," and a third era (1985 to the present) of "biomedicalization." A number of the dominant rationalities of medicine and health care within these eras overlap with the characteristics of nutritionism. For example, as with functional nutritionism, the present era of biomedicalization is characterized by a shift to more individualized and customized bodies and medical therapies, a new emphasis on the enhancement and optimization of bodily health, and the attempt to directly treat and modify disease risk factors.

In the chapters that follow, I explore in more detail how these three paradigms of nutritionism have played out within and across the three historical eras. I identify some of the dominant nutritional theories and concepts and how they have reflected and defined the character of each nutritional era. I also explore these dynamics through a number of case studies, including the battle of the weight-loss diet plans, the margarine and *trans*-fats controversy, and the nutritional engineering and marketing of functional foods.

CHAPTER THREE

The Era of Quantifying Nutritionism

Protective Nutrients, Caloric Reductionism, and Vitamania

Hereafter, you are going to eat calories of food. Instead of saying one slice of bread,
or a piece of pie, you will say 100 Calories of bread, 350 Calories of pie.
—LULU HUNT PETERS, *DIET AND HEALTH,*
WITH KEY TO CALORIES, 1918

Published in 1918, physician Lulu Hunt Peters's *Diet and Health, with Key to Calories* was the first best-selling weight-loss diet book in the United States, going on to sell 800,000 hard-back copies.[1] She was one of the earliest to popularize the practice of counting calories as a weight-loss strategy. But before people could count calories, they had to *think* about food and their bodies in terms of calories, and Peters had to train her readers to do so.

Peters's book listed foods in 100-calorie portions and advised how many calories should be consumed by men or women per day based on their occupations. The rationale for her advice was that people wanting to maintain their weight would consume precisely this quota of calories, while those wanting to lose weight would eat less than that. What mattered most to Peters, though, was that the calories were counted. "You may eat just what you like—candy, pie, cake, fat meat, butter, cream—but—*count your calories!*"[2]

As middle-class people, influenced by the new ideals of the early twentieth century about beauty and the body, began to find a plump figure less attractive, many of them became calorie counters as they sought to lose weight.[3] In addition to Peters's groundbreaking work, in the first two decades of the twentieth century several other weight-reducing diets appeared, all advocating calorie reduction as a key strategy. For example, in his 1916 book *Eat Your Way to Health*, Robert Rose referred to calorie-counting as a "scientific system of weight control."[4] Calorie-counting diet-book authors had clearly tapped—and then helped promote—an emerging way of thinking about food and the body. Some cereal manufacturers also began voluntarily listing calorie counts on cereal boxes as a marketing strategy, and calories began to feature on the menus of some restaurant chains.

The calorie was a means of translating the emerging science of nutrition into everyday and personal terms. In the context of a growing public fascination with modern science, by counting calories people could now not just think scientifically but also eat scientifically. This era of quantifying nutritionism began in the middle to late nineteenth century and waned by the middle of the next. Quantifying nutritionism is characterized by the logic of nutri-quantification, a calculating approach to food, nutrients, and the body. Nutrition scientists borrowed from the quantifying spirit that dominated the physical and chemical sciences in the nineteenth century. The primary concerns of nutrition scientists throughout this era were to identify and quantify the nutritional components of foods, to understand their primary role in the body, and to quantify the body's nutritional requirements. They endeavored to discover and measure the essential nutrients required to prevent nutrient deficiency diseases, to promote normal growth and bodily functioning, and to provide "energy" to fuel the body.

Nutritionists' dietary advice in this period aimed to ensure as far as possible that people consumed an adequate intake of nutrients—particularly protein, vitamins, and calories—by consuming an appropriate balance of various foods or food groups. Following the discovery of vitamins, such nutrients were defined by nutrition experts as "protective," in the sense of affording protection against deficiency diseases. Protective foods were those that contained high concentrations of these protective nutrients. Within the terms of this quantifying or protective nutritionism, the primary aim of dietary advice was to ensure people simply got enough of each of these nutrients to facilitate normal growth and bodily functioning. However, some people also hoped that consuming more of these protective nutrients might afford faster growth, in the case of protein, or enhanced health, in the case of vitamins.

This era was marked by three successive obsessions, each of which is explored in this chapter. The first was the identification of the three macronutrients: proteins, fats, and carbohydrates. Nutrition scientists in the nineteenth and the early to mid-twentieth centuries fetishized protein, in particular, for its capacity to promote bodily growth. The second obsession was with the calorie, which provided a uniform system for quantifying and comparing all foods and measuring the food intake requirements of all bodies. The third stage was the discovery of vitamins, which were valued not only for the protection they afforded from deficiency diseases but also for the promise of other health benefits. However, fueled by advertisements for vitamin supplements, the widespread fascination with vitamins induced public anxieties about the perceived lack of vitamins in modern foods, and promoted a more general perception of a scarcity of nutrients in the food supply.

A number of prominent nutrition scientists shaped the nutritional agenda in this era. In the mid-nineteenth century, the German scientist Justus von Liebig dominated the nutriscape in Europe. In America, Wilbur Atwater—commonly referred to as the father of nutritional science in the United States—was a key researcher and promoter of a reductive understanding and comparison of foods and diets in terms of calories. In the first half of the twentieth century, Elmer McCollum was an important figure in vitamin research who also developed and disseminated the concept of protective nutrients and foods. This chapter examines the three key nutrients of the quantifying era—protein, calories, and vitamins—and how a reductive focus and interpretation of these nutrients by scientists such as Liebig and Atwater, as well as by food and supplement companies and the lay public, established some of the central features of the nutritionism paradigm.

THE PROTEIN FETISH

The beginnings of nutrition science can be traced back to the "chemical revolution" in France in the late eighteenth century.[5] One of the French chemists involved in this revolution, Antoine Lavoisier, declared that "life is a chemical process," and his fellow scientists conceived of nutrition in similar terms.[6] Canadian nutritional biochemist Ross Hume Hall has referred to the "chemistry paradigm" that shaped and was adopted first by the medical sciences and then by the nascent science of nutrition in the late eighteenth and early nineteenth centuries.[7] Hall characterizes the dominant paradigm in chemistry as analytic and reductionist because it involved reducing both living and nonliving things to their essential chemical elements and studying the function of these components in isolation. In adopting this approach, chemists and physiologists set about identifying and chemically classifying the macronutrients and micronutrients in food and identifying the specific biological functions of each of them.

In his 1827 paper "On the Ultimate Composition of Simple Alimentary Substances," the English biochemist William Prout put forward the idea that foods can be divided into the three primary substances: "The principal alimentary matters employed by man . . . might be reduced to three great classes, namely the *saccharine*, the *oily*, and the *albuminous* [i.e., nitrogenous]."[8] Scientists later identified these substances as carbohydrates, fats, and proteins, respectively, and they analyzed them in terms of their composition of carbon, oxygen, nitrogen, and hydrogen atoms.

The German organic chemist Justus von Liebig was the dominant figure in nutrition science for much of the nineteenth century. While many of Liebig's nutritional concepts derived from the work of other scientists, in his 1840 book *Animal Chemistry or Organic Chemistry in Its Application to Physiology and Pathology* he provided the first major synthesis of nutritional ideas.[9] Liebig emphasized the distinction between nitrogenous and non-nitrogenous (or carbonaceous) foods. At the time, scientists considered "nitrogenous molecules" found in animal and plant foods, later identified as protein, to be the only substances able to be converted into blood and capable of forming flesh.[10] Liebig thereby came to regard and promote protein as "the only true nutrient."[11] Other scientists later contradicted his view, finding that carbohydrates and fats are also able to form tissue and flesh in the body.[12]

Protein was the celebrated nutrient of the nineteenth century, with meat considered a necessary source of the concentrated quantities of protein required for bodily growth and functioning.[13] The dominant nutritional theories of this period provided scientific legitimacy for the production and global trade in fresh and canned meat. Given the interest of military planners in providing soldiers with durable and nutritious rations, the emphasis on meat led to the development of meat biscuits and meat juice products that were to be distributed on the battlefields of Europe.[14] But others were not convinced that people needed to eat such quantities of meat; a number of European physicians and specialists in dietetics, for example, instead advocated more "balanced" diets—moderate meat consumption and more vegetables and grains.[15] In his 1841 book *A Treatise on Food and Diet*, the British physician Jonathan Pereira argued that Liebig's focus on protein and the macronutrients was unable to explain the nutritional benefits of fruits and vegetables or of more diverse diets, "which experience has shown to be necessary for the preservation of human life and health."[16]

In addition to being a scientist, Liebig was an entrepreneur who sought to commercialize and capitalize on his nutritional knowledge and scientific authority. In 1865, a product called Liebig's Extract of Meat appeared on the market, which through advertising and favorable publicity achieved considerable commercial success. By the late 1860s, food manufacturers had produced and sold hundreds of thousands of kilograms of the stuff throughout Europe and the Americas.[17] Companies made the meat extract by pressing and boiling cattle flesh into liquid form, removing the fat, and reducing the juice to a thick gravy. Liebig's company promoted the high-protein extract as a nutritious, convenient, durable, and cheap alternative to meat, one that could be added to many dishes to enhance their health-fulness and flavor. As Barbara Griggs notes in her history of the period, many housewives "believed it to be a wonder-food, a concentrated es-sence of pure protein, as it were—an illusion which Liebig did nothing to dispel."[18]

Other scientists and physicians at the time questioned the nutritional value of the meat extract, pointing out that, ironically, it even lacked some of the nutrients found in meat.[19] In a letter to the London *Times*, Liebig responded to some of these criticisms by suggesting that "extract of meat is not nutriment in the ordinary sense. . . . Like tea, it possesses a far higher importance by certain medical properties of a peculiar kind . . . taken in proper proportions it strengthens the internal resistance of the body to the most various external injurious influences."[20] Liebig's claim that the meat extract somehow offered "peculiar" health benefits beyond "ordi-nary" nutrition was perhaps a harbinger of how today's proponents of functional foods claim that such foods provide health benefits "beyond basic nutrition."[21]

Another product that carried Liebig's name was Liebig's Infant Food, or Malt Soup, marketed as a complete substitute for breast milk.[22] Based on his analysis of the protein, fat, and carbohydrate content of human milk, this infant formula was manufactured from cow's milk, wheat flour, malt flour, and potassium bicarbonate but was later found to be deficient in fat, vitamins, and amino acids.[23] Other companies produced their own patented baby milks based on Liebig's formula, including Henri Nestlé in Switzerland.[24] Nestlé's dried milk food was made from "good Swiss milk and bread, cooked after a new method of my invention, mixed in propor-tion, scientifically correct, so as to form a food which leaves nothing to be desired."[25] However, a number of physicians reported that infants failed to thrive on Liebig's formula and advised against its use.[26] The use of these milk formulas, together with the new practice of feeding pasteur-ized cow's milk, may also have contributed to the rising incidence of a number of terrible deficiency diseases, including rickets and scurvy, in babies and young children in the late nineteenth century.[27] Liebig's Infant Food and Extract of Meat products represent the premature translation of scientists' limited and reductive nutritional knowledge into nutritionally engineered food products.

In the late nineteenth and early twentieth centuries, as nutrition scientists' focus shifted to calories and vitamins, their faith in the paramount nutritional importance of protein declined, but it reemerged in the early to mid-twentieth century. Nutrition experts again came to prize meat and dairy foods rich in protein for their capacity to promote and accelerate growth in children and to thereby help build a tall and strong population.[28] In 1956 the *Basic Four* food guide was issued in the United States, which was a simplified version of the *Basic Seven* released in 1943. In the *Basic Four* guide, the "Milk Group" and the "Meat Group" (the latter of which included meat, fish, eggs, or "alternates" such as nuts and legumes) constituted two of the four food categories. This food guide's emphasis on meat and milk in part reflected a continuing fetish for animal protein, as well as the government's attempt to deal with the excess production of these foods after World War II.[29]

In the early 1950s, nutrition experts working in Africa concluded that a newly diagnosed disease called kwashiorkor was caused by a deficiency of protein and found it could be cured with skim milk. The United Nations declared a worldwide deficiency of protein in developing countries and devoted considerable resources to try to "avert the impending protein crisis."[30] "Protein malnutrition" was considered the primary global nutritional problem during the 1950s and 1960s and became the focus of international nutrition research for many years.[31] However, rather than implementing their original idea to devise new crop varieties or simple methods of food processing appropriate for resource-poor villages, government-financed research projects in Europe and the United States were directed toward developing high-tech methods for synthesizing protein, such as using biotechnologies for manufacturing single-cell proteins or high-protein powder extracted from fish protein concentrate. The perceived problem of a single-nutrient deficiency was thereby addressed through the development of a single-nutrient supplement made of highly processed materials.[32] In this sense it represented an attempt at a narrowly framed technological fix to a problem that had already been defined narrowly in terms of a single-nutrient deficiency. It also effectively promoted the use of highly processed foods or supplements to address the limitations of a poor-quality diet, rather than providing people with the whole foods that could remedy these deficiencies.

By the early 1970s, nutrition experts realized that kwashiorkor sufferers typically lived on diets deficient not just in protein but in many other nutrients: they simply weren't getting enough of their otherwise nutritionally adequate local foods. As some nutrition experts had long suspected, the protein deficiency explanation was an oversimplification of the causes of kwashiorkor and ill health in these poor communities. These experts also acknowledged that recommended daily intakes of protein had been overestimated, thereby exacerbating the perception of a global protein crisis.[33] The "world protein gap" and the "protein deficiency paradigm" were instead later dubbed the "Great Protein Fiasco."[34]

CALORIC REDUCTIONISM AND THE QUANTIFIED-MECHANICAL BODY

While a reductive interpretation of the role of protein defined the early to mid-nineteenth-century nutriscape, by the end of the century the nutritional focus had shifted to the calorie. In the 1880s and 1890s, leading European and American nutrition scientists began studying the "energy" content of foods and the expenditure of energy by the body. They used the unit of the calorie to measure the uniform and homogeneous form of energy thought to be contained in foods and then expended or "burned" by the body. These scientists and physiologists assumed that all foods could be measured, reduced to, and meaningfully compared in terms of the quantities of calories they contained—assumptions that many nutrition experts still hold today.

Students of thermodynamics in the nineteenth century used the calorie as a unit to measure mechanical work, defining it as the energy required to raise one kilogram of water by one degree Celsius. In adopting this approach, physiologists in the United States and Germany looked to extend the physical laws of thermodynamics to animal and human bodies.[35] Around 1880, American chemists developed a modified "bomb calorimeter" that they used to combust (burn) foods. The amount of heat released was equated with the energy value of the food.[36] Meanwhile, in Germany, the nutritional chemists Karl Voit and Max Rubner invented the room calorimeter to study human energy expenditure. A person would be placed in these sealed rooms for several days, and their output of heat, respiration gases, and excrements would also be measured in calories.[37]

In the 1880s, American chemist Wilbur Atwater worked with Voit and Rubner in Germany.[38] On his return to the United States, Atwater's research group developed a more precise room calorimeter, and his team established that carbohydrates yield more or less precisely four kilocalories per gram, protein four, and fat nine.[39] In their respective countries, these scientists set about comparing foods in terms of the energy they contained and measuring the amount of energy that workers would consume and expend during various activities. In 1894, Rubner demonstrated that the amount of heat released by a dog after consuming a given quantity of food was the same amount of heat released when that food was combusted, and Atwater was later able to confirm that this law also applied to humans.[40] Atwater also began publishing tables on the protein, fat, and carbohydrate content of foods.[41]

The food calorimeter was a nutritional technology for quantifying the energy contained in foods and the rate at which this energy was expended in the body. The idea of food as "fuel" that is burned by the body is more than a metaphor, for it expresses the very practical sense in which these scientists reduced foods to an undifferentiated mass of nourishment for the body, and the body itself was viewed as a "human motor."[42] Accordingly, these scientists designed experiments to test whether the amount of energy expended by the body was equivalent to the amount of energy it consumed.[43] Sociologist Bryan Turner has observed that "the growth of theories of diet appears to be closely connected with the development of the idea that the body is a machine, the input and output requirements of which can be precisely quantified mathematically."[44] The emergence of these mechanical metaphors and models in nutrition science reflected and reinforced the mechanistic view of the body—this *quantified-mechanical body*—that had infiltrated scientific discourses in the nineteenth century.

The science of the calorie and the technology of the calorimeter also played an important role in introducing the logic of nutri-quantification into the nutritional discourses of the era.[45] As Jessica Mudry argues in *Measured Meals*, "The calorimeter was a cornerstone technology for the application of science to human food, to the organization of new knowledge about food, and to the integration of numeric language for communication about food."[46] It enabled a calculating and scientifically rational mode and language for understanding food and dietary health to take hold, as well as techniques for the scientific management of food and the body. Yet despite Atwater's claims to scientific and nutritional precision, his recommended daily protein and caloric requirements were later found by other scientists to be excessive. His protein recommendation of 125 grams per day, for example, was revised downward to 60 grams per day by Yale University scientist R.H. Chittenden in the early 1900s.[47]

The calorie was and is still talked about as if it had an independent existence, as if it were a nutrient compound in foods that one could literally count up. In practice, the calorie also plays the role of a kind master nutrient, or metanutrient, providing a single value according to which all foods—and all nutrients—can be measured and compared. This caloric value provides a summary of the total quantity of carbohydrates (four calories per gram), protein (four calories), and fat (nine calories) a food contains. Food is thereby represented as an absolutely uniform fuel or energy source. Those who subscribe to this model in turn implicitly assume that the body functions like a machine that uses or "burns" all calories in the same way, regardless of the food source of those calories or of differences among individual bodies. It is captured by the contemporary cliche that "a calorie is a calorie": a calorie from meat is assumed to be the same as one from a grain or a soda. I refer to this reduction of food and the body to uniform caloric values as a form of *caloric reductionism*.

While calorie values provide a weighted measure—perhaps a crude measure—of the total quantity of foodstuff contained in a food product or meal, they tell us little about how the different food components and ingredients are put together within a whole food, or about how these components might have been transformed and reassembled within refined and processed foods. How each of these components is absorbed and metabolized by the body may be affected by the overall matrix of nutrients and other food components they are combined with. In other words, the body may deal with these different types of calories in different ways. The body may also adjust how, and at what rate, it metabolizes calories (or foods) in different circumstances.[48] In this complex interaction of food and bodily metabolism, how meaningful is it to assign a single "energy" value to each food, as well as to all bodies and physical activities? Yet despite nutrition scientists' increasingly complex understanding of food and the body over the past century, the simplified idea that "a calorie is a calorie" continues to dominate dietary discourses around weight management. These contemporary discourses are discussed further in chapter 5.

The Social Life of the Calorie

The unit of the calorie was used by nutrition scientists to compare and contrast on a one-dimensional scale qualitatively different types of foods and dietary patterns, as well as different types of bodies and bodily activities. These experts came to see foods as interchangeable sources of calories and macronutrients, and they compared and valued them on the basis of these quantitative measures.[49] One effect of this nutritional leveling of foods was that the exaggerated importance of meat in the human diet promoted by nutrition scientists in the middle to late nineteenth century was downgraded by Atwater following his realization that plant foods could provide cheaper forms of protein and energy.[50]

In *Never Satisfied: A Cultural History of Diets, Fantasies and Fat*, historian Hillel Schwartz emphasizes how "Atwater's charts reduced the smell, taste, texture and weight of food to an essential nutritional line" and "entirely reconstrue the meanings of food without reference to taste, ethnic tradition, or social context."[51] Atwater's reductive interpretation and application of the calorie abstracted food out of preexisting sensual and cultural settings and experiences. But at the same time, Atwater also used the calorie to reposition foods within the dominant political, economic, and cultural agendas of the day. He designed his research and dietary recommendations, for example, to support the aims of labor reformers, industrialists, and the social progressive movements that had helped to fund his studies.[52] From these studies he was able to determine the most cost-efficient foods in terms of their cost per calorie. "The cheapest food," Atwater wrote, "is that which supplies the most nutrient for the least money."[53] For Atwater, cheap calories were good calories, an approach that now stands in direct contrast to the condemnation of cheap calories by contemporary critics of highly processed foods and by anti-obesity campaigners.[54]

At the turn of the twentieth century, in response to labor unrest in North America and Europe over inadequate wages, employers used Atwater's research to quantify the minimum wages required to purchase a nutritionally adequate diet. In Germany, nutrition scientists were similarly applying this new scientific nutrition to the "problems" of feeding the urban masses and containing political unrest, by devising and promoting economically and scientifically "rational" diets.[55] The emergence of this scientific management of nutrition drew upon and paralleled the rise of "Taylorism" in the early twentieth century. Taylorism was the management system devised by Frederick Taylor for the scientific measurement and management of the labor process and workers' tasks that aimed to increase productivity and to overcome workers' resistance to technological innovation and expert control.[56]

To Atwater and other social reformers at the time, the diets of the poor and the working class were extravagant and wasteful: their nutritional needs could be met within their existing wages if only they would learn to eat in a scientifically and economically efficient manner.[57] His belief in the importance of protein and energy led him to promote foods that delivered these nutrients cost-effectively, such as cheap cuts of meat, beans, and flour.[58] Fruits and vegetables were discouraged because they were deficient in calories and protein and were relatively expensive on a per-calorie basis. They were thus, for the working class at least, seen as a delicacy, a mere flavoring agent—indeed, as a luxury food.[59] Atwater campaigned against "the conceit, let us call it, that there is some mysterious virtue in those kinds of foods that have the most delicate appearances and flavor and the highest price."[60] He even prized sugar as a cost-efficient source of calories and as representing better "fuel value" than beans, mutton, or cheese.[61]

As historian Harvey Levenstein suggests in *Revolution at the Table*, "If America turned *en masse* to follow their advice, rickets, beriberi, scurvy, and other vitamin deficiency diseases may have reached epidemic proportions."[62] The denigration of fruits and vegetables also contradicted the folk knowledge embedded in the cultural traditions of the working class and of the new immigrant populations that had settled in the United States from Europe.[63] Rather than complementing, supporting, and perhaps even learning from this diverse range of cultural traditions and cuisines, these nutrition experts were already demonstrating their nutritional hubris by setting themselves up against lay understandings of food and health.

While the working class largely ignored these dietary recommendations, the middle class showed more interest in what came to be called the New Nutrition movement at the turn of the twentieth century.[64] The social reform movement that arose in the late nineteenth century, initially known as *scientific cookery*, and later as *domestic science*, embraced this burgeoning scientific approach to food.[65] One of the aims of the scientific cookery movement was to educate women about the nutritional composition of foods and about how to prepare nutritionally adequate meals. In

Perfection Salad: Women and Cooking at the Turn of the Century, Laura Shapiro describes the movement's dedication to the ideas of Atwater: "At the height of their reputation teachers of scientific cookery liked nothing better than to take up Atwater's food composition tables and bring them to life in the kitchen. Protein, fat, and carbohydrate became categories to be wielded in the assembly of a meal."[66]

The emergence of calorie counting as a weight-loss dieting strategy was another means by which the calorie was socialized and incorporated into everyday eating practices. Schwartz evokes the hope and anticipation that calorie counting called forth in the 1920s, based on its capacity to predict the future: "As a habit of seeing through and beyond food, calorie-counting gave dieters a power which no scale could equal. Scales measured immediate bodies and dispensed random fortunes, but dieters could truly anticipate the future: so many extra, invisible calories would mean so much extra, visible fat."[67] While interest in dieting died down during the Great Depression, the calorie was again at the center of a growing interest in weight-loss diets from the 1950s.[68]

The quantification of energy intake and expenditure also came to inform the national food and nutrition policies of a number of countries in the first half of the twentieth century. As historian Nick Cullather argues, "The calorie has never been a neutral, objective measure of the contents of a dinner plate. From the first, its purpose was to render food, and the eating habits of populations, politically legible."[69] Beyond regulating personal dietary practices, the calorie could be used to measure, compare, and control the food supply of local populations and foreign countries. Industry and the military could design the most cost-efficient diets not only for workers on minimum wages but also for soldiers on daily rations in the lead up to World War I.

The culturally distinct diets and tastes of different countries could also be compared by the universal measure of the calorie, and the extent of hunger and malnourishment could similarly be calculated and addressed on the basis of minimum caloric requirements. In India in the 1920s and 1930s, for example, dietary statistics alerted the British imperialists to the malnutrition of the local populations but also provided justification for their colonial control under the guise of improving the diets of the locals. They promoted diets rich in meat, milk, and wheat as nutritionally superior to the local dishes of lentil-based dal and rice that they thought could not produce a strong and prosperous local population. Some Indian nutrition experts responded within the terms of the nutritionism paradigm by emphasizing the high nutrient density of lentils and rice. Mohandas

Gandhi—though a keen student of nutrition science—took a different tack, questioning the universal and calculating claims of nutrition science and urging each person to experiment with their own personal dietary practices.[70]

Vitamins Unleashed

The discovery of vitamins was a triumph of science. It demonstrated the power of science to disclose the secrets of nature and to use that knowledge in the service of humanity. Vitamins represented the hope of better things to come.
—RIMA APPLE, *VITAMANIA*, 1996

Scientists' discovery in the early twentieth century of the existence and role of vitamins offered great insights into the prevention and cure of a number of diseases and maladies and helped us to understand and improve inadequate diets. But the vitamin discoveries also highlighted the limitations of earlier scientific theories of nutrition centered on protein and energy, and of the definitive dietary advice upon which they were based.

In the eighteenth and nineteenth centuries, some doctors suspected that poor diets were somehow related to the onset of diseases such as scurvy, rickets, and beriberi. In the case of scurvy—a disease common among sailors—an experiment by British naval medical officer James Lind in 1747 confirmed that citrus fruit could cure scurvy, though the biochemical mechanisms behind the cure were unknown at the time.[71] From the late eighteenth century doctors also prescribed cod liver oil as the standard remedy for rickets.[72] However, the medical community generally viewed these diseases as probably caused by infections or contagion.[73]

Nutrition scientists in the late nineteenth century still assumed that protein, fat, and some minerals in foods provided all the necessary nutrients.[74] But in 1906, Cambridge University physiologist and chemist Frederick Hopkins conducted animal feeding experiments from which he concluded that "no animal can live on a mixture of pure protein, fat and carbohydrate."[75] Hopkins suspected that a deficiency of some unknown food components might be the cause of some of these diseases. He referred to these components as "accessory food factors," since they were accessories to the three macronutrients.[76]

In 1912, Polish chemist Casimir Funk coined the term *vitamines* to refer to those still unidentified factors associated with deficiency diseases, so named because he assumed they were "vital" and were part of the "amine" group of organic chemical compounds.[77] Scientists later shortened the term to "vitamins" when they realized that not all of the vitamins were amines. Other researchers in this period considered the term *vitamin*— suggesting vitality—to be a "stroke of genius" because they thought it "such a captivating word."[78] Years later Funk himself noted that "the name contributed in no small measure to the dissemination of these ideas."[79] The word captured the popular imagination and brought to life these invisible and otherwise inert micronutrients, investing them with almost magical properties.

It was also in 1912 that Elmer McCollum's research team at Yale University first identified a fat-soluble substance they called fat-soluble A or Factor A (later renamed vitamin A) found in butter, liver, and leafy greens. Through his experiments on rats, McCollum demonstrated that a deficiency of Factor A led to impaired vision and stunted growth. The team also identified "water-soluble B" or "Factor B," later renamed vitamin B, the absence of which they linked to the tropical disease beriberi.[80] In the 1920s scientists identified various important relationships between vitamins and human health: they linked deficiency in vitamin C, which they found in citrus fruits, to scurvy, and they linked deficiency in vitamin D, found in various foods and produced by the body in response to sunlight, to rickets. During the 1920s and 1930s, other vitamins and minerals were identified, including riboflavin, folic acid, beta-carotene, vitamin E, and vitamin K.

While scientists linked these vitamins with a number of deficiency diseases, not until the early 1930s did they begin to measure more accurately the quantities of vitamins in foods.[81] It was also a number of years after their discovery that chemists were able to define the chemical structure of vitamins and synthesize and manufacture them in the form of nutritional supplements.[82] In 1941, the U.S. Food and Nutrition Board published the first tables of Recommended Dietary Allowances (RDAs) for vitamins and other nutrients. The RDA tables initially referred only to energy, protein, two minerals, and six vitamins and were set at levels intended to ensure normal bodily functioning and the avoidance of deficiency diseases.[83]

This knowledge of the role of vitamins and the causes of some common nutrient deficiency diseases were important innovations in public health. They could immediately be used to cure deficiency diseases, to address inadequate diets, and to examine the nutritional quality of agricultural products and of refined and processed foods. After companies synthesized some of these nutrients, public health authorities launched a series of national and international vitamin fortification programs, many of which were reasonably successful in eradicating deficiency diseases within particular populations. In the 1940s, for instance, doctors prescribed vitamin B–enriched flour to treat the vitamin B_3 deficiency disease pellagra, iodine-fortified salt for goiter, and vitamin D–enriched milk for children with rickets. Also around this time, public health experts attributed the large decrease in beriberi and pellagra to the government-mandated fortification of flour with the B vitamins thiamin, niacin, and riboflavin. Thiamin and niacin are found in wheat bran but are removed by the milling process during the production of white flour.[84]

While sufferers of vitamin deficiency diseases could cure or ameliorate them by consuming vitamin-fortified foods or supplements, taking vitamin supplements is nevertheless a reductive, one-dimensional, and fragmented approach to food and the body. These technological products may "work" in some respects to address very specific vitamin deficiencies. But they work in a nutritionally reductive manner. The isolated or synthesized vitamins found in many supplements are not necessarily in the same form as those found in foods. Taking vitamins as supplements also doesn't provide the (known and unknown) interactions among vitamins and other food components that occur within foods and food combinations. Nutrient supplements may even be harmful, particularly when taken in large, concentrated, and isolated doses. An overdose of vitamins A and D, for example, can have toxic and potentially fatal effects.[85] Some studies have also found an association between beta-carotene supplements and an increased risk of both cardiovascular disease and certain cancers, and high doses of vitamin E supplements are associated with increased all-cause mortality.[86]

The industrialization of food production practices in the late nineteenth and early twentieth centuries seems to have contributed to a new wave of nutrient deficiency diseases, particularly following the development of mechanical and steam-powered machines for finely milling flour, rice, and corn.[87] People on restricted diets, and those dependent on a narrow range of refined and processed foods—such as sailors on long ocean journeys, soldiers and civilians in times of war, and the urban poor in rapidly industrializing cities—were the most vulnerable to these deficiency diseases. Whereas nutrition scientists' reductive focus and interpretation of calories in the late nineteenth century had been used by industrialists to argue that workers' wages were high enough to purchase an adequate diet in terms of energy needs, the vitamin theory could now be used by social reformers to highlight the nutritional inadequacy of the diets of the poor.[88] Whether it was to support or question the adequacy of the wages and the diets of the working class, nutritional knowledge was being drawn upon by various authorities and interest groups as an objective source of expertise to support particular political agendas.

The discovery of vitamins should have highlighted not only the inadequacy of earlier nutritional theories but also the dangers of nutritionally reductive dietary advice per se, especially where it had so thoroughly contradicted lay knowledge of the relationship between food and health. By the late nineteenth century, nutrition science not only had failed to identify the link between industrial foods and deficiency diseases but in some cases had promoted the nutritional superiority of these industrial foods. Atwater, for example, had devalued fruits and vegetables as poor "fuel value."[89] As Barbara Griggs has noted in her social history of nutrition, "To many Americans the truths now being painfully elaborated in the laboratory were plain, honest, peasant wisdom which had been self-evident for centuries until the march of nineteenth-century mechanized progress and the growing industrialization of food had overwhelmed it."[90]

Following the vitamin discoveries, foods containing these vital components were categorized by nutrition experts as "protective foods," a term probably coined by Elmer McCollum. In 1918 McCollum argued that "milk and the leaves of plants are to be regarded as protective foods and never omitted from the diet."[91] McCollum—who had developed a close association with and received research funding from the National Dairy Council—was to become a key promoter of milk, declaring that "milk is the greatest of all protective foods because it is so constituted as to correct the deficiencies of whatever else we are likely to eat."[92] Americans' consumption of milk soared during the 1920s, partly fueled by the National Dairy Council's intense nutritional marketing of milk on the basis of its vitamin content and claimed protective properties.[93] McCollum's close relationship with the dairy industry was an early instance of the potential influence of commercial interests on the production and dissemination of nutritional knowledge. McCollum was also hired as a spokesperson for General Mills in the 1920s, and contrary to his earlier indictment of white flour for its lack of vitamins, he began promoting white bread as more nutritious than whole wheat bread on the basis that the latter was less digestible.[94]

Members of the lay public were quick to embrace these protective vitamins, partially driven by their anxieties about the deficiency of modern foods and their fears of vitamin deficiency diseases. As Rima Apple argues in *Vitamania*, "Undeniably, the micronutrients produced miraculous cures in cases of gross deficiency diseases. These wonders inspired speculation about vitamin's other health-giving and health-preserving actions, speculation built on public announcements about the role of vitamins in human nutrition. In our consumer culture, vitamins became a symbol of the benefits of science available to all."[95] Apple explores how "vitamania" seized many members of the lay public, convincing them of the curative and magical properties of vitamins, properties that went well beyond any of the modest benefits promoted by nutrition scientists and government authorities.

While nutrition experts generally regarded whole foods as protective against nutrient deficiencies, many also questioned the nutritional adequacy of industrially grown foods and processed foods. Some people feared that the combination of poor crop soils and modern agricultural techniques—as well as modern practices of refining, processing, storage, transportation, and cooking of foods—had stripped foods of some of their vitamins. From the 1930s, the American health food movements also characterized processed foods in particular as vitamin deficient, and these concerns were used to promote the consumption of whole and unprocessed foods, rather than vitamin supplements.[96]

Food manufacturers played on this new fascination with vitamins and concerns over vitamin deficiencies in advertisements that highlighted the health benefits of the vitamins naturally occurring in their foods or those added during processing. Ovaltine was advertised as rich in "growth-promoting vitamins," while Bond Bread gave consumers "sunshine vitamin D."[97] In a sign of things to come, this nutritional promotion was aimed not just at human consumers: Red Heart Dog Biscuits also advertised the importance of vitamin D for dogs.[98] In the 1920s and 1930s, the pharmaceutical industry heavily advertised a new range of vitamin supplements whose claimed curative qualities exploited consumers' growing fears of hidden vitamin deficiency diseases.[99] Some advertisements warned parents that vitamin deficiencies might be undermining their children's growth and that deficiency diseases could be developing that were not immediately visible to the naked eye: "Inside, where it can't be seen, the damage starts!"[100]

In response to this push by the pharmaceutical industry, in the 1920s the American Medical Association (AMA) urged consumers to "get . . . [their] vitamins from the garden and the orchard rather than from the drug counter."[101] Throughout the twentieth century, most mainstream nutrition experts have echoed this approach, insisting that a well-balanced diet is adequate to receive the required vitamins.[102] Yet articles in popular newspapers reported on a regular basis that most Americans were not eating such well-balanced diets.[103] Based on arguably inflated RDAs, surveys conducted by the U.S. Department of Agriculture (USDA) and other institutions during the 1950s and 1960s found that up to half of American households were deficient in least one of the micronutrients, thereby adding scientific legitimacy to popular anxieties.[104] Government-mandated food fortification programs, such as the B vitamin fortification of flour, also implicitly endorsed the idea that either modern foods or the dietary patterns of many people were deficient.

Fueled by a stream of media reports and supplement advertisements, a wave of anxiety swept across the middle class regarding the nutritional inadequacy of industrially produced foods and unbalanced diets. Vitamania contributed to the creation of a more exaggerated *perception of nutrient scarcity* among those with access to a diverse and plentiful food supply. Not only food but also the body was represented and experienced as being nutrient deficient. Yet many of the specific diseases these newly discovered vitamins could cure—such as beriberi and scurvy—were not common in America, and members of the middle class—even anxious ones—generally did not suffer deficiency diseases. But middle-class Americans' enthusiasm for vitamins also went beyond their concerns about deficiency diseases, relating to the hope that by consuming more vitamins they would enhance their health and longevity.[105]

From the 1930s, the supplement industry used the belief that vitamin supplements provided a form of "health insurance" to justify and promote their use.[106] The industry promoted this vitamin insurance policy—or *vitaminsurance*—as a safety net for a range of nutritional threats, such as the occasional lapses in good eating habits by people with busy modern lives, or the invisible deficiencies in modern foods and diets. In recent decades, this vitaminsurance has taken the form of the multinutrient supplement designed to meet a broad spectrum of nutrient requirements.

The rationale of proponents of supplement use has also shifted over the past century, from meeting vitamin deficiencies in the quantitative era, to reducing the risk of chronic disease in the good-and-bad era, to enhancing health and bodily functioning in the functional era.[107] Today, many nutrition experts commonly endorse the taking of supplements as a nutritional insurance policy.[108] For example, in his 2005 book *Eat, Drink, and Be Healthy*, leading nutritional epidemiologist Walter Willett of the Harvard School of Public Health promotes multivitamin, vitamin D, and calcium supplements, which he justifies as "a cheap and effective genuine 'life nutritional insurance' policy."[109]

In the late 1960s and early 1970s, Nobel Prize–winning chemist Linus Pauling—who had no recognized expertise in nutrition science—promoted megadoses of vitamin C as a cure for the common cold, based on his review of the scientific literature rather than his own nutrition studies.[110] Medical experts and institutions such as the AMA belittled Pauling's ideas, arguing that the studies cited by Pauling failed to support his contentions. But Pauling's theories received much publicity in the popular media, and the idea of the preventive and curative power of vitamin C became widely recognized and accepted by the lay public at the time. Sales of vitamin C supplements skyrocketed.[111] A belief in the preventive or curative power of vitamin C for the common cold is still held by many people today.[112]

In the quantifying era of nutritionism, the promotion of megadoses of vitamin supplements and claims for a range of health benefits beyond the avoidance of nutrient deficiencies were associated with alternative health practitioners and the supplements industry, but in some respects these alternative ideas have now assumed some mainstream respectability. Very high doses of vitamin D as well as omega-3 fat supplements—beyond those required to protect against more immediate deficiency diseases—are now promoted by some nutrition experts, who consider the long-term inadequate intake of these nutrients as contributing to a range of chronic diseases.[113] The discourse of functional nutritionism similarly promises people an enhanced state of health and bodily functioning if they consume an optimal amount of these functional nutrients.

Having unleashed vitamins, nutrition experts have had trouble containing the public's expectations. From the 1920s these experts advised the public to *think* of the vitamins and nutrients that their bodies required but to eat food in order to receive adequate quantities of them. Yet many people decided to take control of their own vitamin intake to address their own perceived nutritional requirements and deficiencies, and to consume their vitamins directly in the form of fortified foods and supplements. By the 1980s, an apparent gap had also opened up between nutrition experts' use of supplements and the advice they gave about them to the public. A survey of dieticians in Washington State in 1981, for example, revealed that 60 percent of them used some kind of nutritional supplement.[114] As public health nutritionists Joan Gussow and Paul Thomas commented at the time, "Even as nutrition professionals seek to teach Americans to 'eat well' and avoid 'pills,' they themselves are swallowing supplementary nutrients. 'Do as I say,' nutritionists seem to be telling the public, 'not as I do'; and few of them dare to defend their own pill practices before their fellows."[115]

Food regulators have also struggled to contain the commercial exploitation of vitamania by the food and supplement industries. From the 1940s, the U.S. Food and Drug Administration (FDA) had attempted to impose greater regulation over the vitamin supplement industry, and particularly to limit the health claims in advertising. Yet each time, the FDA was met with resistance not only from the industry but also from a public that demanded access to these supplements. Rima Apple has observed that the social, scientific, and regulatory struggles around vitamins continued through the second half of the twentieth century:

> Decade after decade . . . the same scenario is repeated: scientists report on the beneficial effects of vitamins; the media and particularly manufacturers publicize the claims; skeptical scientists declare that the American consumer is being hoodwinked; government agencies propose regulations to control the advertising, labeling, and sale of vitamin pills; and concerned consumers assert their right to take vitamins without government interference.[116]

Vitamania—and the earlier obsession with calorie counting—signaled the rise of a wider nutritional consciousness in members of the lay public in the first half of the twentieth century. The nutricentric person had arrived. Everyday food discourses had begun to be suffused with nutri-speak. The public was growing familiar with the language of nutrients, learning to select and eat foods with some of this nutritional knowledge in mind, and becoming more open to the nutritional marketing of the food and supplement industries.

Despite the public's growing familiarity with the science and the language of nutrients, much of the government's dietary advice to the public during this nutritional era primarily referred to foods. The first food guide published by the USDA in 1917 contained five food groups: milk and meat, cereals, vegetables and fruits, fats and fatty foods, and sugars and sugary foods.[117] These food-based dietary guides went through several revisions throughout the first half of the twentieth century. The *Basic Seven* guide, for example, released in 1943, included three groups of different fruits and vegetables, and the milk/dairy, meat/beans, bread/grains, and bread/margarine groups. Nutritionists intended that their recommended number of servings of each food group would ensure a nutritionally adequate diet, based on the quantities specified in the first RDAs released in 1941.[118]

By the 1950s, many nutrition experts considered that all of the important nutrients in foods had been discovered, that their roles in the body were well understood, and that most of the important questions concerning nutrition had been answered. As evidence of this nutritional hubris, in 1946 Oxford University in the United Kingdom was offered a large sum of money to establish an Institute of Human Nutrition but reportedly turned down the offer because its directors believed that after ten years "there would be no human nutrition problems to study."[119] However, by the early 1960s, nutrition scientists had begun to rethink their enthusiastic promotion of meat and dairy products, following a rise in the incidence of heart disease and its claimed association with saturated fat intake. This reevaluation signaled the transition to the new paradigm and era of good-and-bad nutritionism.

Even if some of the specific nutritional hypotheses of the era of quantifying nutritionism have since been discredited, a number of its features live on, such as the myth of nutritional precision, caloric reductionism, and the perception of nutrient scarcity. The history of vitamania also illustrates how easily the food and supplement industry could exploit scientific knowledge as a strategy to market their products, and the willingness of members of the lay public to embrace these scientific claims and scientifically marketed products.[120]

CHAPTER FOUR

The Era of Good-and-Bad Nutritionism

Bad Nutrients and Nutricentric Dietary Guidelines

Foods are subjected to binary moral judgments like characters in a detective story, as if the problem were to designate a culprit for the eventual eater's death. In the "theater of food," fiber is currently cast in the leading role. Sugar, once a popular hero, became a major villain in the seventies ("pure, white and deadly") and is currently being reluctantly rehabilitated. Fat has now taken over the part of the ultimate villain, with a Jekyll-and-Hyde personality: unsaturated, admirable; and saturated, heavy and deadly.

—CLAUDE FISCHLER, "A NUTRITIONAL CACOPHONY," 1993

The defining characteristic of the good-and-bad era of nutritionism beginning in the 1960s was scientists' differentiation of nutrients into "good" and "bad" types. While talk of good and bad foods has a long history, the extension of what French sociologist Claude Fischler calls "binary moral judgments" to the scientific discourse around nutrients was new.[1] Biomarkers also became subject to this binary logic, particularly the distinction between good and bad blood cholesterol.

The good-and-bad era of nutritionism was dominated by the negative nutritional messages of nutrition experts and dietary guidelines, emphasizing the need to eat less of the bad nutrients and the implicitly bad foods that contained them.[2] Food scholar Warren Belasco refers to the "negative nutrition" that pervaded guidelines and food cultures in the United States in the 1970s and 1980s and the negative terminology of "avoid," "reduce," "limit," and "decrease" that were its watchwords.[3]

The shift to this new era of nutritionism was in part precipitated by an emerging crisis in the quantifying nutritionism paradigm in the middle of the twentieth century. Nutrition scientists' entreaties during the quantifying era that people consume an adequate quantity of protective and growth-promoting nutrients, to assist their bodily growth and to avoid deficiencies, were giving way to new concerns about the overconsumption of certain nutrients and foods and about their contribution to the new epidemics of heart disease and other chronic diseases. Americans had apparently become *overnourished* due to the consumption of too many bad nutrients as well as to just too many calories. The meat, eggs, and dairy products that had been the celebrated foods of the quantifying era were now cast as a significant threat to our health. Mainstream nutrition experts, as well as countercultural whole food advocates, also derided the highly processed foods that had proliferated since the 1950s, particularly for their high levels of added fats, sugar, and salt.[4]

In this era, government and public health institutions, such as the U.S. Department of Agriculture (USDA) and the American Heart Association (AHA), became the primary drivers and promoters of the nutritionism paradigm as they translated nutricentric scientific research into population-wide dietary guidelines aimed at reducing chronic disease risks. By the 1970s the dietary guidelines they formulated and promoted began to speak the language of nutrients rather than foods, but this merely reflected the nutricentric character of most scientific research at the time. It was these nutricentric guidelines, and an obsessive focus on the harmfulness of fats in particular, that were pivotal in shifting nutritionism from the margins to the center of everyday food discourses.

This chapter explores the emergence of the distinction between good and bad nutrients that framed much of the scientific research and dietary advice of this era, and how it was disseminated through the diet-heart hypothesis, the *Dietary Goals for the United States*, the *Dietary Guidelines for Americans*, and the *Food Guide Pyramid*.

Good and Bad Nutrients, Foods and Biomarkers

In *Food and Health: The Experts Agree*, a report published in the United Kingdom in 1992, public health nutrition expert Geoffrey Cannon summarized the findings of one hundred "authoritative scientific reports" produced by governments around the world between 1961 and 1991. Cannon claimed that despite the outward appearance of disagreement among nutrition experts, there was an overwhelming global consensus among them about what constituted healthy and unhealthy diets:

> The experts agree on food, nutrition and health. The analysis of one hundred reports . . . shows a clear consensus amounting to practical unanimity, on what is wrong with the Western industrialized diet

and how to put it right. Expressed in terms of nutrients, the general healthy eating advice is: eat more complex carbohydrates and fibre as contained in starchy and other plant foods; eat less total fat and a lot less saturated fat, and thus dietary cholesterol, and also switch from saturated to polyunsaturated fats; eat a lot less refined sugar and salt; and drink alcohol sparingly if at all. These changes will have the effect of boosting vitamin and mineral intake. The general advice for people, except for those who are decidedly overweight, is not to cut calories but to be physically active throughout life instead.[5]

This summary statement is a fair reflection of the specific recommendations regarding fats, carbs, cholesterol, calories, sugar, and salt promoted by national dietary guidelines in the United States and a number of other countries in the era of good-and-bad nutritionism. More important, this expert agreement was almost entirely framed in terms of nutrients, with only euphemistic references to types of foods and levels of processing.

Prior to the 1960s, nutrition scientists understood nutrients as essentially good, protective, and literally nutritious. Nutrients promoted good health and protected against deficiency diseases. Government-endorsed dietary advice in the first half of the twentieth century aimed to ensure that people consumed an adequate intake of all nutrients. This approach largely meant promoting "eat more" messages so people would increase their intake of particular nutrients. The idea that nutrients found in common whole foods might be bad was novel, with the exception of concerns about excessive calorie intake or an overdose of vitamin supplements.

In the good-and-bad era, the overwhelming emphasis of dietary guidelines and nutritional discourses shifted to the need for people to avoid, reduce, or eat sparingly the more harmful nutrients, particularly fat, saturated fat, and cholesterol. By the late 1950s nutrition scientists had already identified dietary fat as a cause of the perceived epidemic of heart disease that had swept America and other highly industrialized countries, and consequently, leading nutrition scientist Ancel Keys called on people to steeply reduce their total intake of fat. By the 1960s, the focus of nutrition scientists shifted to the role of saturated fats and dietary cholesterol in increasing heart disease risk. Polyunsaturated fat became a good, protective fat because it helped to lower blood cholesterol levels and, by extension, heart disease risk. By the 1970s, nutrition scientists further differentiated the carriers of blood cholesterol into LDL (low-density lipoprotein)— the "bad cholesterol"—and HDL (high-density lipoprotein), the "good cholesterol."

The general anti-fat rhetoric that persisted throughout the era was distilled and entrenched in the 1980 *Dietary Guidelines for Americans* directing people to "avoid too much fat, saturated fat, and cholesterol."[6] The low-fat advice was partially an attempt by nutrition and public health experts and policy makers to simplify the good- and bad-fat advice that they considered far too complex for the lay public to comprehend. In the 1990 version of the *Dietary Guidelines*, the low-fat recommendation was given the more precise numerical goal of reducing fat to 30 percent of total calories. Salt and sugar were also included in the category of bad nutrients and often translated into their biochemical constituents: salt as sodium chloride, and sugar as a type of "simple" carbohydrate.

Dietary guidelines urged Americans to replace fat with carbohydrates, particularly the "complex," fiber-rich carbohydrate foods such as whole grains and vegetables. British scientist Denis Burkitt was best known for championing the beneficial attributes of fiber.[7] The 1977 *Dietary Goals for the United States* introduced for the first time a chemically defined distinction between "complex carbohydrates" (starches found in grains and vegetables) and "simple carbohydrates" (sugars, whether from fruit or sugar cane).[8] The language of "good and bad carbs," however, would not become common until the 1990s.[9]

The labels "good" and "bad" suggest a precise, black-and-white, one-dimensional understanding of the role of nutrients and of biomarkers with respect to their relationship to bodily health. It implies that certain isolated nutrients are either harmful or beneficial to one's health, rather than acknowledging that they may be involved—either in isolation or combination with other nutrients and food components—in multiple and complex metabolic processes that are not easily reduced to such simplistic characterizations. For example, cholesterol plays an essential role in the functioning and repair of every cell in the body, yet its classification as a bad nutrient reduces it to its assumed role in promoting atherosclerosis.

The language of good and bad *foods* also became a distinctive feature of the American nutriscape of this era.[10] However, nutrition experts differentiated these good and bad foods primarily on the basis of the quantities of the good and bad nutrients they contained, rather than on the basis of epidemiological or clinical trials directly linking these foods to particular health outcomes. The bad foods during this period were red meat, whole milk products, and eggs due to their fat, saturated fat, and cholesterol content; refined grains and flour due to the removal of fiber and other nutrients; and processed and convenience foods high in fat, sugar, and salt. Items in the good foods basket included not only whole grains, fruits, and vegetables but also reduced-fat milk, refined vegetable oils, and margarine high in unsaturated fats.

One of the consequences of the decontextualized focus on good and bad nutrients was the blurring of the distinction between whole and technologically reconstituted foods and ingredients in terms of their health effects. Whole foods once celebrated as "protective foods"—such as red meat, whole milk, and eggs—were now condemned as artery cloggers and promoters of so-called Western diseases.[11] The naturally occurring components contained within these whole foods, such as saturated fat and cholesterol, were similarly vilified. American biochemist Raymond Reiser observed in 1978 that "they have made cholesterol appear to be a toxic substance similar to dangerous additives."[12]

At the same time, fabricated ingredients such as artificial sweeteners, and chemically modified fats and starches, began to receive a level of nutritional legitimacy for their role in displacing naturally occurring food components such as fat and sugar. In *Empty Pleasures*, Carolyn De La Pena documents some nutrition experts' tolerance of artificial sugars such as NutraSweet during the 1970s and 1980s.[13] British nutrition scientist John Yudkin, for example, who in *Pure, White and Deadly* attributed the rise in incidence of a range of chronic diseases to sugar consumption, gave his tacit support to low-calorie soft drinks containing artificial sweeteners and dismissed the growing concerns regarding the health risks associated with them.[14]

CHRONIC DISEASE, RISK FACTORS, AND THE AT-RISK BODY

The era of good-and-bad nutritionism was partly precipitated by changing disease patterns during the twentieth century in the United States and in other highly industrialized countries.[15] By the middle of the twentieth century, heart disease, stroke, and a range of cancers had overtaken infectious diseases as the leading cause of death, while diabetes and obesity were also on the rise.[16] Age-adjusted death rates from heart disease had peaked by the 1950s, and these rates have steadily declined since then.[17] Nevertheless, medical and nutritional researchers in the United States and Europe began to focus on heart disease, a focus that has since the 1960s been very influential in shaping dietary guidelines for the entire population.

In changing the focus from deficiency to chronic diseases, the gaze of medical and nutrition experts also shifted from treating and curing diseases to more proactively preventing and reducing their incidence. Medical re-searchers used the relatively new science of epidemiology to identify the risk factors associated with chronic diseases. The insurance industry first developed the risk factor approach in the late nineteenth century, drawing on new statistical methods for the calculation of probabilities.[18] Insurance companies used their comprehensive population statistics to identify the correlation between lifestyle factors and the incidence of diseases. This enabled them to determine policies and premiums based on these correla-tions, regardless of whether a causal relationship existed between the iden-tified risk factors and the disease. Life insurance companies, using these statistical techniques, were even able to confirm and quantify the associa-tion between high blood pressure and heart disease incidence in the early twentieth century.[19]

By the middle of the twentieth century, medical and nutrition scien-tists such as Ancel Keys began to use epidemiological data to determine risk factors, generate hypotheses for disease causation, and thereby pre-scribe changes in diet and lifestyle. Some medical researchers considered the risk factor approach a way of moving beyond a narrow biochemical model for understanding disease causation. The biomedical model had been relatively effective for understanding and treating infectious dis-eases, because these diseases often have single causes—usually bacteria—that can be identified and treated. Unlike infectious diseases, chronic diseases seemed to medical researchers to have multiple contributing causes, and some thought that the risk-factor approach would enable a broader range of factors to be taken into account, producing a better understand-ing of ill health.[20]

However, as medical historian Robert Aronowitz argues in *Making Sense of Illness*, these risk factors have often been interpreted in a reductive manner.[21] He suggests that there has been a continual slippage and blur-ring of risk factors and disease determinants, such that risk factors have been treated by medical experts as if they were causal factors. These risk factors have even been interpreted as diseases or health conditions in their own right and therefore require treatment. Risk factors for coronary heart disease, such as hypertension (high blood pressure) and hyperlipidemia (high blood cholesterol), are now directly treated with blood pressure drugs and cholesterol-lowering statins.[22] Medical and nutrition research has also tended to focus on risk factors that could be easily measured and quantified—such as specific food or nutrient intake data, blood choles-terol levels, body weight, or the number of cigarettes smoked—but at the expense of less easily measurable factors such as exercise or stress.[23]

Sociologists Alan Petersen and Deborah Lupton have argued that since the 1970s, public health and health promotion discourses have represented individuals and individual bodies as being *at risk*: "To be labelled 'at risk' means entering a state in which an apparently healthy body moves into a sphere of danger."[24] Otherwise healthy looking, well-fed, and symptom-less people may thereby be recategorized as being at risk of chronic diseases.[25] The risk factor approach contributes to the production of at-risk individuals, and more specifically *at-risk bodies*—bodies that are perceived to be at increased risk of chronic diseases due, in part, to the overconsumption of bad nutrients and foods. It was over-nourished individuals in particular—those who ate too many bad nutrients or just too many calories—whose overnourished bodies were now deemed to be most at risk.

Epidemiologists extended the quantifying logic of the earlier nutritional era into the understanding of the relationship between nutrients and the body, though this time in the form of statistical probabilities. The combination of this risk factor approach to disease, on the one hand, and a more proactive approach to preventing disease and promoting good health, on the other, encouraged researchers and policy makers to translate some of these emerging scientific theories into medical and nutritional guidelines, even without solid evidence that their policies and interventions would be effective. Dietary interventions for the prevention of heart disease exemplified this new discourse of health promotion.[26]

The Diet-Heart Hypothesis and the Vilification of "Artery Clogging" Saturated Fats and Cholesterol

The diet-heart hypothesis has for more than fifty years been central to nutrition research and dietary guidance. The AHA has promoted it since the early 1960s, and it has been enshrined in U.S. dietary guidelines since the late 1970s. This hypothesis is based on a causal chain of associations linking dietary fats to blood cholesterol levels, and in turn linking blood cholesterol levels to atherosclerosis and cardiovascular disease. In its classical form, the diet-heart hypothesis states that saturated fats and dietary cholesterol raise the levels of total cholesterol in the blood, which in turn clogs the arteries and causes heart disease. The diet-heart hypothesis was also the basis for nutrition experts' campaigns for the reduction in total fat consumption from the 1970s. But while the underlying scientific understanding of the role of fat, dietary cholesterol, blood cholesterol, and the causes of cardiovascular disease has changed significantly since the 1960s, the vilification of the supposedly "artery-clogging" saturated fats within the dominant nutritional paradigm has been consistent throughout this period.

The chief researcher and promoter of the diet-heart hypothesis in the 1960s and 1970s was American physiologist and epidemiologist Ancel Keys. Following the apparent increase in coronary heart disease after World War II, Keys designed an epidemiological study comparing six carefully selected countries that showed an association between high-fat diets and higher rates of heart disease. Despite acknowledging a lack of evidence for this hypothesis, he advocated a reduction of total intake of dietary fat from animal- and plant-based foods by one-third.[27] In 1959 Keys and his wife published a popular nutrition and recipe book, *Eat Well and Stay Well*, that promoted a low-fat diet, noting that with respect to the causes of the "plague" of coronary heart disease at the time, "the case for dietary fats being an important factor is impressive and the inferences are obvious."[28] However, by the late 1950s, Keys had also shifted his attention from total fats to the different types of fats and their effect of total blood cholesterol levels.

In the early 1950s medical researchers such as L.W. Kinsell and E.H. Ahrens had shown in clinical trials on hospitalized patients that, while monounsaturated fats were considered neutral (neither raising nor lowering cholesterol levels), saturated fats raised blood cholesterol levels and polyunsaturated fats lowered them.[29] Meanwhile, medical researchers working on the Framingham Heart Study—a study conducted in the factory town of Framingham, Massachusetts, that began in 1950—reported a strong association between very high blood cholesterol levels and heart disease incidence in young and middle-age men, though not in women. These findings gave support to the emerging "lipid hypothesis," which proposed that high cholesterol levels in the blood is a risk factor for heart disease. However, the Framingham study failed to show a correlation between the types of fat consumed and blood cholesterol levels.[30] Nevertheless, the lipid hypothesis became an important plank of the diet-heart hypothesis, and it was simply assumed that if saturated fats raised blood cholesterol levels, then they also increased the risk of heart disease.

In 1960 Keys began his famous seven-country epidemiological study to test this reformulated diet-heart hypothesis, and a decade later he published preliminary results that identified a correlation between saturated fat intake and heart disease in the countries he selected.[31] But Keys's cross-country studies have been criticized for the way he seemingly selected countries whose data fitted his hypothesis, while leaving out countries that did not.[32] The so-called French paradox identified by French researchers in the 1980s is an example of a cross-country anomaly that contradicted Keys's hypothesis, since the French ate a diet high in saturated fat yet had relatively low rates of heart disease.[33]

In 1957 a report by the AHA first suggested that intakes of fat, calories, and saturated fat are "probably important factors" in the development of atherosclerosis.[34] In 1961 the AHA published a more strongly worded report implicating the role of fats, though by this time Keys and another scientist supportive of the diet-heart hypothesis had joined the AHA's Committee on Nutrition.[35] This report recommended that people at high risk of heart disease reduce their intake of fat to no more than 25–35 percent of total calories, substitute polyunsaturated for saturated fats, and reduce their total calorie intake.[36] This advice was directed at those considered at high risk of heart disease, rather than for the whole population.[37] But Keys himself considered it good advice for everyone. When he made the cover of *Time* in 1961, the magazine reported his recommendation that *all* Americans reduce their total fat consumption from 40 percent to 15 percent.[38]

During the mid-1970s the diet-heart hypothesis underwent further modification. New techniques to measure blood cholesterol enabled medical researchers to differentiate among the types of lipoprotein molecules— such as LDL and HDL—that carry cholesterol through the bloodstream and to study their association with cardiovascular disease. These studies showed that higher levels of LDL cholesterol carriers were associated with a marginally higher risk of heart disease, while higher levels of HDL were associated with lower risks of heart disease.[39] The eventual description of HDL cholesterol carriers as good cholesterol and LDL as bad cholesterol implied a definitive understanding of the role of these lipoproteins in the development of cardiovascular disease, even though medical researchers still did not understand the precise biological mechanisms involved. This differentiation of good and bad blood cholesterol carriers led nutrition scientists to slightly reorder their fat hierarchy. Polyunsaturated fats remained good fats because they lowered both HDL and LDL levels. Saturated fats remained bad fats because they raised LDL levels, though they also had the beneficial effect of raising HDL levels. But a study published in 1985 demonstrated that monounsaturated fats raised HDL and lowered LDL, giving it the title of best fat of all with respect to heart disease risk factors.[40]

While blood cholesterol levels could be altered through dietary changes, there was still little direct evidence at that stage—in the form of controlled trials—that reducing saturated fat intake or raising unsaturated fat intake actually decreased the incidence of heart disease.[41] This is, arguably, still the case today. For example, a 2008 expert collaboration, jointly sponsored by the Food and Agriculture Organization of the United Nations and the World Health Organization, reviewed the evidence on fatty acids and heart disease and concluded that "the available evidence from cohort and randomized controlled trials is unsatisfactory and unreliable to make judgment about and substantiate the effects of dietary fat on risk of CHD [coronary heart disease]."[42]

Since the 1970s nutrition experts and associated health institutions have also consistently stigmatized the cholesterol that naturally occurs in animal foods. Dietary cholesterol is metabolized into blood cholesterol in the body, yet scientists have long known that increases in dietary cholesterol only modestly increase blood cholesterol levels.[43] The liver produces most of the cholesterol found in the blood and adjusts bodily production and absorption of cholesterol in response to changes in dietary cholesterol intake. There are also considerable differences among individuals in their response to cholesterol intake.[44] Nevertheless, the recommendation to reduce cholesterol was being promoted by the AHA in the 1970s, as well as by the 1980 *Dietary Guidelines*.

The diet-heart hypothesis was first translated into U.S. population-wide dietary advice in the 1977 *Dietary Goals for the United States* released by Senator George McGovern's Senate Select Committee on Nutrition and Human Needs. It recommended that everyone reduce their saturated fat to 10 percent of total calories and reduce dietary cholesterol to 300 milligrams per day.[45] But many scientists at the time questioned whether there was adequate scientific evidence to warrant translating the diet-heart hypothesis into dietary advice for the whole population. The American Medical Association, for example, argued for more targeted medical advice for those falling into "risk categories" based on individual blood lipid profiles.[46] Nutrition scientist Raymond Reiser described the universal advice to reduced saturated fat consumption as an "oversimplification" and "exaggeration."[47]

There were also rival theories to Keys's diet-heart hypothesis, though they ultimately attracted only limited support from nutrition and cardiovascular experts. Beginning in the late 1950s, British nutrition scientist John Yudkin and British surgeon Thomas Cleave focused on sugar and refined grains, rather than fat, as the chief nutritional culprits. Cleave had argued in his book *The Saccharine Disease* that it was the steep rise in the consumption of "refined carbohydrates" (i.e., refined flour and sugar) in the twentieth century that explained the rise in the incidence of a range of chronic diseases and obesity.[48] Cleave attributed these effects primarily to the absence of fiber in these refined carbohydrate foods and the consequent speed at which these foods were digested and absorbed into the bloodstream, thereby raising blood sugar levels.[49]

By contrast, Yudkin argued that it was primarily high sugar consumption that caused heart disease and other chronic diseases, rather than refined grains.[50] He focused on factors such as the way sugar raised triglyceride levels in the blood, since triglycerides, like blood cholesterol, are another biomarker of heart disease risk. Yudkin also pointed to the role of sugar in increasing insulin insensitivity, the latter a characteristic of diabetes.[51] However, since sugar and saturated fat intake were both associated with heart disease risk in a number of countries, Keys's fat hypothesis and Yudkin's sugar hypotheses were situated as competing single-nutrient explanations.[52] The possibility that the combination of a high-fat *and* high-sugar diet might explain the rise of various chronic diseases seems not to have been seriously entertained in this debate.[53] In any event, Yudkin's sugar theory was dismissed by most nutrition experts at the time as lacking evidence.[54] Both Cleave and Yudkin were also no less definitive than Keys in attributing the heart disease epidemic and a range of other diseases to one nutrient or food component.

Other critics of the diet-heart hypothesis argued that the wrong dietary fats were being indicted for the rise in heart disease and cancer. In the 1970s American biochemist Mary Enig and colleagues argued that unsaturated fat consumption had increased at four times the rate of saturated fat consumption since 1909 and that unsaturated fats accounted for most of the increase in total fat intake over this period.[55] The ratio of polyunsaturated to saturated fats had increased from 0.2 in 1900 to 0.4 in 1970, the period in which heart disease rates had climbed.[56] Enig argued that refined vegetable oils, and particularly partially hydrogenated oils, were more probable causes of these chronic diseases. Some studies in the 1960s and 1970s had reported that polyunsaturated vegetables oils seemed to promote cancer more than saturated fats.[57] *Trans*-fat consumption had also risen from four to twelve grams per day since 1910.[58] Keys himself had published a paper in 1961 that argued that hydrogenated oils raise blood cholesterol levels more than nonhydrogenated oils do.[59] But not until the 1990s did mainstream nutrition scientists take seriously the possible role of *trans*-fats in heart disease.

Whether it was refined grains, sugar, or refined and reconstituted vegetable oils, these counterhypotheses were pointing to the rising consumption in the twentieth century of more highly refined and processed foods and ingredients, rather than to the overconsumption of the whole animal foods and naturally occurring nutrients vilified by Keys. Enig also questioned the "strong tendency to identify saturated fat with animal fat and unsaturated fat with vegetable fat."[60] She estimated that "more saturated fat in the diet has come from vegetable fat than from beef since 1929," thereby questioning the basis for the vilification of red meat.[61]

The evidence supporting the diet-heart hypothesis was, and still is, largely based on bringing together two separate correlations: first, between dietary fats and blood cholesterol levels, and second, between blood cholesterol and atherosclerosis (the lipid hypothesis). But few studies have examined whether reducing saturated fats directly reduces heart disease incidence, and the results from these studies have been mixed.[62] Over the past two decades, research has further complicated, and arguably undermined, the classical diet-heart hypothesis. A number of studies and reviews of the literature have suggested that any benefits of reducing saturated fat intake depend upon the type of nutrients they are replaced with.[63] These studies have claimed that replacing saturated fats with polyunsaturated fats may modestly reduce the incidence of cardiovascular disease and may also reduce LDL cholesterol. However, according to these same studies the replacement of saturated fats with carbohydrates—particularly in the form of refined grains and sugar—seems to offer no benefits in terms of cardiovascular disease incidence and may even increase heart disease risk.[64] For example, studies have shown that, compared with carbohydrates, higher consumption of saturated fat increases LDL but also increases HDL and decreases triglycerides, with the latter two biomarkers associated with lower heart risk.[65] One of the authors of these studies, Frank Hu of the Harvard School of Public Health, argues that "the time has come to shift the focus of the diet-heart paradigm away from restricted fat intake and toward reduced consumption of refined carbohydrates."[66]

Nutrition scientists have also found that types of saturated fatty acids—such as lauric, palmitic, and stearic acid—can be differentiated in terms of their relative health effects on blood cholesterol levels. Stearic acid, for example—which makes up half the saturated fats in beef—is considered not so bad, because it is converted into monounsaturated fat in the body and does not significantly increase LDL levels. A study published in 2012 has also suggested that the association between saturated fats and cardiovascular disease risk identified in epidemiological studies may in fact vary when the *food source* of the saturated fats is taken into account.[67] This study found that higher intakes of saturated fat from dairy foods are associated with a slightly lower risk of heart disease compared with intake of saturated fats from meat. The authors of the study speculated that this difference may be due to the different types of saturated fats, or the other accompanying nutrients and food components, found in meat and dairy foods.

With respect to blood cholesterol levels, some researchers now consider the distinction among different types of LDL particles, in terms of their size and density, to be a better predictor of heart disease risk than total LDL concentrations.[68] According to this theory, the smaller and denser types of LDL particles have been found to be more strongly associated with elevated heart disease risk than the larger, less dense, or "fluffier," types of LDL particles—though such an association does not prove causality.[69] Nevertheless, to be consistent with the logic and language of distinguishing between good and bad cholesterol, this research suggests that there may be "good" and "bad" types of LDL cholesterol. Importantly, high-carbohydrate diets—at least when they take the form of diets high in refined grains and sugar—appear to raise concentrations of the small, dense LDL particles, thereby increasing heart disease risk, while higher saturated fat intake has the opposite effect, increasing the concentration of the large, fluffy LDL particles (thereby contradicting the long-standing advice to replace saturated fats with carbohydrates).[70]

Another scientific development challenging the classical diet-heart hypothesis is the theory that oxidized LDL particles, rather than LDL particles per se, may have a causal role in atherosclerosis.[71] The significance of this theory is that polyunsaturated fats are much more susceptible to oxidation than are monounsaturated and saturated fats. Refined vegetable oils—which are now the primary source of polyunsaturated fats in the American food supply—may suffer oxidative damage as a result of the extraction and refining process, as well as during high-temperature frying. Processing and frying oils also deplete them of the antioxidants that some medical experts believe might protect the body against oxidized fatty acids.[72] Many refined vegetable oils are high in omega-6 polyunsaturated fats and have a high ratio of omega-6 to omega-3 fats, which some experts believe may be another contributor to heart disease risk.[73] High-carb foods—and particularly so-called refined carbs, as well as the fructose in sugar—may also promote "oxidative stress" and the oxidation of LDL particles.[74]

Some lipid experts argue that the diet-heart hypothesis and the dominant discourse of "artery clogging saturated fats" has been decentered—if not undermined—by these and other developments in the understanding of diet and heart disease. Biochemist Glen Lawrence, for example, argues that biomedical research over the past twenty years has shattered the "pervasive popular belief that cholesterol clogs the arteries, with cholesterol buildup eventually becoming so great that blood flow to the heart or brain becomes blocked, causing heart disease or stroke."[75] Instead, coronary heart disease is now more commonly characterized as a condition of chronic inflammation in the arteries, since inflammation is now considered to play an essential role in the development and progression of atherosclerosis, as well as in other conditions such as insulin resistance and type-2 diabetes.[76]

We should, of course, welcome this increasingly sophisticated and nuanced scientific understanding of the complex relationships among nutrients, biomarkers, and cardiovascular disease, including the further differentiation of types of fats and biomarkers. As scientists have implicated ever more possible dietary contributors to heart disease risk—from *trans*-fats, sugar, and refined flours and vegetable oils, to insufficient omega-3 fats, vitamin D, and antioxidants—our efforts to adjust our diets at the level of nutrients, particularly in a one-nutrient-at-a-time manner, become correspondingly more difficult. However, despite the complexities, uncertainties, and unknowns surrounding the dietary causes of heart disease, the single-nutrient explanation that saturated fats increase heart disease risk via their effects on blood cholesterol levels is still promoted by most nutrition experts and institutions.[77] The 2010 *Dietary Guidelines* not only continues to recommend that intake of saturated fats be limited to 10 percent of total calories (which isn't far below the current average of 11 percent), but also encourages a further reduction to 7 percent with the claim that this would further reduce heart disease risk.[78]

One way to interpret the recent evidence and hypotheses is that they increasingly point toward the quality of foods consumed. Many of the suspect food components, such as *trans*-fats and sugar, have been extracted, refined, concentrated, reconstituted, or further degraded through various processing techniques. At the same time, many of these food components are often combined within highly processed foods and desserts. For example, some of the major sources of saturated fats in Americans' diets are convenience foods such as pizza, grain-based desserts (e.g., cakes and cookies), ice cream, and processed meats (e.g., sausages and salami), and these foods often also contain sugar, refined flour, and other processed ingredients and additives.[79] But few nutrition experts seem game to admit that when it comes to heart disease, we may not yet know enough to give any more specific advice than to eat a good-quality diet made up of good-quality, minimally processed foods.

THE 1977 *DIETARY GOALS FOR THE UNITED STATES*: THE SHIFT TO NUTRICENTRIC DIETARY ADVICE

The translation of the good and bad fats and low-fat advice into population-wide, government-endorsed eating guidelines can be traced to the publication of the *Dietary Goals for the United States* in 1977. The *Dietary Goals* were the first guidelines to embody a number of characteristics of the era of good-and-bad nutritionism. These characteristics include the shift in orientation from tackling nutritional deficiencies to addressing chronic diseases and obesity, the new concern with addressing risk factors for the prevention of these chronic diseases, and the shift from "eat more" to "eat less" dietary advice.[80]

The greater significance of the *Dietary Goals*—yet one barely commented on at the time of their introduction—was that it materialized and accelerated the transition that had been taking place since the early 1960s from food-level to nutrient-level dietary advice. In terms of specific nutrient-level guidelines, the *Dietary Goals* were the first government-backed guidelines to specify quantitative goals for fat, carbohydrate, and protein. Importantly, this report also helped to galvanize expert consensus behind the diet-heart hypothesis and to stigmatize fat, saturated fat, and cholesterol.

Senator McGovern's Senate Select Committee on Nutrition and Human Needs held hearings over five years involving a range of food and nutrition experts. The committee was therefore well aware of the debates and lack of consensus among the experts on some key issues, particularly on the dietary contributors to heart disease and other chronic diseases. Yet the draft document they released in 1977 strongly reflected the views of just one expert, Mark Hegsted from the Harvard School of Public Health, a strong promoter of the diet-heart hypothesis. Hegsted's position was summed up in his foreword to the first edition of the *Dietary Goals*: "The diet of the American people has become increasingly rich—rich in meat, other sources of saturated fat and cholesterol and in sugar. . . . It should be emphasized that this diet which affluent people generally consume is everywhere associated with a similar disease pattern—high rates of ischemic heart disease, certain forms of cancer, diabetes and obesity."[81]

The *Dietary Goals* report painted a picture of what science journalist and low-carb proponent Gary Taubes refers to as the "changing American diet story"—the story that the American diet had changed radically over the previous fifty years, from a primarily grain-based diet to one high in meat, animal products, and fat, and that this change accounted for the rise in the incidence of chronic diseases.[82] For the authors of the *Dietary Goals*, the main culprits in the poor American diet were the animal-based foods—red meat, dairy, and eggs—stigmatized particularly for their high levels of fat, saturated fat, and cholesterol. Yet the report itself acknowledged that the rise in fat consumption over this period was largely due to people consuming more vegetable oils, rather than animal products.

The *Dietary Goals* promoted the idea that the average American diet was inherently unhealthy and that public health had deteriorated over the course of the twentieth century. By contrast, some critics of this view defended the typical American diet and the general health of the population. Leading nutrition scientist Alfred Harper, for example, argued that "changes in our food supply during this century have been associated with improved health rather than with deteriorating health."[83] He noted that life expectancy had increased by twenty years since 1900, that nutritional deficiencies were rare, and that age-adjusted incidence of heart disease and stroke had already begun to decline. Another outspoken scientific critic of the report, Robert Olson, argued that changes in the consumption of eggs, butter, and beef did not even correlate with changes in cardiovascular disease mortality, because consumption rates had largely remained steady or had decreased over the fifty-year period between 1900 and 1950, during which time heart disease deaths had climbed steeply.[84]

The first edition of the guidelines released by the McGovern committee in 1977 contained six dietary goals that referred primarily to nutrients and food ingredients (see table 4.1). The emphasis of the guidelines was on getting people to increase their consumption of carbohydrates and unsaturated fats and to decrease their consumption of fat, saturated fat, cholesterol, salt, and sugar. The report stated that reducing fat consumption would lower the incidence of obesity and cancer, and that reducing saturated fat and cholesterol intake would reduce cardiovascular disease. It also suggested that lowering sugar intake may reduce tooth decay, diabetes, and cardiovascular disease, and that lowering salt would reduce hypertension.

These nutrient-level goals were also translated into seven food-level goals (table 4.1). The emphasis of these goals was generally to eat more plant-based food and less saturated fat–rich animal food, while avoiding

TABLE 4.1
Dietary Goals for the United States, First Edition, February 1977

1. Increase carbohydrate consumption to account for 55–60 percent of energy (caloric) intake.
2. Reduce overall fat consumption from approximately 40 percent to 30 percent of energy intake.
3. Reduce saturated fat consumption to account for about 10 percent of total energy intake, and balance that with polyunsaturated and monounsaturated fats, which should account for about 10 percent of energy intake each.
4. Reduce cholesterol consumption to about 300 milligrams per day.
5. Reduce sugar consumption by about 40 percent to account for about 15 percent of total energy intake.
6. Reduce salt consumption by about 50–85 percent to approximately 3 grams per day.

Changes in food selection and preparation suggested by the goals

1. Increase consumption of fruits and vegetables and whole grains.
2. Decrease consumption of meat, and increase consumption of poultry and fish.
3. Decrease consumption of foods high in fat, and partially substitute poly-unsaturated fat for saturated fat.
4. Substitute nonfat milk for whole milk.
5. Decrease consumption of butterfat, eggs, and other high-cholesterol sources.
6. Decrease consumption of sugar and foods high in sugar.
7. Decrease consumption of salt and foods high in salt.

SOURCE: U.S. Senate Select Committee on Nutrition and Human Needs, *Dietary Goals for the United States,* 1st ed. (Washington, D.C., 1977).

foods with a high sugar or salt content.[85] While the *Dietary Goals* purportedly separated the nutrient-level and the food-level recommendations, even most of the food selection goals were qualified in terms of the nutrients they contained, such as "decrease . . . foods high in total fat," "substitute poly-unsaturated fat for saturated fat," "substitute nonfat milk for whole milk," and decrease "other high-cholesterol sources." The food selection goals also largely repeated the nutrient/ingredient goals of reducing sugar and salt intake rather than referring to the common food sources of these ingredients.

The guidelines' overwhelming message—repeated several times within these thirteen nutrient and food recommendations—was the need for people to reduce their total fat and saturated fat intake. The guidelines also clearly recommended that fat be reduced from all food sources, with no distinction made between the fats found in whole foods and those in processed foods. It was this stigmatizing of fats in general that was perhaps the most significant innovation in dietary guidance in America and had the greatest impact on the nutriscape of the following two decades.

While the *Dietary Goals* sometimes recommended that people increase or decrease their consumption of particular whole foods, there was no explicit reference to processed foods. The recommendation to cut down on any foods with high salt, sugar, and fat content was clearly a nutritional euphemism for confectionery and other highly processed foods and beverages. The body of the report identified the high intake of processed foods and soft drinks as one of the sources of nutrient deficiencies and excesses in the average diet, such as its large amounts of sugar and the lack of fiber. There was a reference to "processed sugars" in the second edition of the *Dietary Goals*, but the term *processed foods* did not appear in any of the stated goals, which would have pleased the food manufacturing industry. At the same time, the report promoted reduced-fat—that is, refined—milk, thereby undermining any clear whole food messages.

In a later commentary on the *Dietary Goals*, Mark Hegsted rejected the matter of processed foods as an issue in determining a healthy diet: "The issue is *not* natural vs. processed foods. We don't really know how to make that distinction—some people consider such items as pasteurized milk and frozen vegetables as processed foods. The issue is: How to apply the best nutritional knowledge."[86] For Hegsted and other nutrition scientists, certainty existed only at the level of nutrients, rather than at the level of foods, since much of the research had been directed at the nutrient level. We therefore should not—or could not yet—distinguish between foods on the basis of levels of processing, at least with respect to their health consequences.

This first edition of the *Dietary Goals* was extremely controversial for two main reasons. The first was the food industries' intolerance of any government-endorsed guidelines recommending that the consumption of any of their products be reduced. The meat and livestock industry in particular lobbied to remove the guideline calling for a reduction in meat consumption. The second was the lack of scientific consensus among nutrition and public health experts regarding the specific recommendations of the committee, particularly concerning the advice for people to eat less meat, fat, and saturated fat.[87] While in his foreword Hegsted acknowledged that there was no scientific consensus on the guidelines, he justified them by saying there was no time to lose in addressing the dangers of the American diet and by reassuring readers that it would not do people harm to follow them:

There will undoubtedly be many people who will say we have not proven our point; we have not demonstrated that the dietary modifications we recommend will yield the dividends expected.... The question to be asked ... is not why should we change our diet but why not? What are the risks associated with eating less meat, less fat, less saturated fat, less cholesterol, less sugar, less salt, and more fruits, vegetables, unsaturated fat and cereal products especially whole grain cereals. There are none that can be identified and important benefits can be expected.[88]

The *Dietary Goals* received enthusiastic support from bodies such as the AHA, the American Society for Clinical Nutrition, and the consumer advocacy group Center for Science in the Public Interest—organizations that already backed dietary recommendations against fat and animal foods.[89] While there was much controversy over the content of the dietary goals, there seems to have been little if any questioning of the nutricentric focus and language of these goals in general, or much reflection on how the lay public might interpret and respond to this nutrient-level advice.

The Senate committee convened several more public hearings in 1977 to listen to expert and industry responses to the draft report. Despite the intense political lobbying and scientific debate, only a few relatively minor changes were made to the final set of guidelines published later that year (table 4.2).[90] A new dietary goal to "avoid overweight" was added to the second edition, a goal to be achieved by balancing energy intake and expenditure. The more significant change was the replacement of the guideline to "decrease consumption of meat and increase consumption of poultry and fish" with the less prohibitive and somewhat more obscure nutricentric advice to "decrease consumption of animal fat, and choose meats, poultry, and fish, which will reduce saturated fat intake."[91] Rather than suggesting that individuals simply eat less meat, they were encouraged to continue eating meat, and even in the same quantities, as long as they "choose" meats with lower fat or saturated fat content. Marion Nestle argues that this transformed a negative "eat less" message into a more positive "choose" message designed to placate food producers.[92]

In his preface to the report Mark Hegsted suggested that reducing meat consumption was a key aim of the *Dietary Goals*, so he was less supportive of a changed wording. Yet years later he admitted that there was not sufficient scientific evidence against meat, other than its saturated fat content.[93] In other words, the revised guideline was consistent with the

TABLE 4.2

Dietary Goals for the United States, Second Edition, December 1977

1. To avoid overweight, consume only as much energy (calories) as expended; if overweight, decrease energy intake and increase energy expenditure.

2. Increase the consumption of complex carbohydrates and "naturally occurring" sugars from about 28 percent of energy intake to about 48 percent of energy intake.

3. Reduce the consumption of refined and processed sugars by about 45 percent to account for about 10 percent of total energy intake.

4. Reduce overall fat consumption from approximately 40 percent to about 30 percent of energy intake.

5. Reduce saturated fat consumption to account for about 10 percent of total energy intake, and balance that with polyunsaturated and monounsaturated fats, which should account for about 10 percent of energy intake each.

6. Reduce cholesterol consumption to about 300 milligrams per day.

7. Reduce the intake of salt to about 5 grams per day.

Changes in food selection and preparation suggested by the goals

1. Increase consumption of fruits and vegetables and whole grains.

2. Decrease consumption of refined and other processed sugars and foods high in such sugars.

3. Decrease consumption of foods high in total fat, and partially replace saturated fats, whether obtained from animal or vegetable sources, with polyunsaturated fats.

4. Decrease consumption of animal fat, and choose meats, poultry, and fish, which will reduce saturated fat intake.

5. Except for young children, substitute low-fat and nonfat milk for whole milk, and low-fat dairy products for high-fat dairy products.

6. Decrease consumption of butterfat, eggs, and other high-cholesterol sources. Some consideration should be given to easing the cholesterol goal for premeno-pausal women, young children, and the elderly in order to obtain nutritional benefits of eggs in the diet.

7. Decrease consumption of salt and foods high in salt content.

SOURCE: U.S. Senate Select Committee on Nutrition and Human Needs, *Dietary Goals for the United States*, 2nd ed. (Washington, D.C., 1977).

scientific evidence regarding saturated fat rather than meat and was there-fore justified in its focus on nutrients rather than foods. As noted earlier, a significant portion of saturated fat in the American diet was in fact consumed in the form of vegetable oils. In the second edition of the *Dietary Goals*, the nutrient goal for saturated fat was also changed to read that saturated fats must be reduced "whether obtained from animal or vegetable sources," thereby reinforcing the decontextualized focus on saturated fat. This nutritional guideline was also consistent with the dietary goal for milk in the first edition, which merely suggested switching from full-fat to low-fat milk in order to reduce fat consumption, rather than reducing milk consumption per se.

This revised wording certainly pushed the *Dietary Goals* a little further in the direction of nutricentric language. However, it is important not to overemphasize, as some commentators have done, the food industry's role in the formation of the nutricentric character of these guidelines. For example, Michael Pollan has mistakenly suggested that the first edition of the *Dietary Goals* was "a fairly straight-forward set of dietary guidelines" that consisted of "plain talk about foodstuffs," and that only after pressure from the food industry did the language of the *Dietary Goals* shift to that of nutrients.[94] Yet this focus was in fact already dominant in the first edition of the report, which in turn reflected the nutrient-level focus of scientific research and of the dietary advice emanating from institutions such as the AHA.

The nutricentric focus of these dietary recommendations was, however, not necessarily very meaningful or useful for the lay public. Given that a significant proportion of the total fats and saturated fats in Americans' diets at that time was derived from animal foods such as meat and dairy products, by not explicitly recommending less consumption of these foods the *Dietary Goals* potentially undermined any serious attempt to reduce fat consumption. The meat and dairy industries, as well as the food manufacturing industry, seem to have immediately recognized that dietary messages framed in terms of nutrients rather than specific food products would be less damaging to consumer demand for their products. Eventually they also realized the commercial potential of exploiting these nutrient-level messages so that they could more positively market their products in health terms, such as by emphasizing the high iron and protein content of red meat.

THE NUTRICENTRIC *DIETARY GUIDELINES* AND THE WHOLE FOOD-CENTRIC *FOOD GUIDE PYRAMID*

The *Dietary Goals* report was never adopted as an official government document.[95] Nevertheless, throughout the 1980s and 1990s both the form of these dietary guidelines (i.e., their nutrient-level focus) and their particular content (e.g., the recommendations on fat and cholesterol) were more or less directly adopted in later reports and dietary recommendations.

The seven key recommendations in the first set of *Dietary Guidelines for Americans* released in 1980 (see table 4.3) included the advice to "avoid too

TABLE 4.3
Dietary Guidelines for Americans, 1980

1. Eat a Variety of Foods
2. Maintain Ideal Weight
3. Avoid Too Much Fat, Saturated Fat, and Cholesterol
4. Eat Foods with Adequate Starch and Fiber
5. Avoid Too Much Sugar
6. Avoid Too Much Sodium
7. If You Drink Alcohol, Do So in Moderation

SOURCE: U.S. Department of Agriculture and Department of Health and Human Services, *Nutrition and Your Health: Dietary Guidelines for Americans* (Washington, D.C., 1980).

much fat, saturated fat, and cholesterol," "eat foods with adequate starch and fiber," and "avoid too much sugar."[96] As a guide for the lay public, the *Dietary Guidelines* were shorter and punchier than the *Dietary Goals* and made no reference to quantified dietary targets. Yet they reproduced and even extended the nutricentric focus of the *Dietary Goals* by referring almost exclusively to nutrients and food components, such as fat, cholesterol, starch, and fiber. Sugar is a food ingredient as well as a component of foods. Even salt was referred to by its chemical classification, sodium. In the body of the *Dietary Guidelines* document, some of the food sources of the targeted nutrients were discussed, and it mentioned the need for people to "limit" foods such as butter, coconut oil, and sodas and to "choose" foods such as "lean meat" and whole grain breads. Yet its take-home message was wrapped up in its seven short nutricentric recommendations.

The *Dietary Guidelines* have been reissued every five years since 1980, with the seven recommendations largely unchanged up to the 2000 report. The most significant change in this period was in 1990, when Americans were no longer asked to "avoid too much" fat, saturated fat, cholesterol, sugar, and sodium but—in a more positive and encouraging tone—to "choose" foods containing lower quantities of these supposedly harmful nutrients and ingredients. The guideline "avoid too much fat, saturated fat, and cholesterol" became "choose a diet low in fat, saturated fat, and cholesterol." The guideline for people to "avoid too much sugar" was changed in 1990 to "use sugars in moderation," and then in 1995 to "choose a diet moderate in sugars."[97]

The *Dietary Goals* and the *Dietary Guidelines* have also had a much wider international influence on other countries' dietary guidelines, including those in Europe, Canada, Japan, and Australia.[98] Scandinavian countries

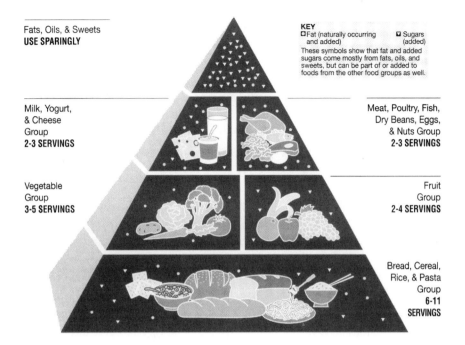

FIGURE 4.1
Food Guide Pyramid
SOURCE: U.S. Department of Agriculture, *Food Guide Pyramid* (Washington, D.C.: Center for Nutrition Policy and Promotion, 1992).

had already in the late 1960s begun recommending a reduction in fat, with the official Norwegian dietary guidelines released in 1975 recommending as one of its "ten good eating rules" to "cut down on fat—choose lean/low fat foods."[99] The first Australian guidelines released in 1981 included "avoid eating too much fat," and in 1985 the Japanese guidelines recommended that people "avoid excess fats" and "use vegetable oils rather than animal fats."[100]

Not until 1992 did the USDA release, as the long-awaited successor to the *Basic Seven* and *Basic Four* food guides of the 1940s and 1950s, its famous *Food Guide Pyramid* (see figure 4.1), a food-based visual guide intended to complement the *Dietary Guidelines*. The *Food Guide Pyramid* created a hierarchy of food categories.[101] The food groups at the bottom were identified as the healthier foods, for which a larger number of servings were recommended than the food groups at the top. The pyramid clearly advocated a plant-based diet, with the grains, vegetable, and fruit groups dominating the base, and the animal foods toward the top.

In contrast with the *Dietary Goals* and *Dietary Guidelines*, the *Pyramid* refers primarily to foods rather than nutrients and in this sense appears to be a food-based dietary guide. Yet at the top there is the "fats, oils, and sweets" group, which is essentially the bad nutrients and food components group that the public is advised to "use sparingly." Symbols representing fat and sugar are also scattered throughout the other food groups of the *Pyramid*, indicating that all foods may be contaminated by both "naturally occurring and added" fats and sugars. The entire pyramid is in fact structured in terms of the hierarchy of macronutrients within mainstream nutrition science, with the carbs dominating the base of the pyramid, protein-rich foods in the middle, and fats at the top. As such, it visually illustrated and translated into food-level advice the low-fat/high-carb diet that dominated nutritional recommendations throughout the 1980s and 1990s.

While the *Pyramid's* graphics primarily represent foods and food groups rather than nutrients, like the *Dietary Guidelines* it makes no explicit reference to processed foods or to the level of refining and processing that the depicted foods are typically subjected to.[102] The *Pyramid* can therefore be understood as a form of whole food-centric dietary advice that is blind to the processed realities of the food supply and of many people's diets. As Ross Hume Hall has argued, the *Pyramid's* graphics "give no indication that much of the food people eat has been processed. . . . One can follow the Food Guide Pyramid to the letter while selecting white bread in the grain category, French fries in the vegetable category, canned fruit cocktail in the fruit category, ice cream for dairy, and hot dogs for meat."[103] The *Pyramid* therefore implies that the problem with contemporary diets is an imbalance in the quantities of foods among the various food groups that people consume, rather than the quality of the foods within each group, particularly in terms of levels of processing.

Over the years, some nutrition experts have also criticized the *Pyramid* because of its specific food-level advice and for its failure to provide more nuanced nutrient-level advice. Walter Willett from the Harvard School of Public Health has been one of the most vocal critics of the original *Pyramid*, arguing that it was "built on shaky scientific ground"[104] and was "really out of date from the day it was printed."[105] Willett's main concerns have been that the *Pyramid* failed to distinguish between good and bad fats and good and bad carbs, and that it therefore oversimplified the science of fats and carbs.[106] The grains group makes no distinction between whole grain foods and rapidly digested carbohydrates, such as white bread and pasta. Willett also observes that the directive to eat fat sparingly does not distinguish between good and bad fats or between the food sources of good and bad fats. He also considers the number of servings of red meat and dairy to be excessive. Willett essentially argues that the *Food Guide Pyramid* does a poor job of translating the *Dietary Guidelines'* nutrient-level advice into food-level recommendations. Other experts, such as Marion Nestle, have largely defended both the form and content of the original *Pyramid*.[107] Nestle nevertheless emphasizes that the serving sizes specified for each food group are an attempt to appease the interests of powerful sectors within the food system, such as the meat and dairy industries.

While nutrition scientists shaped the form and content of the dominant nutritional paradigm in this era, the key drivers and promoters of nutritionism were government agencies such as the USDA and the U.S. Food and Drug Administration, as well as public health organizations such as the AHA and the Center for Science in the Public Interest. Underpinned by the new health promotion paradigm and an urgency to stem the rising incidence of chronic diseases, these institutions have been proactive in translating controversial scientific hypotheses into definitive nutrient-level advice for the lay public. They have also encouraged the simplification of the science of food and nutrients for the sake of presenting what they considered to be easily understandable dietary messages for the public.

This era was one in which governments attempted to exert greater control over food production and consumption. Government agencies shaped and modified both the form and the content of dietary guidelines in an attempt to meet the conflicting aims of protecting public health while not impeding the commercial interests of the food industry. In the 1970s and 1980s, the food industry also began to recognize the benefits and to embrace the idea of promoting its foods on the basis of their nutrient contents.

By the mid-1990s, some of the nutritional certainties of this era were being challenged. The promotion of margarine over butter came unstuck when the *trans*-fats in margarine were found to have detrimental effects on blood cholesterol levels. The vilification of eggs on the basis of their cholesterol content was also softened after experts acknowledged that dietary cholesterol was not a significant contributor to blood cholesterol levels. The low-fat guideline in particular was starting to be discredited, both because of the lack of scientific evidence supporting the supposed benefits of this guideline, and because it had seemingly failed to prevent—and some commentators claimed it may have contributed to—the "twin epidemics" of obesity and diabetes in America. The decline of the low-fat campaign opened up a space for other macronutrient approaches and weight-loss diets to flourish, but also marked the transition to a new era of functional nutritionism.

CHAPTER FIVE

The Macronutrient Diet Wars

From the Low-Fat Campaign to Low-Calorie, Low-Carb, and Low-GI Diets

Eating fat makes you fat, even if you take in fewer calories.
—DEAN ORNISH, *EAT MORE, WEIGH LESS*, 1993

It's the calories, stupid!
—ALICE LICHTENSTEIN,
TUFTS UNIVERSITY SCHOOL OF NUTRITION, 2003

Dietary fat, whether saturated or not, is not the cause of obesity, heart disease, or any other chronic disease of civilization. . . . The problem is the carbohydrates in the diet.
—GARY TAUBES, *GOOD CALORIES, BAD CALORIES*, 2007

On February 24, 2000, the U.S. Department of Agriculture (USDA) hosted the Great Nutrition Debate, a forum bringing together various popular weight-loss diet-book doctors and nutrition experts to discuss "approaches to dieting, nutrition, and long-term health effects." Opening the debate, then U.S. Secretary of Agriculture Dan Glickman admitted that "as a society, I'm convinced that we remain very confused and conflicted about what it is that we should eat."[1] This was a disarming admission from the head of the department that oversees much of the government-sponsored nutrition research and that had been producing and promoting the *Dietary Guidelines for Americans* and the *Food Guide Pyramid* over the previous two decades.[2]

Glickman thought that even if the Great Nutrition Debate would "not clear up the confusion" about what we should eat, it might "at least bring the issues out in an objective way so that the country can make up its own mind."[3] So Glickman and his department took the bold step of inviting diet-book authors whose views had previously been ridiculed and dismissed by mainstream nutrition experts. Among them was Robert Atkins, whose low-carb diet books had caused a sensation in the 1970s and were once again in vogue. Glickman also invited authors who promoted other variations on the low-carb, high-fat, high-protein theme, such as Morrison Bethea, author of *Sugar Busters! Cut Sugar to Trim Fat*, and Barry Sears, whose book *The Zone* emphasized the effects of carbs on insulin regulation. Also present was Dean Ornish, author of the best-selling *Eat More, Weigh Less* and a promoter of a low-fat, plant-based diet that was fairly compatible with the *Dietary Guidelines*. The debate itself was orderly, if robust, with the speakers lining up predictably on the side of the national dietary recommendations or else backing alternative low-carb, high-protein diets.

By bringing these people together for a debate over what we should eat, the USDA acknowledged that not all was well with the recommendations the U.S. government had been promoting since 1980. The *Dietary Guidelines* and the *Food Guide Pyramid* advocated as a core dietary recommendation that people should reduce their fat consumption. Yet the United States was in the midst of the recently diagnosed "obesity epidemic," with the upward trend in obesity as well as diabetes beginning at about the same time as the start of the low-fat campaign twenty years earlier. By the late 1990s, some nutrition experts began to suggest that the low-fat campaign may have contributed to—or even been a major cause of—the "twin epidemics" of obesity and diabetes. Perhaps Atkins and the low-carb diet gurus had been right after all?

The decline of the low-fat campaign since the late 1990s has allowed a number of alternative weight-loss dietary approaches to flourish. Most nutrition experts have responded to the discrediting of the low-fat advice by returning to a very nineteenth-century understanding of the calorie and advocating a reduction in calorie intake. Low-carb diets have become very popular again since the early 2000s, but they have now also gained a degree of scientific legitimacy among nutrition experts. Low-GI (glycemic index) diets also enjoy widespread popularity and expert support, especially because they provide one method for distinguishing between so-called good and bad carbs.

Most of these popular dietary approaches embody a form of macronutrient reductionism—the idea that we can adequately describe foods and dietary patterns in terms of their macronutrient profiles, regardless of the foods in which you find these macronutrients. *The Zone* diet, for example, quantifies the ideal macronutrient ratio in the most precise terms: 40 percent fat, 40 percent carbs, and 20 percent protein. Alternatively, dietary guidelines and many nutrition experts now reemphasize calories and the energy balance equation as the key to understanding weight gain and weight loss, in what amounts to a return to the caloric reductionism of the nineteenth century. Each of these dietary approaches reduces foods and their effects on bodily health to one or two key nutrients, biomarkers, or nutritional concepts, whether fat, carbs, calories, glycemic levels, or insulin. In doing so, they typically present simplified, decontextualized, and deterministic explanations of the causes of weight gain and chronic diseases.

This chapter begins with an examination of the science, the consequences, and the public debates regarding the low-fat campaign that dominated the nutriscape of the 1980s and 1990s, before considering three alternative nutritional theories and weight-loss diet plans—low-calorie, low-carb, and low-GI diets.

THE LOW-FAT CAMPAIGN

The contemporary concern with dietary fat primarily dates back to nutrition studies published in the 1950s that examined the links between types of fat and heart disease, but it was not until the 1980 *Dietary Guidelines* that the public was officially advised to "avoid too much fat" (see chapter 4). The 1988 *Surgeon General's Report on Nutrition and Health* also placed a strong emphasis on the dangers of total fat consumption with the first of its dietary recommendations: "Reduce consumption of fat (especially saturated fatty acids) and cholesterol." This report identified fat as the chief nutritional threat to the nation's health: "The Report's main conclusion is that overconsumption of certain dietary components is now a major concern for Americans. While many food factors are involved, chief among them is the disproportionate consumption of foods high in fats, often at the expense of foods high in complex carbohydrates and fiber that may be more conducive to health."[4] Similarly, the National Academy of Science (NAS) 1989 report *Diet and Health: Implications for Reducing Chronic Disease Risk* recommended that the "highest priority is given to reducing fat intake" and set a maximum limit of 30 percent fat, though the report admitted that "no studies in humans have yet examined the benefits of changing to low-fat diets."[5] The 1990 *Dietary Guidelines* also set a maximum of 30 percent fat of total caloric intake.[6] The USDA's 1992 *Food Guide Pyramid* placed fats and oils at the very top and recommended that they be used only "sparingly."[7]

Many public health and consumer advocacy organizations also supported the low-fat guideline. The prominent consumer advocacy group

Center for Science in the Public Interest referred to fat as the "greasy killer."[8] In 1981, the center's director, Michael Jacobson, claimed that there is a "mountain of scientific evidence that indicts the high-fat diet as a major killer, a killer of far more Americans than all our nation's wars combined."[9] Despite this broad level of support for the low-fat guideline, the recommendations were also strongly contested, particularly when they first appeared in the *Dietary Goals* in 1977. Institutions such as the American Medical Association and the National Research Council's Food and Nutrition Board questioned whether there was adequate scientific evidence for the effectiveness and safety of these low-fat dietary goals.[10]

While the language of these dietary guidelines and reports clearly pointed to the need to reduce the quantity of total fat consumed, most guidelines specified targets in terms of a proportion of energy intake.[11] These quantified targets, such as 30 percent fat, gave the low-fat advice a veneer of scientific precision. Yet there were no studies that identified this percentage of fat as a safe or optimal proportion.[12] Instead, experts seem to have arbitrarily chosen 30 percent as an achievable target, given that in the late 1970s the average American's diet contained around 40 percent fat. At the height of the low-fat campaign in the late 1980s and early 1990s, some experts and popular commentators were suggesting that the less fat eaten the better.[13] Dean Ornish, for example, advised a diet of just 10 percent fat, echoing the proportion recommended by the very low fat, very high carb, plant-based Pritikin diet.[14] The flip side of the "all fats are bad" message was that all carbohydrates are good, and the low-fat/high-carb diet became the dominant nutritional mantra of the 1980s and 1990s. Many experts and lay Americans alike came to see the low-fat/high-carb diet as a simple, universal, one-size-fits-all healthy diet that would address obesity and a range of chronic diseases.

In terms of heart disease, scientific studies had pointed to saturated fats rather than total fats as being associated with increased risk due to their effects on blood cholesterol levels. But since saturated fat represented a large fraction of the total dietary fat in the American diet, reducing total fat consumption was considered an indirect means of reducing saturated fat intake.[15] The low-fat message deliberately simplified the scientific understanding of the relationship between fats and heart disease and was based on the assumption that the public would have difficulty understanding the distinctions between types of fats.[16] Evidence from the Framingham Heart Study that obesity was an independent risk factor for heart disease provided another indirect justification for the low-fat approach—if a low-fat diet could reduce obesity, then it would also indirectly reduce the risk of heart disease.[17]

But since the early 2000s, many experts have backed away from recommending the low-fat guideline as a way to prevent heart disease and have instead shifted back to the good-and-bad fats discourse and the indictment of saturated fats. A number of studies have also demonstrated that replacing saturated fats with carbohydrates—particularly in the form of refined grains and sugar—may in fact have a detrimental effect on blood triglycerides, HDL cholesterol levels, and the density of LDL particles, and therefore—from the standpoint of the diet-heart hypothesis discussed in chapter 4—may increase the risk of heart disease.[18] Nutritional epidemiologist Walter Willett has also suggested that by simplifying the fat message, the low-fat guideline may have led to a reduction in the intake of what he considers the good unsaturated fats.[19] Since 2006, the American Heart Association has also reemphasized the good-and-bad fats message for reducing heart disease risk, though it still recommends that total fat intake should contribute no more than 35 percent of total dietary energy.[20] It also continues to publish its *Low-Fat, Low-Cholesterol Cookbook*.[21]

In terms of cancer risk, the 1982 NAS report on *Diet, Nutrition and Cancer* recommended a reduction of dietary fat to 30 percent of dietary energy to reduce the risk of cancer, and breast cancer in particular.[22] It mainly justified this guideline on the basis of a small number of epidemiological studies comparing fat consumption and cancer rates in different countries, as well as based on evidence from animal studies. However, the NAS report admitted that the "epidemiological data are not entirely consistent."[23] According to Willett, the evidence in the early 1980s linking total fat intake and various forms of cancer was always "meager."[24] Two large prospective studies were partly designed to test the relationship between fat consumption and cancer: the dietary component of the Nurses' Health Study, led by Willett from the Harvard Medical School, and the Women's Health Initiative, conducted by the National Institutes of Health. Neither study reported a significant association between reduced fat consumption and reduced cancer risk.[25] These studies should not necessarily be accepted as definitive evidence of the lack of a causal relationship between fat and cancer, because they too are subject to the limitations associated with all epidemiological studies. More recent studies have differentiated between the role of different types of fats in cancer risk, with some researchers suggesting that saturated fats and omega-6 polyunsaturated fats increase the risk or promote the growth of particular cancers, while omega-3 fats may reduce the risk or hinder the growth of cancer.[26] However, nutrition experts have largely abandoned the low-fat guideline as relevant for cancer prevention.[27]

For the treatment and prevention of diabetes, the advice of diabetes experts over the past century has swayed back and forth, from restricting carbohydrates to restricting fat consumption.[28] Prior to the discovery and synthesis of insulin in the 1920s, the standard advice for people with diabetes was to severely limit their intake of starchy and sugary foods and to be on diets in which as much as 75–85 percent of their total energy comes from fat.[29] From the 1930s, some leading diabetes experts also recommended reduced-fat diets, though the recommendations that people restrict their consumption of high-carbohydrate foods and avoid sugar also remained standard practice.[30] Following the more general shift to low-fat/high-carb dietary guidelines in the 1970s, diabetic dietary recommendations drifted further in the low-fat direction. At the time, the American Diabetes Association began to advocate that people with diabetes increase their carb consumption to 50–60 percent of total calories, though coming mainly from "complex carbs" and fiber-rich foods.[31] In practice, however, most carbohydrates are eaten in the form of refined foods, so the expectation that people with diabetes would suddenly start eating whole grain products or legumes was perhaps unrealistic. The aim of this low-fat guideline was primarily to decrease the very high risk of cardiovascular disease associated with diabetes.[32]

Over the past decade, mainstream diabetes experts and institutions have backed away from the low-fat directive and have more openly acknowledged the dangers of those high-carb diets that include high levels of refined carbohydrate foods.[33] The American Diabetes Association emphasizes the importance of people monitoring their carbohydrate intake, such as through carb counting, and now accepts that lower-carb diets may be an effective short-term weight-loss strategy.[34] However, they are still reluctant to advocate severe carbohydrate restriction for people with diabetes, despite the acknowledgment that the quantity of carbohydrates consumed is an important determinant of blood sugar and insulin levels.[35] The American Diabetes Association also continues to refer to the idea that sugar causes diabetes as a "myth" and portrays sugar as just another source of calories.[36] But given the other possible deleterious effects of sugar on the body's metabolism, and the enormous quantities of sugar in the food supply, this characterization of sugar as mere calories seems rather oversimplified and understated. Mainstream diabetes dietary guidelines also continue to recommend reductions in saturated fat intake, based on the assumption that these fats not only increase heart disease risk but also decrease insulin sensitivity.[37]

The most widely recognized justification for a low-fat/high-carb diet has been its claimed weight-management benefits. The case against fat was largely based on the fact that it contains more than twice as many calories per gram as protein or carbohydrate. It follows that high-fat foods also tend to be relatively high in total calories. The low-fat advice was therefore an indirect strategy for reducing calorie intake. Another assumption of low-fat proponents was that high-fat foods might promote the passive overconsumption of food, because they were assumed to be both highly palatable and less satiating than carbs and protein.[38] Animal studies also supported the idea that fat is more readily converted into body fat than are carbs and protein. The low-fat guideline was thereby used as a proxy for low-calorie advice, and fat counting came to displace calorie counting as the primary nutrient-level approach to weight management in the 1980s and 1990s.[39]

In his best-selling 1993 diet book *Eat More, Weigh Less*, the high-profile doctor and clinical researcher Dean Ornish adopted this view of fats as the especially fattening macronutrient: "Not all calories are alike. A fat calorie is not the same as a calorie from protein or carbohydrate.... The *type* of calories you eat is more important than the *amount*.... Simply put, eating fat makes you fat, even if you take in fewer calories."[40] Yet no studies at the time had demonstrated that a high-fat diet was a cause of obesity, or that a low-fat diet was the most effective route to weight loss. Subsequent studies have also largely failed to support the benefits of a low-fat diet over other macronutrient ratios.[41]

Regardless of the scientific evidence underpinning the low-fat campaign, the low-fat guideline was nutritionally reductive in the way it decontextualized fat and promoted the idea that the quantity and ratio of fats and carbs are the ultimate determinants of the quality and healthfulness of a food. Mainstream dietary guidelines made no distinction between the fats that naturally occur in whole foods, on the one hand, and the added, reconstituted, or degraded fats found in many processed and convenience foods, on the other. In either case, the quantity of fat had to be reduced. The low-fat recommendations also failed to distinguish between eating fewer high-fat foods, on the one hand, and eating reduced-fat varieties of these high-fat foods, on the other. Nutrition experts often used the term "high-fat foods" as a euphemism for highly processed and poor-quality foods, such as deep-fried, fast-food meals. Yet the low-fat guideline also tended to blur the distinction between whole foods and highly processed foods, and it endorsed the processing of whole foods to reduce the fat content, as in the case of reduced-fat milk. The lay public seemed to go further and interpreted the low-fat guideline as a stamp of approval for reduced-fat versions of highly processed, convenience foods, such as low-fat Oreo cookies, Frito Lay's low fat potato crisps, and the short-lived McDonald's McLean Deluxe burger. The American Heart Association also promoted this view through its endorsements of low-fat products, such as Kellogg's Low-Fat Pop-Tarts.[42]

This obsession with reducing the fat content of foods and meals ignores the potentially beneficial ways in which fat may interact with other nutrients within foods or in food combinations. For example, while most dietary guidelines promote reduced-fat milk, the fat in milk plays an important role in facilitating the absorption of some of the other nutrients, such as the fat-soluble vitamins, and may moderate the effects of the milk's lactose on blood sugar levels.[43] The combination of high-fat and high-carb foods—such as butter with bread—is also a means of regulating the rise in blood sugar levels compared with consuming the refined, high-carb food in isolation.

The 1990 U.S. Department of Health and Human Services report *Healthy People 2000* encouraged the food industry to respond to the low-fat challenge, in the hope that by the end of the decade the industry would increase to "at least 5,000 brand items [in] the availability of processed food products that are reduced in fat and saturated fat."[44] The food industry did its duty by translating this nutritionally reductive dietary advice into a flood of nutritionally engineered food products and nutritionally reductive marketing practices. Marketing foods on the basis of their fat content was a simple and powerful strategy, with "low fat," "no fat," "reduced fat," and "97 percent fat free" some of the dominant nutritional marketing slogans of the good-and-bad era. Nutrition claims relating to total fat content rose from an average of 5 percent of all nutrient-content claims in the early 1980s to more than a third of nutrient claims by the late 1990s.[45] However, a food marketed as "reduced fat" is not necessarily much lower in fat content than other comparable food products. For instance, reduced-fat Oreo cookies contain 140 calories of fat per 33 grams, versus 160 calories of fat in the full-fat variety.[46]

Reducing the percentage of just a single nutrient allowed food manufacturers great scope to adjust the types and quantities of ingredients and of other nutrients, particularly in highly processed foods. This reduction in fat was often achieved by adding sugar, chemically modified starches, or artificial fat replacers, such as olestra—ingredients that have a taste, texture, or "mouthfeel" similar to that of fat.[47] In this way, the low-fat guideline has either directly or indirectly endorsed the replacement of some whole food ingredients with highly refined and reconstituted ingredients. Some nutrition experts have openly promoted the use of low-fat foods produced with olestra as a means of weight loss.[48] As with all nutrient-content claims, the marketing of foods as low fat also serves to conceal the level of processing of the food product and to distract people's attention from the ingredients and additives used in its production. To some extent, the focus on fat may even have overwhelmed the public's concerns over both the calorie content and sugar content of foods. The International Sugar Research Foundation was so confident of this that at the hearings of the McGovern Senate committee for the *Dietary Goals for Americans* in the 1970s, it defended sugar on the basis that it consisted of "pure calories with no fat and no cholesterol."[49]

By the mid-1990s, commentators had already observed the so-called Snackwells phenomenon. Named after the popular Snackwells line of fat-free, high-sugar cookies, this phenomenon referred to people eating more low-fat foods because they considered them healthier than regular, full-fat foods. For example, they might have been tempted to eat two low-fat chocolate cookies instead of eating just one regular chocolate cookie.[50] Based on controlled studies testing low-fat claims on nutrition labels, Cornell University marketing professor Brian Wansink argues that "all people—particularly those who are overweight—eat more calories from snack food when it is labeled as 'low fat' than when it is labeled as 'regular'."[51] Wansink suggests that low-fat claims reduce guilt and so encourage increased consumption of those foods. Even low-fat advocate Dean Ornish observed the Snackwells phenomenon among his patients in the 1990s: "The week that Entenmann's rolled out its fat-free desserts, a number of our patients gained weight. They thought that as long as they were eating something fat free, they could eat as much as they wanted."[52]

LOW-FAT PARADOXES AND THE LOW-FAT DEBATE

By the mid-1990s, many nutrition experts began to realize that the low-fat campaign was not exactly going to plan.[53] The period of the low-fat campaign happened to coincide with a steady rise in obesity levels. Some nutrition experts came to refer to this as the "low-fat paradox" and even as the "American paradox."[54] Between 1971 and 2004, the prevalence of obesity increased in men from 11.9 percent to 31.1 percent and in women from 16.6 percent to 33.2 percent.[55]

The other apparent paradox of the low-fat campaign—though one much less acknowledged or debated—is that it does not seem to have translated into significant reductions in total fat consumption![56] Dietary surveys based on consumer recall data suggest that between 1971 and 2001 the proportion of fat calories in the diets of men and women decreased respectively from 37 percent to 33 percent and 36 percent to 33 percent. But while the proportion of fat in the diet decreased, the absolute quantity of fat consumed did not decrease significantly. Rather, there was an increase in carbohydrate consumption and of total caloric consumption over this period, which accounts for the decrease in the proportion of fat in the diet.[57]

Regarding how Americans changed what they ate during the low-fat campaign, USDA food supply data suggest that the 12 percent (300 calorie) increase in average daily calorie consumption was largely due to the increased consumption of refined grains (46 percent increase), added fats (24 percent), and added sugars (23 percent). While Americans ate 12 percent less red meat, this was more than offset by a 90 percent increase in poultry consumption. Their consumption of dairy products remained largely unchanged, with a steep decline in whole milk consumption largely replaced by an increased consumption of reduced-fat milk and cheese.[58] Children consumed less milk but drank more sodas and other sweetened beverages.[59]

But neither the nutrient intake data nor the food intake data adequately reveals the extent to which the foods consumed had become increasingly processed. In this period many people's eating and living patterns were changing dramatically. For example, from 1977 to 1995, the number of meals and snacks consumed in both non-fast-food and fast-food restaurants increased by 150 percent and 200 percent, respectively.[60] The production and availability of a range of processed and convenience foods had greatly expanded, particularly in the form of semiprepared, ready-made, and packaged foods and beverages, fast foods such as pizza, breakfast cereals, snack foods, and sugary drinks.[61] Many of these convenience foods are high in refined grains, added fats, added sugars, and calories. There was also a corresponding shift in consumption from the visible fats found in oil and full-fat milk to the "hidden fats" in mixed meals and snacks.[62]

The coincidence of the low-fat campaign with rising obesity and diabetes rates has prompted a lively expert and public debate over the causes of these "twin epidemics." A number of commentators have specifically blamed the low-fat campaign—and, more generally, the *Dietary Guidelines for Americans* and the *Food Guide Pyramid*—for contributing to, or being largely responsible for, the rise in the prevalence of obesity.[63] Nutrition scientist

John Allred was one of the first to reflect on this low-fat paradox, arguing in 1995 that the "overemphasis on consumption of low-fat foods has contributed to the current widespread increase in body weight."[64] Allred identified both biological and behavioral explanations for this paradox. He suggested that the emphasis on fat reduction had given the public the idea that caloric consumption was not important, and they had subsequently indulged in "too much of a good thing" by eating more of these low-fat foods. But he also argued that reduced-fat foods were less satiating than high-fat foods and could therefore lead to increased consumption of low-fat/high-carb foods. Allred noted that this excess carb consumption also increases insulin levels, which in turn increases the amount of fat stored in the body.

Some of Allred's concerns were echoed in the report of the USDA's Dietary Guidelines Advisory Committee that prepared the 2000 edition of the *Dietary Guidelines for Americans*—the dietary guide that had ushered in the low-fat campaign twenty years earlier. Their report acknowledged that the low-fat advice could distort public understandings of a healthy diet and lead to an overconsumption of carbohydrates, while limiting the consumption of unsaturated fats:

> The committee further held the concern that the previous priority given to a "low-fat intake" may lead people to believe that, as long as fat intake is low, the diet will be entirely healthful. This belief could engender an overconsumption of total calories in the form of carbohydrates, resulting in the adverse metabolic consequences of high-carbohydrate diets. Further, the possibility that overconsumption of carbohydrates may contribute to obesity cannot be ignored. The committee noted reports that an increasing prevalence of obesity in the United States has corresponded roughly with an absolute increase in carbohydrate consumption. Finally, with a "low-fat" recommendation, the potential benefit to be derived from the several forms of unsaturated fats may not be realized.[65]

Some of the comments of members on the Dietary Guidelines Advisory Committee reflect this more critical attitude. Regarding obesity, one committee member suggested that "[perhaps] our emphasis on low percentage of fat may have backfired on us, and that perhaps we would be wiser to go forth with a message that was across the board calories rather than just emphasizing fat."[66] Despite such frank admissions from the advisory committee about the failure of the form and content of the low-fat recommendation to improve human health, the revised 2000 *Dietary Guidelines* merely made a subtle change in wording from "low" to "moderate" total fat recommendations, and continued to advise people to limit their total fat, saturated fat, and cholesterol consumption.

The debate over the consequences of the low-fat campaign became much more public and inflamed following the publication of science journalist Gary Taubes's controversial and widely read 2002 *New York Times Magazine* cover story, "What If It's All Been a Big Fat Lie?" His essay unequivocally blamed the low-fat campaign for the "obesity epidemic." As he interprets it, "We ate more fat-free carbohydrates, which in turn, made us hungrier and then heavier. . . . [Such] a diet cannot help being high in carbohydrates, and that can lead to obesity, and perhaps even heart disease."[67]

Taubes, who has since become a leading proponent of low-carb diets, claimed that low-fat/high-carb foods are more fattening and yet less satiating. He pointed to the decline in the proportion of fat in the American diet over the previous two decades, yet mischievously he mentioned neither that total fat consumption in the period had remained fairly stable nor that the rise in total calories, and carb calories in particular, was largely responsible for the drop in the percentage of fat.[68] Taubes's claim that the low-fat advice caused the shift in eating patterns toward a low-fat/high-refined-carb diet also ignored all the other changes in the food supply, in food marketing, and in eating habits, such as the dramatic expansion in the number and variety of processed and convenience foods, spreads, and beverages being produced and consumed. Even so, he acknowledged that perhaps Americans were not following the dietary guidelines after all and were just eating more of the cheap, tasty, processed foods that had flooded the food supply:

> Surely, everyone involved in drafting the various dietary guidelines wanted Americans simply to eat less junk food, however you define it, and eat more the way they do in Berkeley [California]. But we did not go along. Instead we ate more starches and refined carbohydrates, because calorie for calorie, these are the cheapest nutrients for the food industry to produce, and they can be sold at the highest profit. It is also what we like to eat.[69]

Michael Pollan, in his book *In Defense of Food*, follows Taubes by presenting the low-fat campaign as a "historical disaster" and as having "made us less healthy and considerably fatter."[70] He claims that this single-nutrient dietary guideline was a major cause of the "obesity epidemic":

"Americans got really fat on their low-fat diet." For Pollan, the low-fat advice was based on "bad science."[71] He suggests that the public dutifully followed this bad advice but that they were also confused by it. Unlike Taubes, Pollan acknowledges that Americans did not in fact reduce their fat intake, only the percentage of fat consumed, due to an increase in carbohydrate consumption. However, he seems to blame the increase in carbohydrate consumption for this rise in obesity and suggests that the low-fat campaign tricked the public into thinking they could eat more low-fat/high-carb foods: "It was easy for the take-home message of the 1977 and 1982 dietary guidelines to be simplified as follows: eat more low-fat foods. And that is precisely what we did."[72] Pollan thereby offers a one-to-one causal explanation for the change in eating patterns and the rise in obesity, and directly blames the low-fat dietary guideline for the rise in obesity rates.[73] He also assumes that the defective dietary guideline was the problem—that is, that the science on low-fat diets itself was flawed—rather than acknowledging that the public could misunderstand, and the food industry could exploit, any nutricentric guideline, such as low carb or low calorie. Nor does he consider the possibility that these changes in the food supply and eating patterns—particularly the rise in processed and convenience food consumption—as well as the rise in obesity rates, might have occurred without the low-fat campaign.

While the engineering and marketing of low-fat foods may have had an influence on consumer behavior and consumption practices, it is important not to exaggerate this effect. To expect a one-to-one relationship between nutrient-specific advice and changes in dietary patterns, or between this advice and the rising incidence of obesity and diabetes, represents another type of nutritional reductionism—in this case a nutritionally reductive sociological or behavioral explanation—one that ignores the other variables and contexts that shaped dietary patterns and the interpretation and application of this advice. While dietary guidelines framed and shaped the eating habits of the public in various ways during this period, the changes in nutrient and food consumption patterns were products of many profound changes and transformations in the food environment and in living and working patterns. The rise in consumption of convenience and fast foods, for example, is associated with an increase in meals eaten outside of the home.

The real failure of the low-fat campaign, and of nutricentric dietary guidelines in general since the 1970s, may have been that they seem to have done little to *prevent* people from eating more of these poorer quality, highly processed foods. While a low-fat label may have swayed the purchasing decisions of consumers choosing between similar products—say, between low-fat and full-fat milk, or between low-fat and full-fat cookies—it seems unlikely that they will have switched from a minimally processed (good quality) to a highly processed (poor quality) food in many instances just because the latter was perceived to be lower in fat.

One of the ways nutrition experts have responded to the failures of the low-fat campaign has been to deflect attention from the low-fat guideline itself and instead attribute these failures to the lay public's "confusion" and "misinterpretation" of the guideline. Leading Dutch nutrition scientist Martijn Katan, for example, pointed to the public's apparent misunderstanding of the low-fat guideline as an explanation for people eating more junk foods and drinks that are also high in carbohydrates, a situation that he dubbed the "great carbohydrate fiasco":

> In the 1990s people were told that foods low in fat and high in carbohydrate prevented chronic diseases. That led to the "great carbohydrate fiasco" during which Americans stuffed themselves with low-fat chips and sugary drinks, to the detriment of their waistlines and their blood lipids. The origin of this fiasco was the fuzzy definition of what constitutes a healthy diet. The scientists who introduced the term *low fat* intended beans, vegetables, and whole-wheat bread. However, low fat also applies to low-fat cookies and soda drinks.[74]

Did Americans really stuff themselves with chips and sodas because of the low-fat guideline? Katan echoes the claim by other nutrition experts that the public was confused by the low-fat guideline and had misinterpreted the dietary recommendations to eat less fat. But while some people may have taken liberties in the way they interpreted the low-fat guidelines, in many ways they were just following the decontextualized advice of nutrition experts to reduce the intake or proportion of fat in their diets as an end in itself.

CALORIC REDUCTIONISM: THE RETURN OF THE NINETEENTH-CENTURY CALORIE

While some nutrition experts continue to promote a low-fat diet, the decline of the low-fat campaign since the late 1990s has created space for a range of alternative dietary approaches to flourish.[75] But most mainstream nutrition experts have returned to the energy-balance equation as the only nutritional concept required to explain the causes of, and the solutions to, the "obesity epidemic" and as a strategy for weight loss. The rise in people's caloric consumption between 1980 and 2000—estimated at anywhere between 200 and 500 calories per person—is used to explain the increase in body mass index (BMI) over this period.[76] To the extent that this rise in calorie intake is accurate, and reflects an increase in the sheer quantity of food consumed, then it seems a very plausible way of explaining the rise in the percentage of overweight and obese individuals. Nevertheless, I argue that the singular focus on and interpretation of calories as a way of measuring food quantity, bodily activity, and weight fluctuations is another form of nutritional reductionism—one that exaggerates the precision that experts claim for this explanatory concept, simplifies the complex ways in which different types of foods may be metabolized by the body and affect body weight, and blurs qualitative differences between foods.

For Tufts University nutrition scientist Alice Lichtenstein, the singular biological cause of obesity is obvious: "It's the calories, stupid."[77] Similarly, Marion Nestle argues that "when it comes to obesity . . . it is the calories that count. Obesity arises when people consume significantly more calories than they expend in physical activity."[78] The solution to losing weight is similarly framed in terms of the need to limit calorie intake and/or increase energy expenditure. Nestle describes just how simple dieting is when we understand it in terms of the energy-balance equation: "The science of dieting is easy. Diets are about calories. Eat too many, and weight goes up. To lose weight, you have to eat fewer calories than your body needs ('eat less'), use up more calories than usual by increasing your physical activity ('move more'), or even better, do both."[79] She also suggests that as long as the calories stay in balance, it hardly matters what you eat: "Once you balance calories from food against activity levels, and make sure that enough calories come from fruits and vegetables but not too many from junk foods, other aspects of your diet matter much less. You can eat what you like as long as you don't eat too much."[80] Given that Nestle suggests that calories are all that counts when it comes to weight gain or weight loss, limiting the junk food or sweetened beverages within your daily calorie allocation is presumably just to make sure that you consume an otherwise nutritionally adequate diet, rather than because junk foods are any more fattening than other foods on a per-calorie basis.

Mainstream dietary guidelines have redoubled their focus on calories and on the need for people to restrict their calorie intake. The 2010 *Dietary Guidelines for Americans*, for example, has placed weight management at the top of its recommendations, with "balancing calories" the only variable that the public is required to keep their eyes on for this purpose. It states: "Control total calorie intake to manage body weight. For people who are overweight, this will mean consuming fewer calories from foods and beverages."[81] Public health experts have campaigned for calorie labeling on the front of food packaging and on restaurant and fast-food menus, to enable consumers to more carefully monitor their caloric intake. The food industry has pledged to do its bit by slimming a few calories off of some its food products. In 2010 a coalition of food manufacturers calling itself the Healthy Weight Commitment Foundation, which includes Coca-Cola, PepsiCo, and many other large corporations, pledged to remove 1.5 trillion calories from the food supply by 2015 through the development of "new lower-calorie options, reduced calorie content of current products, and reduced portion sizes of existing single-serving products."[82]

Obesity expert George Bray summarizes the caloricentric explanation of weight gain when he says that "obesity is the result of a prolonged small positive energy surplus with fat storage as the result."[83] For the energy-balance equation to be useful as a weight-management strategy, energy intake and energy expenditure need to be fairly accurately measurable in terms of calories, so that the difference between the two can explain any consequent weight gain or loss. In their accounts of the dietary causes of the obesity epidemic, or of the enormous effort supposedly required to work off a fast-food meal, many obesity experts invoke such a claim to caloric precision. For example, Martijn Katan and David Ludwig claim that "walking an extra mile a day expends, roughly, an additional 60 kcal compared with resting—equal to the energy in a small cookie."[84] Similarly, obesity researchers Christina Baker and Kelly Brownell have suggested that "expending the calories of a single meal from a fast-food restaurant consisting of a large hamburger, fries and a milkshake would require half a marathon."[85] Eating a steak, baked potatoes, and a glass of wine would presumably also require a half a marathon to prevent much of this meal being stored as fat.

In 2003, obesity expert James Hill and colleagues produced a back-of-the-envelope calculation that decreasing food intake or increasing energy expenditure by a mere 100 calories per person per day may close the "energy gap" that has caused the rapid increase in obesity in the United States over the past two decades—although they admitted that this idea "remains to be empirically tested."[86] The 2005 *Dietary Guidelines for Americans* similarly suggested that "for most adults a reduction of 50 to 100 calories per day may prevent gradual weight gain."[87] The types of foods adding up to the 100 calories responsible for putting on this weight, or that could be cut to lose this weight, are also apparently irrelevant. More recent estimates have been that a much higher "energy gap" has been responsible for such increases in average weight of the population. For example, Katan and Ludwig calculate that for a person to go from normal weight (BMI < 25) to obese (BMI > 35) over a period of twenty-five years would require an extra 680 calories per day, either from increased food intake or decreased physical activity.[88]

Most nutrition experts support the assumption that a calorie is a calorie, regardless of the kind of macronutrients, foods, or food combinations they are contained in. In this respect, nothing much has changed since the late nineteenth century. According to the energy-balance equation, a calorie from a high-fat fast-food hamburger is no different from a calorie from a carrot, or from a candy bar, in terms of their effects on weight management. As Harvard nutrition scientist Fred Stare put it in the early 1980s, "Calories are all alike, whether they come from beef or bourbon, from sugar or starch, or from cheese and crackers."[89] Similarly, many nutrition experts once again consider the macronutrient source of the calories irrelevant for the purposes of weight management. In what amounts to a return to the nutritional orthodoxy of the pre-low-fat era, they assume that a fat calorie is equivalent to a protein calorie and a carbohydrate calorie. While some experts continue to implicate high-fat foods in weight gain, they do so only on the basis that these foods tend to be higher in calories.

The return of the calorie into the contemporary obesity discourse is in many respects a return to a very nineteenth-century understanding of calories (described in chapter 3) and to the caloric reductionism of that earlier era. Despite a century of further scientific research and an increasingly sophisticated understanding of food, nutrients, and the body at the molecular level, most nutrition experts still represent food as an undifferentiated mass of calories and the body as a "black box," such that the calories-in/calories-out equation is all we need to explain fat accumulation and weight management. Even though the same experts acknowledge that there are important differences between foods when it comes to their effects on all other aspects of dietary health, in the case of fat storage it is as if only the calories count.

Caloric reductionism can be defined as the assumption that all foods and all bodies can be reduced to, and precisely quantified in terms of, the uniform unit of the calorie, that the body uses or "burns" all calories in the same way and at the same rate, and that weight gain or loss can be predicted in advance on this basis. Caloric reductionism thereby assumes that the type or the quality of the food that delivers these calories is essentially irrelevant when it comes to weight management and fat storage. It simplifies and decontextualizes food quantity and exaggerates the precision with which it can be used to measure the way the body uses or stores this food. It also continues to rely on the mechanical concept of food as a uniform "fuel" that feeds the mechanical body.

In some respects caloric reductionism goes further than other forms of nutritional reductionism, since calories—unlike nutrients—do not actually exist as material entities. They are just a way of measuring energy that is released when a given quantity of food is literally burned. In this sense, the calorie can be described as a highly abstract concept—one that abstracts certain properties of a food. Yet while there may be a uniform calorie of energy released when a food is combusted, we know that different foods and food components are not uniformly metabolized by the body in the same way. The energy-balance equation—calories in equals calories out—may be accurate as a way of measuring food and the body at the abstract level of pure energy or heat transfers, but it tells us little about how the body metabolizes different food substances.

Nutrition experts often speak of calories as if they have some kind of independent existence. For example, in *Why Calories Count*, Marion Nestle and Malden Nesheim suggest that "calories are invisible and devoid of taste. You cannot tell how many are in a food just by looking at it or even tasting it."[90] This comment is certainly applicable to nutrients, such as vitamins, but it implies that—like nutrients—calories do exist in some substantive sense, except that they, too, cannot be seen or tasted. Similarly Nestle and Nesheim argue that "if you eat too many calories for the number you expend, most of them will end up as body fat. Fatty tissue is an ideal place to store calories."[91] Here, too, they imply that calories are real entities that we eat and that are either expended or stored as fat in the body. While these may be considered turns of phrase, they reflect the way this abstract concept of the calorie has assumed a very concrete form—as if they are material entities that exert deterministic, uniform, and precisely calculable effects on body weight.[92]

To question the calorie hypothesis is not to deny that how much one eats, or how much one exercises, has a significant bearing on one's weight gain or weight loss over a long period of time—if you start eating twice as much of the same types of foods you are already eating, you will probably eventually put on weight. But it is to question whether such weight fluctuations can simply be reduced to the calories-in/calories-out equation and can be precisely predicted and measured with this equation.

The calorie value of a food is a simplified way of measuring the total quantity of food. It is calculated on the basis of the values Wilbur Atwater determined in the late nineteenth century: a gram of fat yields nine calories, while carbohydrate and protein yield four calories per gram. Certain deductions are made to arrive at the metabolizable energy intake value, which is the calories available for the body to metabolize. However, the way in which the body metabolizes actual foods is not accurately captured by these generalized values.[93] Scientists acknowledge that the available energy from these macronutrients may vary considerably depending on the *source* of the food. For example, they estimate the available energy from protein in animal products such as meat, dairy, and eggs (between 4.25 and 4.35 calories) is higher than from the protein found in plant foods such as cereals and legumes (between 2.9 and 3.7 calories).[94] Some food components, such as protein, require considerably more energy to be broken down into a form usable by the body compared with fat and carbohydrates.[95] The available energy in high-fiber foods is also overestimated by standard Atwater values.[96] Despite claims to caloric precision, studies show that the calculated calorie values based on current standards can be off as much as 10 percent, yet food regulatory agencies do not consider this grounds to modify these standards.[97]

However, even these qualified calorie conversion values do not adequately account for the various ways nutrients and food components may be metabolized by the body, how different combinations and quantities of nutrients found in different foods may affect this metabolism, or how different individual bodies may metabolize foods differently and in different situations. For example, the impact of certain foods on bodily hormones that produce or regulate the storage and release of fat in cells may vary considerably. A mashed potato may raise your blood sugar or insulin levels much more rapidly than a same-size potato baked in its jacket, though these two forms of potato may have the same quantity of calories. Sugar, and fructose in particular, has been implicated by some experts as promoting weight gain through various metabolic pathways.[98] Sugary foods and drinks may therefore do more than simply contribute to excess calorie intake.[99]

The body also seems to be able to self-regulate its weight, such that a person's weight can remain stable over long periods of time despite great variations in daily consumption and activity levels. This counters the extremely simplified and mechanical view of the body implicit in the energy-balance equation. Caloric reductionism continues to treat the body as an energy-burning machine and acknowledges the benefits of physical exercise only for its immediate calorie-burning effects. However, some experts have also argued that physical activity may assist in reducing food intake.[100] This is one of the ways in which energy intake and energy expenditure may be interconnected, rather than being two independent variables.[101]

The calorie value of a food also does not tell us how satiating a food is and how it might meet our nutritional needs in a way that may reduce hunger cravings and increase the gap between meals. While the question of satiety is independent of the energy-balance equation, it has practical significance in terms of the quantity of food we eat. If calorie values do not determine how full we feel after a meal or drink, then selecting lower calorie foods is not necessarily the best strategy to weight loss. We also need other strategies for selecting foods, which may at times contradict a narrow (i.e., reductive) focus on calories and the accompanying "eat less" messages. Some highly processed foods may be more easily or quickly consumable, potentially overriding the body's satiety mechanisms. On the other hand, some whole foods—such as nuts or full-fat milk—may be relatively energy dense yet may have a number of beneficial nutritional qualities that ultimately promote satiety and limit excessive food consumption.[102] Being told to eat more good-quality foods may turn out to be a more effective public health message than to eat less calories.

To refer to the calorie hypothesis as a form of reductionism is not to deny that it can be useful as a way to measure food quantity, and in some cases may be a guide to the quality of a food or meal. First, when comparing two identical foods or meals, the calorie difference is a direct measure of the size of each meal. If, for example, you compare two different-size serves of French fries from the same restaurant, or two different-size bottles of soda, the calorie count of each will be proportional to the size or quantity of food or drink. When comparing two foods or meals of the same general type but made with different ingredients, a high calorie count may also be an indicator of a poor-quality food. With processed and fast-food meals, for example, a high calorie count may reveal the existence of so-called hidden calories, that is, ingredients hidden in the food and so not immediately apparent to the consumer. These hidden ingredients may take the form of "hidden fats" (e.g., refined vegetable oils), "hidden carbs" (e.g., flour, chemically modified starches, or sugar), or "hidden protein" (e.g., soy isolates). In these ways, the caloric value of a food can act as a nutrient marker of both the quantity and the quality of a food.

At the same time, however, the calorie count can blur the distinction between foods in terms of their quality and the levels of processing they have undergone. A low-calorie or reduced-calorie food is not necessarily a healthy or healthier option. As with the nutritional engineering of fat-reduced products, calorie-reduced foods have been developed through the application of a number of food processing techniques and additives. This includes the replacement of fat and carbohydrates with noncaloric synthesized ingredients, such as artificial fats and artificial sugars. By manipulating the chemical structure of ingredients, food manufacturers can increase the air and water content of foods while also changing the texture, thereby increasing the creaminess of a product in order to offset the reduction in fat content. Food scientists are also engineering ingredients that may inhibit the absorption or utilization of fats and carbohydrates in the body.[103] These are some of the ways the food industry is able to at least partially respond to caloricentric dietary guidelines and consumer demands. The use of noncaloric and artificial sweeteners has also been endorsed by the American Heart Association and the American Diabetes Association as a means of reducing sugar and calorie intake.[104]

Over the past decade, the assumption that "a calorie is a calorie" has been challenged by some nutrition experts. Much of the scholarly and public debate on this theme has focused on whether fat calories, carb calories, and protein calories are metabolized or turned to fat in the way or at the same rate. However, this macronutrient qualification of calories can be understood as just a more nuanced form of caloric reductionism, in that it assumes that all carb calories or all fat calories are uniform and have similar effects on the body, regardless of the types of foods in which they are contained.

A number of weight-loss studies over the past decade have compared "isocaloric" diets (those with the same number of calories) with different macronutrient ratios. Some report that all such diets produce a statistically similar amount of weight loss in studies lasting more than one year, thereby affirming the energy-balance equation. For example, a study by Frank Sacks and colleagues published in the *New England Journal of Medicine* in 2009 compared isocaloric diets with different ratios of fat, protein, and carbs. They concluded that "reduced-calorie diets result in clinically meaningful weight loss regardless of which macronutrients they emphasize."[105] A number of studies, however, have countered this assumption by reporting slightly better weight-loss benefits from low-carb diets, but these studies have usually been carried out on diets that are not calorie restricted, that is, the participants were eating to appetite.[106] Thus, any benefits of these particular diets may be due to the way they promote satiety and reduce overall food intake, rather than their direct impact on fat storage. Nevertheless, with most weight-loss studies, the differences in weight lost among the various diets tend to even out after a year.[107] One survey of the trends in macronutrient intake between 1971 and 2006 has also claimed that those people who consumed higher protein diets tended to have a lower calorie intake.[108]

Proponents of low-carb diets have been the most vocal critics of the energy-balance hypothesis and the assumption that a calorie is a calorie. In his 1961 diet book *Calories Don't Count*, Herman Taller argued that the body burns fat calories more readily than carb calories, and he thus advocated a carb-restricted diet.[109] In *Dr. Atkins' Diet Revolution*, Atkins urged dieters to "cut carbohydrates not calories."[110] As his book title suggests, low-carb proponent Gary Taubes's *Good Calories, Bad Calories* also challenges the idea that all calories are alike, and he instead distinguishes the so-called quality of calories, by which he means their macronutrient source. Taubes argues that "obesity is caused by the quality of the calories, not the quantity, and specifically by the effect of refined and easily digestible carbohydrates on the hormonal regulation of fat storage and metabolism."[111] Like most other critics of the energy-balance equation, Taubes seems to accept the idea that calories can be counted—that is, he does not seem to question that there are such things as carb calories, fat calories, and protein calories. Nevertheless, he rejects the idea that these uniform carb calories and uniform fat calories have the same metabolic effects in the body. For Taubes, only carbohydrates significantly increase blood sugar and insulin levels and therefore promote fat storage and weight gain. In effect, Taubes argues that while carb calories do count, fat calories do not. But he also takes the next—and quite implausible—step and argues that not just the total number of calories but even the quantity of food consumed is more or less irrelevant to the question of weight gain or loss. In his more recent book *Why We Get Fat*, Taubes tells us that he is "going to argue that this calories-in/calories-out paradigm of adiposity is nonsensical: that we don't get fat because we eat too much and move too little, and that we can't solve the problem or prevent it by consciously doing the opposite."[112]

The critique of the "calorie is a calorie" assumption has been slowly gaining a wider following beyond the low-carb community. In 2010, Weight Watchers redesigned its weight-loss program in recognition that a calorie may not be a calorie any more. Under its old points system, foods were given a point value primarily based on their calorie content, with some adjustments also made for the food's fat and fiber content. It was therefore a simplified means of calorie counting. But Weight Watchers' new ProPoints plan is based on a more complex formula of protein, carbs, fiber, and fat and seems to penalize refined carbohydrate foods more than under the old system.[113] Eating foods that the "body works harder to convert to energy," such as ones higher in fiber, is encouraged under the new points system. As the chief scientific officer for Weight Watchers International, Karen Miller-Kovach, revealed when launching their new program: "Fifteen years ago we said a calorie is a calorie is a calorie. If you ate 100 calories of butter or 100 calories of chicken, it was all the same. Now, we know that is not the case, in terms of how hard the body has to work to make that energy available. And even more important is that where that energy comes from affects feelings of hunger and fullness."[114]

The new Weight Watchers points plan is still based on the idea that the only way to lose weight is to create an energy deficit, but the type of calories also seems to count: "The bottom line is that an energy deficit is still at the heart of weight loss. The issue is that calorie-counting has become unhelpful. When we have a 100-calorie apple in one hand and a 100-calorie pack of cookies in the other, and we view them as being 'the same' because the calories are the same, it says everything that needs to be said about the limitations of just using calories in guiding food choices."[115]

THE LOW-CARB CHALLENGE: FROM FAT REDUCTIONISM TO CARB REDUCTIONISM

It is only because of grains and starches that fatty congestion can occur . . . and it can be deduced, as an exact consequence, that a more or less rigid abstinence from everything that is starchy or floury will lead to the lessening of weight.
—JEAN BRILLAT-SAVARIN, *THE PHYSIOLOGY OF TASTE*, 1859

In *Good Calories, Bad Calories* Taubes argues that carbohydrate restriction was the default approach to preventing and treating obesity, as well as for diabetes management, for much of the nineteenth and early twentieth centuries. Many physicians and members of the lay public recognized the importance of restricting consumption of starchy, floury, and sugary foods, such as bread and potatoes. This knowledge was based primarily on the direct experience of restricting these foods, rather than on a nutrient-level or biochemical understanding of their role in the body. Taubes also documents the scientific evidence accumulated throughout the twentieth century for what he calls the "carbohydrate hypothesis" and the counterevidence for the fat hypothesis.

Taubes characterizes the shift in the 1960s and 1970s from the idea of restricting carb-rich foods to promoting such foods for weight loss as "one of the more remarkable conceptual shifts in the history of public health."[116]

However, he does not also acknowledge the nutricentric shift that paralleled the rise of the low-fat campaign and the new tendency of experts to describe these various dietary regimes in terms of their macronutrient composition. Prior to the 1960s, experts and popular commentators framed the so-called low-carb diet primarily in terms of types of foods to be avoided, such as bread, pasta, potatoes, and sweets, rather than in terms of their carbohydrate content. The expression "low-carb" became widely used only after Atkins's first diet book appeared in the early 1970s.

The 1972 book *Dr. Atkins' Diet Revolution* (and its sequels such as *Dr. Atkins' New Diet Revolution* and *Atkins for Life*) sparked the popularity of low-carb diets.[117] Atkins promoted the idea that "carbohydrates—not fat—are the principal elements in food that fatten fat people" and that overweight people needed to "cut carbohydrates, not calories."[118] Atkins also claimed that "many of today's diseases have one predisposing factor in common: carbohydrate intolerance," and he blamed "carbohydrate poisoning" for most of the killer diseases of the twentieth century. He particularly indicted those high-carb diets that are predominantly composed of so-called refined carbohydrates.[119]

Atkins's weight-loss solution advised people to adopt a very low-carb/high-fat diet that included ample quantities of meat, dairy, and eggs—the very foods that had come to be stigmatized within mainstream nutrition circles. Atkins promised that on this diet "you will never feel a hunger pang."[120] The Atkins diet is extremely low in carbs in its initial phases, before adding modest amounts of some carb-based foods in the later stages. The original Atkins diet was also very low in vegetables and fruit, though Atkins promoted the consumption of more vegetables in later versions of his diet books. In the 2002 book *Dr. Atkins' New Diet Revolution*, Atkins acknowledged that "not all carbohydrate found in food is created equal," adopting the glycemic index as a tool to help people to choose "carbohydrate foods" that could safely be eaten.[121] In this respect, at least, his approach began to converge with the mainstream expert advice to limit the consumption of refined grains and sugar.

Popular interest in the low-carb diet rose again in the late 1990s as the low-fat campaign started to wane, and it has remained popular throughout the past decade.[122] Other low-carb/high-fat/high-protein diet books released since the 1990s include Arthur Agatston's *South Beach Diet*, Barry Sears's *The Zone*, and Leighton Steward's *Sugar Busters*.[123] Since the early 1970s, low-carb diets have been stigmatized by mainstream nutrition experts and dismissed as fad diets that pose long-term health dangers, particularly due to their high proportion of fat, saturated fat, cholesterol, and red meat. In 1974, the American Medical Association referred to the At-kins diet as a "bizarre regimen" that is "without scientific merit."[124]

While into the early 2000s mainstream nutrition experts continued to ridicule low-carb diets, in recent years their hostility and intolerance has softened significantly, particularly because they now take more seriously the detrimental effects of a diet high in refined grains and sugar.[125] A num-ber of studies have been published that demonstrate that low-carb diets can be effective for weight loss, at least in the short term.[126] Walter Willett, for example, has also bluntly acknowledged that it is the high-carb foods in the American diet, rather than the fat, that have caused the greatest prob-lems: "Fat is not the problem," he noted in a recent interview. "If Ameri-cans could eliminate sugary beverages, potatoes, white bread, pasta, white rice and sugary snacks, we would wipe out almost all the problems we have with weight and diabetes and other metabolic diseases."[127]

Although most nutrition experts advise people to eat fewer refined grain and sugar products, many reject the strategy of reducing the overall quantity or percentage of carbs consumed or of increasing fat or animal food intake. The 2010 *Dietary Guidelines for Americans*, for instance, empha-sizes more than ever before the need for people to limit their intake of refined grains and sugars, though it studiously avoids referring to these foods as "carbohydrate" foods or "refined carbohydrates," and it does not endorse the strategy of reducing carbohydrate intake.[128]

The scientific justification for low-carb diets focuses on the role of car-bohydrates in raising both blood sugar and insulin levels. Taubes summa-rizes the relationship among carbs, glucose, insulin, and fat storage as follows: "Since glucose is the primary stimulator of insulin secretion, the more carbohydrates consumed—or the more refined the carbohydrates—the greater the insulin secretion, and thus the greater the accumulation of fat."[129] For weight loss, some low-carb proponents, such as Taubes, believe not only that it is more important for people to restrict their intake of carbs than their intake of calories but also that to some extent it can make the restriction of calorie intake unnecessary. In their view, this is partly because a low-carb diet is more satiating than a higher-carb diet, thereby restricting overconsumption of calories, and also because they assume that it is primarily carbs that promote fat storage within the body. Only in the past decade have low-carb diets been the subject of controlled weight-loss studies. Some, though not all, of these studies have concluded that low-carb diets are at least as effective as other dietary approaches at re-ducing people's weight, improving their lipid profiles with respect to heart disease risk, and controlling their blood glucose levels.[130] Other studies, however, report that all isocaloric (i.e., calorie equivalent) diets produce a comparable amount of weight loss.[131]

The fluctuations in insulin levels promoted by either high-carb foods or foods high in refined grains and sugar may contribute to the development of insulin resistance—and therefore to type 2 diabetes—though the precise causes of insulin resistance and diabetes are still unknown. For the management of diabetes, low-carb proponents therefore recommend severe carb restriction, which is in line with, but goes further than, the mainstream recommendation that people with diabetes moderate their total carbohydrate intake.[132] High insulin and sugar levels may also increase triglyceride levels and reduce HDL cholesterol levels, which many experts believe increases the risk of heart disease.[133]

In a number of respects, the low-carb ideology produces a mirror image of the low-fat/high-carb dietary recommendations, by framing the diet exclusively in terms of its macronutrient profile and by stigmatizing carbs. Low-carb approaches—by simplifying and decontextualizing the types, sources, and effects of carbohydrates—promote a form of carbohydrate reductionism. Their stigmatization of all "high-carb" foods, or even of just "refined-carb" foods, blurs the important nutritional differences among foods and takes these foods out of the contexts in which they are consumed. By focusing almost exclusively on blood sugar levels and on insulin to explain the biochemical pathways through which carbs inflict their damage, they also adopt a kind of glycemic reductionism and insulin reductionism. Their descriptions of how isolated carbohydrates stimulate blood sugar, insulin, and fat storage at the cellular level may be accurate. However, as their argument moves from the microlevel to the macrolevel of food and the body, they interpret this cellular and molecular level of knowledge in a way that stigmatizes all carbohydrates in all foods, thereby exaggerating the role of these foods within the context of the total diet.

Taubes's approach represents an extreme version of this carb reductionism. He argues that when a person eats carbohydrates, the rise in insulin levels causes the glucose and fatty acids in the blood to be stored as fat, rather than to be made available and utilized for other metabolic processes. For Taubes, this reduction in available energy makes the high-carb eater lethargic and less able to get off the couch and get some exercise.[134] In other words, the carbs not only determine fat storage via their action on hormones but also to a significant degree control human behavior. Taubes's explanation of the relationship among nutrients, fat storage, and exercise is an indication of how much further he is prepared to travel down the road of nutritional and biochemical reductionism. Within his fat cell–centered view of the world, carbs determine everything.

Despite the rhetoric of some low-carb proponents, the average American diet of the last thirty years can hardly be described as "high-carb." Generally speaking, it is high in refined grains, refined flour, sugar, and highly processed potatoes, but it is also high in red and white meats, milk, cheese, and vegetable oils. Often these foods and ingredients are processed to varying degrees and are consumed in various combinations. While any additional carb-rich foods consumed since the early 1980s may be accentuating the overall rises and fluctuations in Americans' blood glucose and insulin levels, these carbs—largely in the form of highly processed foods—have been added to a diet already rich in fat, carbs, and protein (a good proportion of which came from animal products). This is particularly true of poorer people in the United States, and around the world, whose diets are high in refined, carb-rich foods, usually because they are the more highly processed and cheapest foods in the supermarket.[135]

Low-carb proponents of the "carbs made us fat" theory would have us believe that the main cause of obesity and diabetes is the bun rather than the hamburger patty, the pizza crust rather than the cheese and pepperoni toppings, the potatoes rather than the old oil in which they are deep-fried, the white sourdough bread holding together the bacon and egg sandwich, or the plain white rice on the side of the plate next to the steak—rather than the entire combination, and the overall quantity and quality of foods and nutrients being consumed. Within the low-carb paradigm, the poor-quality, quickly consumable, easily digestible, fat-concentrated hamburger patties between the bun, the processed-reconstituted chicken nuggets, and the large quantities of vegetable oil used to process and fry these foods, apparently have little to do with any of the weight or health problems of those who consume them.

The low-carb discourse also suggests that the anti-saturated fat and anti-meat rhetoric of the *Dietary Guidelines* and *Food Guide Pyramid* has transformed America into a vegetarian nation. Yet there has not been a significant decline in meat or dairy consumption since the early 1980s. Nor do low-carb proponents seem to admit that many vegetarians, vegans, and people who eat little meat—and who typically consume very high-carb diets—also manage to remain slim and to maintain good health relative to the wider population. To question low-carb proponents' depiction of all high-carb foods and diets as unhealthy and fattening is not to deny that low-carb dietary plans can be a very healthful way to eat, for low-carb diet plans—like most other weight-loss diets—generally promote good quality whole foods; they just happen to be largely animal-based, high-fat whole foods.[136]

Low-GI Diets and Glycemic Reductionism

Since the early 2000s, mainstream nutrition experts, instead of blaming all carbs for weight gain and a host of chronic diseases, have reemphasized the distinction between good and bad carbs and the overconsumption of bad carbs. One common way to define good and bad carbs is in terms of the level of processing or refinement of the food. In these terms, refined grains and sugars—the so-called refined carbs—are designated as the bad carbs, while whole grains, as well as fruits, starchy vegetables, and legumes, are categorized as whole carbs and good carbs. Running alongside this distinction between whole and refined carbs—but to some extent undermining it—is the concept of the glycemic index (GI). The GI has become another widely accepted scientific way to distinguish between good and bad carbs, but one defined in terms of the physiological impacts of carb-rich foods on the body, rather than in terms of the level of processing or chemical composition of the food itself.

The GI was first introduced by David Jenkins and his colleagues in 1982 as a tool to assist people with diabetes in choosing carbohydrate-rich foods that produce modest rises in blood sugar levels.[137] Jenkins and colleagues found that when they actually measured blood glucose levels following the consumption of various foods, the form of the food, the nature of the carbohydrate, and the quantity of fiber were not accurate predictors of their impact on glycemic response. Great differences between foods were observed even within the same food groups. They therefore developed the GI as a more precise measure of the rate at which single foods raise blood glucose in the two-hour period following its consumption. Based on a value of 100 given to a reference food (usually glucose), individual foods are given a comparative value for their relative impact on blood glucose levels, with low-GI foods scoring 0–55, medium-GI foods at 56–69, and high-GI foods at 70 and above.

A high-GI food is defined as one that produces a sharp rise in blood glucose concentrations, which in turn may lead to an increase in insulin released by the pancreas to bring down the blood glucose levels. High insulin levels may in turn promote fat storage and prevent the release of fat from cells to be burned as "fuel." At the same time, a sharp drop in blood sugar levels can stimulate hunger cravings.[138] Nutrition experts intended the GI to be used as a nutritional tool to directly target and manipulate glycemic levels in the body and to thereby indirectly target insulin response. In these respects, the science of the GI is similar to that of low-carb diets, and many low-carb proponents and dietary plans incorporate the GI concept to support their arguments. However, many GI proponents tend to promote high-carb diets that are based on low-GI foods, rather than recommend cutting out high-carb foods per se. The GI is thereby presented as a means of fine-tuning food selections within the category of carb-rich foods, and as a way to optimize dietary choices for glycemic control.

The GI concept is compatible with many other nutritional hypotheses and approaches and has been incorporated in a number of weight-loss, diabetes, and heart-health management plans. Many promoters of the dominant good-and-bad fats and good-and-bad carbs approaches accept the GI premise. Dean Ornish, for example, adopts this concept in his reconstructed low-fat dietary plan *The Spectrum*.[139] The GI concept is also compatible with low-carb diet plans and was taken up in the later Atkins diet books. There are also stand-alone low-GI and low-glycemic-load diet plans, such as Jennie Brand Miller's popular New Glucose Revolution series. The GI logo features on food labels and enjoys a significant following, although it is more widely used and accepted by experts and the lay public in countries such as the United Kingdom, Canada, and Australia than in the United States. In the United Kingdom, leading supermarket chain Tesco has adopted a GI labeling scheme for its products.[140] The American Diabetes Association, on the other hand, offers only qualified support for the GI concept as a means of "fine-tuning blood glucose management" and instead recommends monitoring and limiting excess carbohydrate intake through "carb-counting," which it considers "a better predictor of blood glucose response than the GI."[141]

One of the limitations of the GI score of a food is that it is calculated by measuring the effect on blood sugar from an amount of food that contains fifty grams of available carbohydrate, yet this amount can be much more or less than a typical serving size for that food. While the GI score of a carrot is high (71), the actual glycemic impact of eating one carrot is very low because a single carrot contains a relatively small quantity of carbohydrate.[142] For this reason, in the 1990s researchers at the Harvard School of Public Health developed the concept of the glycemic load (GL), calculated by multiplying the GI of a food by the quantity of available carbohydrates.[143] The designers of the GL intended it to reflect more accurately the glycemic impact of a typical serving size of a food. The GL is more closely related to the quantity of carbohydrates in a food; therefore, a high-carb food also tends to be a high-GL food. There is some debate among GI/GL advocates over which tool is preferable for consumers to use to guide their food choices. For example, Australian nutrition scientist Jennie Brand-Miller, one of the world's foremost GI experts, favors the GI concept and argues that the GL concept inappropriately promotes total carb restriction: "The problem with the GL is that it does not distinguish between foods that are low carb (and thus higher in fat and/or protein) or slow carb (that is, low GI carbs). Some people whose diets have an overall lower GL are consuming more fat or protein and fewer carbohydrates of any kind, including healthy, low GI carbs."[144] Proponents of the GI concept list many benefits that they claim have been demonstrated in epidemiological and clinical trials, including improved insulin resistance and blood cholesterol profiles, reduced inflammation, and a lower risk of developing diabetes, obesity, cardiovascular disease, and cancer.[145] Other studies, however, have failed to support all of these claims, and many experts remain skeptical that a low GI diet has such wide-ranging benefits.[146]

The GI concept is yet another single-nutrient concept that some nutrition experts use to tell a story about what is wrong with the contemporary American or "Western" diet. Harvard Medical School pediatrics specialist David Ludwig, for example, characterizes in the following fashion the developments in the American diet and obesity since the 1970s:

Many high-glycemic carbohydrates became staples of the American diet over the past four decades because we thought they were healthy. Bread, rice, and potatoes enjoyed star billing at the base of the Food Guide Pyramid as foods that should make up the bulk of our diet.... Food manufacturers eagerly met the increased demand for carbohydrates with cheap, high-glycemic products such as chips, crackers, cookies, and other refined starches and sweets labeled "reduced fat" or "fat-free." We guiltlessly ate them and served them to our children because they tasted good and seemed wholesome. But most were the nutritional equivalent of table sugar.[147]

Ludwig's claim that "high-glycemic products" are the nutritional equivalents of sugar is consistent with the low-carb discourse. He suggests we ignore what our taste buds are telling us and instead accept that, in terms of its effects on the body, a bagel is ultimately no different from table sugar: "Once a refined starchy food is swallowed and moves down the digestive tract, it melts into sugar. A bagel and a bowl of sugar may taste different in the mouth, but below the neck, they are virtually the same."[148]

This GI discourse embodies and perpetuates a number of characteristics of the quantitative, good-and-bad, and functional forms of nutritionism. The GI extends the logic of nutri-quantification and is presented as a scientifically precise and quantified measure of the extent to which carbohydrates are converted into blood glucose in the body and, by extension, how it affects a range of other bodily processes and health outcomes. The GI encapsulates the spirit of good-and-bad nutritionism by providing a new means to differentiate between "good" and "bad" carbs. Low-GI foods are described not only as "good carbs" but also as "smart carbs" and "slow carbs" because they release glucose into the body more slowly. In line with the logic of functional nutritionism, the GI also opens up internal bodily processes to the nutritional gaze of the lay public, inviting them to visualize the way in which a food releases glucose slowly or rapidly into their bloodstream. The GI thereby takes attention away from the physical characteristics of the food per se and instead focuses on the body and its internal processes.

The expression "low-GI foods are absorbed more slowly than high-GI foods" has become an everyday nutritional expression—an everyday nutritionism. It seems to offer members of the lay public a simple explanation for how digestion and satiety work in the body, one that is easy to understand and can be readily repeated by them. It thereby allows people to take ownership of the GI concept, a concept that has intuitive appeal in much the same way that "eating fat makes you fat" made sense to many people in the low-fat era. The GI seems to add scientific validation and precision to the popular knowledge that highly refined and sugary foods are unhealthy and give you "sugar spikes."

To question the usefulness of the GI concept is not to deny the importance of people, especially people with diabetes, managing or avoiding spikes in their blood glucose or insulin levels, or of avoiding the overconsumption of carb-rich foods or food combinations that may cause blood sugar and insulin fluctuations. Rather, it is to question whether the GI concept can accurately capture this functional effect of food on blood glucose and insulin levels, and the definitive attribution of a wide range of health effects to these blood sugar fluctuations. Importantly, the GI concept also seems to undermine other useful ways of distinguishing the quality of different types of foods.

Many nutrition experts present the GI as an alternative measure of "carbohydrate quality." Nutrition scientists usually classify carbohydrates in terms of their chemical composition, with the three main classes being sugars, oligosaccharides, and polysaccharides.[149] The now largely abandoned distinction between "complex carbohydrates" (starches) and "simple carbohydrates" (sugars) that came into use in the 1970s was based on such a chemical classification. By contrast, the distinction between "whole carbohydrates" (whole grains and vegetables) and "refined carbohydrates" (refined grain and sugar) is based on the types of processing the food has undergone. While I have been critical of the term "refined carbs," in part for the way it obscures important differences between types of high-carb foods (see chapter 2), the distinction between whole carbs and refined carbs at least gestures toward the quality of foods based on levels of processing. However, the GI concept refers to neither the chemical composition nor the levels of processing of carbohydrate-containing foods, only to the physiological effects of eating them.[150]

One might expect the GI values of foods to correlate with the degree of processing of a food. But this is not always the case, since measured GI values can vary widely within and between food groups, cutting across and undermining any clear distinctions among foods based on levels of processing, freshness, or other markers of food quality.[151] The GI cuts across and undermines the distinction between "whole-carb" foods (e.g., whole grains, vegetables) and "refined-carb" foods (containing refined grain and refined sugar). For example, many long-grain white rice varieties have an average GI of about 60, while brown rice varieties can average between 50 and 87. Similarly, some whole wheat breads (74) score about the same as white breads (75). These GI scores suggest that there is little benefit to blood sugar levels from eating whole grains. At the same time, the GI scores also suggest there is considerable variation between different varieties of white rice: basmati rice (57) registers close to a medium GI, while jasmine rice (between 89 and 109) is clearly a high-GI food.[152] Some highly processed convenience foods, including those high in added sugars and fats, may also have lower GI scores than raw fruits and vegetables. Coke has a moderate GI score of 58, a Snickers candy bar and sugar-coated Kellogg's Frosted Flakes both score a low 55, apple muffins with sugar register 44, while porridge from rolled oats scores an average of 58.[153] One of the reasons why some processed foods and beverages fare so well is that the fats added to them can improve their GI scores.[154] Fat has been shown to delay gastric emptying, slowing down the digestion and absorption of carbs in the body. This may explain why potato chips fried in fat (54) have a lower GI than a baked potato (85).

A particularly worrying aspect of the GI concept is how generously it treats sucrose, or white table sugar, which receives only a moderate GI score of 65, less than the scores for some fruits and vegetables. This is because half of the sucrose molecule is made up of glucose (100) and the other half is fructose (19). Consuming fructose not only raises blood sugar levels but also has been shown to have other potentially detrimental effects that the GI does not measure, such as its effects on the liver.[155] Jennie Brand-Miller downplays health concerns over sugars, other than worrying about their contribution to an excess consumption of calories: "There really isn't a big difference between sugars and starches, either in nutritional terms or in terms of the glycemic index."[156] This is worrying advice given the large quantities of added sugars (sucrose and fructose) in many processed foods. Brand-Miller has also lent her promotional support to a new low-GI variety of refined sugar, commercialized in 2009 by the Australian sugar company CSR, called LoGiCane. This sugar has a GI score of 50, rather than the usual 65, and the company claims that this has been achieved by adding back to the sugar minute quantities of some of the molasses removed from it during the conventional sugar refining process.[157] To suggest that such minor modifications in sugar composition would make any meaningful difference to health outcomes—especially for those people already consuming very high levels of sugar—seems fanciful.

The GI values of foods do often correlate with food quality and degrees of food processing. The GI concept draws much of its legitimacy from this correlation, by appearing to add scientific precision to the general advice to eat minimally processed foods. But the benefits attributed to low-GI foods and diets could be an *effect* of this correlation, rather than a function of the GI score per se. That is, it may simply be that minimally processed foods in general deliver the range of benefits attributed to low-GI foods. In dietary studies that test for the benefits of a low-GI diet, the foods used are invariably minimally processed low-GI foods, rather than highly processed low-GI foods.[158]

Another limitation of the GI concept is that GI values are calculated for individual foods rather than mixed meals. By awarding scores to single foods or food products, the GI score simplifies the complex realities of how food combinations may affect glycemic impact.[159] Some studies have suggested that you cannot deduce the glycemic response of mixed meals simply by adding up the GI values of the individual foods in a meal. This may be because, as noted earlier, the quantity of fats and protein present may affect the rate at which carbs in a meal are digested and absorbed.[160] When foods high in fat or protein are eaten with high-carb foods, the glycemic response is generally lower than eating the high-carb food alone. This suggests that common food combinations—such as beans and rice, or meat and potatoes—may nullify the sugar spikes expected from eating high-GI foods on their own. If spreading some butter on white bread reduces the glycemic response of a food, is this not a beneficial outcome? Attempting to use the GI as a dietary tool to quantify the countless variations of food combinations and mixed meals is rather impractical. Studies have also demonstrated that glycemic responses may also vary greatly among individuals, and even for the same individual at different times of the day.[161]

The argument of some GI advocates that, within the context of broad dietary patterns, the choice of particular foods within a food category based on their GI scores—such as the choice of one type of fruit, one type of rice, or even one type of sugar over another—would make a meaningful difference to one's blood glucose levels over the course of a day, as well as a meaningful difference to one's long-term health outcomes, is at best another case of nutritional exaggeration. When a lot of current dietary advice encourages people to eat more whole foods, and fewer highly processed foods, the GI concept places a question mark over some whole foods while at the same time dangerously blurring the distinction between minimally and highly processed foods.

Since the 1970s, different groups of nutrition experts and diet-book authors have promoted one of the macronutrients or nutritional concepts I have discussed so far, either as an explanation for the "obesity epidemic" or as the key to weight loss and healthy eating. Some experts have also combined two or more of these nutritional concepts. For example, the best-selling weight-loss diet book of all time in Australia, the CSIRO *Total Wellbeing Diet*—released in 2005 by the country's leading and publicly funded scientific research organization—calls itself a high-protein, moderate-carb, low-fat diet, as well as touting the benefits of low-GI foods.[162]

While each of these dietary plans is primarily framed in terms of their macronutrient profiles (i.e., fat, carbs, and protein, as well as calories), the actual foods promoted are almost exclusively whole foods, with very few refined, highly processed, and reconstituted foods featured in their recommended foods and meal plans. This may be the unspoken secret of the success of all these diets at achieving weight loss, at least in the short term. In this respect, the low-fat, low-carb, low-calorie, and low-GI dietary plans have much more in common than the very loud and public debates regarding these diets would suggest.

CHAPTER SIX

Margarine, Butter, and the *Trans*-Fats Fiasco

As for butter versus margarine, I trust cows more than chemists.
—JOAN GUSSOW, *NEW YORK TIMES*, 1986

Which is healthier, butter or margarine? Beginning in the 1960s, many nutrition experts leaned heavily toward margarine. They did so entirely on the basis of their relative ratios of polyunsaturated and saturated fats, while ignoring the presence of highly processed ingredients used to manufacture margarine, including the artificial *trans*-fats produced by the partial hydrogenation process used to harden vegetable oils. However, a potential crisis for the reputation of margarine emerged in the early 1990s when new scientific studies published by two Dutch nutrition scientists highlighted the harmful effects of these *trans*-fats. These scientists found that *trans*-fats had an even more detrimental effect on blood cholesterol levels than saturated fats and therefore—within the logic of the dominant diet-heart hypothesis—would pose a greater risk of heart disease.

The take-home message of this *trans*-fats fiasco could have been that we should place our trust in cows rather than chemists after all, and that we should question the reductive evaluation of these foods on the basis of their so-called good and bad fat content.[1] However, nutrition experts have responded to this new scientific evidence by recategorizing *trans*-fats as a bad fat, while the chemists and margarine manufacturers have sought new chemical processing techniques to produce a "virtually *trans*-fat-free" margarine. In doing so, the experts have maintained our focus on the nutrient composition of margarine, rather than opening up to scrutiny the types of processing techniques and additives now being used in its production.

This chapter analyzes the history of margarine and its rivalry with butter, and the continual reengineering of margarine across the three eras of nutritionism in response to changing nutritional fears and fetishes. I trace the transformation of the public profile and nutritional facade of margarine from a cheap imitation of butter in the era of quantifying nutritionism, to a "hyperreal" spread boasting a superior fatty acid profile in the good-and-bad era, and then to a cholesterol-lowering and omega-3-enriched functional food in the functional era. I also examine the research and the debate over *trans*-fats since the 1960s, and how the discourse of good and bad fats continues to obscure the underlying ingredients and processing quality of margarine and other spreads.

MARGARINE AS CHEAP IMITATION: CHEMICALLY RECONSTITUTED FATS AND OILS

French chemist Hippolyte Mège-Mouriès invented margarine in 1869. Mège-Mouriès had accepted an assignment from the French government to develop a cheap substitute for butter and an alternative source of fat, in response to butter shortages prevailing in France at the time.[2] His proto-margarine was produced using beef tallow—a plentiful by-product of meat production—mixed with skim milk. This food product was markedly different from contemporary margarines in terms of its ingredients, manufacturing techniques, and nutrient profile. Mège-Mouriès called it *margarine*, since margaric acid (a type of saturated fat) was one of the key fatty acid constituents. It later became known as *oleo margarine* after the Latin word for beef.[3] By the mid-1870s this beef tallow margarine was being sold in Europe, the United States, New Zealand, and Australia.

The next advance came in 1902 when German scientist Wilhelm Normann developed the hydrogenation process for solidifying liquid vegetable oils, a process that manufacturers began to use around 1910.[4] In the following decades, margarine manufacturers mixed into their products a combination of hydrogenated (i.e., hardened) vegetable oils, liquid vegetable oils, and animal fats. The use of animal fats was not phased out by the U.S. margarine industry until 1950.[5]

In the first half of the twentieth century, margarine was considered by the public—and by the dairy industry—as a cheap imitation of butter. Margarine manufacturers such as Unilever largely aimed to simulate some of the characteristics of butter, such as its taste, texture, color, and nutritional profile. In the late nineteenth century, several countries and U.S. states introduced laws prohibiting the use of yellow coloring in margarine; indeed, some states required it to be colored pink. These coloring regulations remained in place until the late 1960s.[6] Canada's federal government also prohibited the production, importation, and sale of margarine for most of the period between 1886 and 1949, and lifted regulations prohibiting the use of yellow coloring only in 2008.[7] Legislators largely used coloring restrictions, as well as production quotas and taxes levied on margarine producers, to protect the commercial interests of the dairy industry, and particularly to prevent the sale of what some considered to be "counterfeit" margarines masquerading as butter.

In keeping with the nutritional imperatives of the era of quantifying nutritionism, as well as the requirements of food regulatory authorities, margarine manufacturers merely attempted to replicate the type and quantity of the nutrients that would otherwise have been obtained from butter, and to thereby achieve "nutritional equivalence."[8] The primary nutritional and culinary role of margarine was as a more affordable source of fat and energy to be placed on the table of the poorer classes.[9] To simulate the nutrient profile of butter, manufacturers fortified margarine with the fat-soluble vitamins A and D. This occurred from the 1920s in the United Kingdom and somewhat later in other countries.[10] As Siert Riepma notes in his history of margarine, "By 1940 the nutritional equivalency of the two 'spreads' had been established as far as nutritional knowledge then went."[11]

HYDROGENATION AND THE PRODUCTION OF NOVEL *TRANS*-FATS

The process of hydrogenation involves mixing vegetable oils with a catalyst, such as finely ground nickel, subjecting the oil to high temperatures and pressures, and then pumping hydrogen gas through the liquid. Complete hydrogenation results in a very solid and largely inedible fat, so manufacturers prior to the 1990s typically made margarines by only partially hydrogenating the vegetable oil in order to achieve a soft and spreadable texture. The smelly, gray, unpleasant-tasting substance that emerges from the hydrogenation process requires steam cleaning under high temperature and pressure to remove the foul odor. Manufacturers bleach this substance to remove the gray color and later add chemical colorings and flavorings to mimic the appearance and taste of butter. Emulsifiers are added to integrate the oil with water and to create the desired texture and consistency. With some margarines, manufacturers also blend in skim milk powder for flavor and texture and add vitamins A and D to mimic the vitamin profile of butter. Hydrogenated oils may also contain trace elements of the metal catalysts used to produce them.[12]

The partial hydrogenation of vegetable oils chemically transforms some of the unsaturated fats into novel forms of *trans*-fatty acids and also leads to an increase in the proportion of saturated fats in these oils. When oils are fully hydrogenated, on the other hand, all of the unsaturated fats become fully saturated, producing a very solid product that contains no *trans*-fats. Table margarine and cooking oils have typically been either partially hydrogenated or produced by blending fully hydrogenated, partially hydrogenated, and liquid vegetable oils. In the 1970s and 1980s, margarines and spreads usually contained between 15 and 25 percent *trans*-fats, and margarines produced before that time may have had even higher ratios.[13] The hydrogenation process also eliminates from margarine most of the omega-3 fats found in vegetable oils, and this benefits food manufacturers—if not consumers—by increasing its stability and shelf life.[14]

Some naturally occurring types of *trans*-fatty acids can also be found in low concentrations in dairy and meat products, typically making up between 2 and 5 percent of dairy and beef fats.[15] However, some of the industrial or artificial *trans*-fats created by the hydrogenation process are novel and have been produced and consumed in much larger quantities than ruminant *trans*-fats from meat and dairy sources. Another source of these industrial *trans*-fats—though one that is very rarely acknowledged or publicized by nutrition experts or by the food industry—is the process of extracting and refining vegetable oils. When extracting vegetable oil, processing companies use a technologically intensive process that involves extreme heating, mechanical extraction, and chemical solvents. The high temperatures involved in deodorizing the oils may produce between 1 and 4 percent *trans*-fats out of the total fat content.[16]

Partially hydrogenated oils have been useful not only for margarine production but also for meeting the various needs of the food-processing and fast-food industries, as well as for use in the home. In 1911, U.S. company Procter and Gamble introduced Crisco, the first hard shortening made entirely from vegetable oil.[17] Crisco was initially marketed by Procter and Gamble as a cheap alternative to lard and butter for the manufacture of processed foods and for frying.[18] For many years the food industry has used partially hydrogenated vegetable oils extensively for deep frying, because they improve the stability and the longevity of oils subjected to high temperatures, and they make chips and other deep-fried foods appealingly crunchy.

Manufacturers of a wide range of processed foods—including ice cream, cookies, potato chips, sauces, frozen foods, confectionaries, and baked goods—have also used hydrogenated oils to cheaply bulk up their products, to provide good texture and mouthfeel, to make baked goods crispy, and to impart heat tolerance and a longer shelf life. By the 1990s the largest source of *trans*-fats in the American diet was not directly from margarines and spreads but from the partially hydrogenated oils used for deep-frying or added to processed and baked foods.[19]

TRANS-FATS RESEARCH AND THE INVISIBILITY OF *TRANS*-FATS

The undermining of butter's perceived superiority over margarine is a key marker of the shift from the quantitative era to the good-and-bad era of nutritionism and follows the rise of the diet-heart hypothesis linking saturated fats to heart disease put forward by Ancel Keys from the late 1950s. As discussed in chapter 4, beginning in the early 1960s nutrition scientists attributed the perceived increase in coronary heart disease in the post-World War II era to foods and diets high in cholesterol and saturated fats, because of their contribution to higher blood cholesterol levels. By contrast, they found that polyunsaturated fats lowered total cholesterol levels.

In the earliest of these studies, nutrition scientists did not distinguish *trans*-fats from saturated fats, because they thought that they acted similarly in the body. Consequently, they may have blamed on saturated fats some of the cholesterol-raising effects actually due to *trans*-fats.[20] From the late 1950s, a number of human and animal studies also found that when polyunsaturated fat–rich vegetable oils were hydrogenated, they lost their ability to lower cholesterol levels, although some other studies failed to confirm this relation.[21] For example, a 1961 study by Keys himself, in which he measured the cholesterol-raising effects of hydrogenated corn and safflower oils compared with nonhydrogenated oils, found little difference between saturated fats and *trans*-fats.[22]

In the late 1950s and early 1960s, the American Heart Association (AHA) remained less than enthusiastic about margarine, and in reports published in 1957 and 1961 it noted that hydrogenated vegetable fats both raised cholesterol levels and decreased the amount of polyunsaturated fats in oils.[23] Until the late 1960s, the AHA continued to caution against the consumption of hydrogenated oils. In 1968, biochemist Fred Kummerow sat on an AHA committee that was revising its position paper on diet and heart disease. In Kummerow's account of events, the committee was concerned about the health effects of hydrogenated oils, but the vegetable oil industry had objected to the AHA's new draft position paper that made reference to trans-fats and their effects on blood cholesterol. The industry later agreed to lower the levels of trans-fats in margarine and shortening, and indeed, after 1968 the trans-fat content of margarines fell from around 40 percent to 27 percent. However, in return, the AHA modified its position paper so that it only warned against the use of "heavily hydrogenated" oils, and omitting any reference to trans-fats. From that time and up until the 1990s, the AHA was largely silent on the effects of trans-fats on blood cholesterol levels while continuing to promote the benefits of soft margarines that contained lower levels of trans-fats than hard margarines.[24]

Given that nutrition experts were promoting partially hydrogenated polyunsaturated fats over saturated fats precisely because of their claimed effects on blood cholesterol levels, it is surprising that research into the health effects of these fats was not more urgently pursued. It was therefore largely on the basis of scientific ignorance of the health effects of partially hydrogenated oils and trans-fats that nutrition experts and manufacturers promoted margarine as being healthier than butter, rather than on the basis of comprehensive knowledge of their safety or beneficial effects.

As Canadian biochemist Ross Hume Hall put it in his 1974 book *Food for Nought: The Decline in Nutrition*, "In spite of the lack of information, medical scientists for a generation have promoted the eating of commercially processed vegetable fat in lieu of butter and other animal fats, knowing nothing of what they recommend."[25] Hall emphasized that hydrogenation and other oil processing techniques transformed the fundamental chemical structure and physical properties of many of the polyunsaturated fats in the vegetable oils. Yet nutrition scientists continued to describe these chemically modified fats as polyunsaturated fats: "[To nutrition scientists] polyunsaturates are polyunsaturates. They do not seem to care about the fact that these are unnatural polyunsaturates whose biological properties remain unknown. . . . The original molecular architecture of the vegetable oil has been reorganized: The product is completely unnatural, yet no hint of the changes appears on the label of the final product."[26]

Hall cited studies showing that hydrogenated oils seemed to raise cholesterol levels. However, he was also critical of the narrow focus in most of these studies, because they considered only the effects of these fats on heart disease or, more narrow still, on blood cholesterol levels as a marker of heart disease risk. For Hall, the failure of these kinds of studies to adequately examine the broader health consequences of these oil processing techniques meant that "North Americans have been subjected unwittingly to a massive experiment involving consumption of *trans* and other unnatural fats ever since about 1914."[27] Hall was also concerned about the degradation of vegetable oils subjected to modern refining and extraction processes, even prior to the oils being put through the hydrogenation process.

Biochemist Mary Enig has been the most consistent critic of *trans*-fats since the 1970s and has examined the possible role of refined vegetable oils and partially hydrogenated oils in heart disease and cancer. In the late 1970s and 1980s, Enig reported that much of the increase in fat consumption during the twentieth century was in the form of unsaturated fats from vegetable oils, and that since 1910 per capita *trans*-fat consumption in the United States had risen from four to twelve grams per day.[28] Enig also noted that since margarine contains a proportion of saturated fat, the switch from butter to margarine meant that margarine has accounted for a large portion of the saturated fat consumption over this period.[29]

Not until new research published in 1990 did the nutrition and public health communities take seriously the possible health hazards of *trans*-fats and partially hydrogenated oils. In a landmark study that was partly sponsored by the margarine manufacturer Unilever, Dutch scientists Ronald Mensink and Martijn Katan reported that *trans*-fatty acids had been found both to increase LDL cholesterol levels and to decrease HDL cholesterol levels.[30] Within the terms of the diet-heart hypothesis, this meant that *trans*-fats were now classified as the most harmful fats of all, worse than the vilified saturated fats. Importantly, this new understanding of *trans*-fats did not itself arise from any paradigm shift or revolution in the methodologies of nutrition science at the time, but rather emerged from within the terms of the dominant nutritional paradigm.

The Mensink and Katan study was followed by a 1993 report by Walter Willett and colleagues, based on the food consumption questionnaire in the Nurses' Health Study, that showed a positive association between *trans*-fat intake and heart disease risk.[31] Other studies have since confirmed the association between *trans*-fats and blood cholesterol levels and have linked *trans*-fats—via a number of biochemical pathways other than those related to blood cholesterol—to the increased risk not only of cardiovascular disease but also of other conditions, such as obesity, diabetes, cancer, and allergies.[32] A number of studies, for example, have reported that *trans*-fats promote inflammation and may worsen insulin sensitivity.[33] *Trans*-fats are also incorporated into cells and have been found to disrupt cellular functioning in a number of adverse ways.[34]

Some of the evidence against *trans*-fats has come from epidemiological studies that estimated *trans*-fat consumption from food-frequency questionnaires. However, in the 1990s epidemiologist Samuel Shapiro warned against prematurely interpreting as causal relationships these associations between a high consumption of *trans*-fats and increased heart disease risk.[35] Shapiro noted that because of the claimed heart-health benefits of margarine prior to the 1990s, many individuals with preexisting heart conditions or with cardiovascular disease risk factors may have been more likely to consume margarine, and therefore to have increased their *trans*-fat intake. If that were the case, then the positive association between heart disease and *trans*-fat intake may have been exaggerated by, or was a by-product of, the people in this high-risk group changing their behavior. Shapiro refers to this type of confounding in epidemiological studies as "confounding by indication."[36] This does not necessarily mean that *trans*-fats do not contribute to heart disease risk. Rather, it highlights another difficulty when scientists attempt to isolate the effects of a single nutrient from epidemiological data on broader dietary patterns, particularly when consumption patterns for this nutrient have been confounded by the nutrition experts' own dietary advice.

HYPERREAL MARGARINE:
THE IMITATION SURPASSES THE ORIGINAL

Margarine has been one of the earliest and most successful examples of a nutritionally engineered and nutritionally marketed food—a food explicitly advertised in terms of its nutrient content and whose ingredients and nutritional profile manufacturers have specifically designed for this purpose. By 1957 Americans were already consuming more margarine than butter, though largely because of its cheaper price. However, by this time margarine and vegetable oil producers had also recognized the great marketing potential offered by the emerging diet-heart hypothesis.[37]

From the late 1950s, margarine was reformulated by manufacturers to reduce its saturated fat content and to increase the proportion of polyunsaturated fat, thereby also producing a softer, more spreadable product that could be sold in tubs rather than as solid sticks.[38] The polyunsaturated fat came from vegetable oils such as sunflower, safflower, and soy oils. Margarine manufacturers effectively constructed a nutritional facade around margarine, a particular image of its nutritional content and health benefits. Those who marketed this nutritional facade were able to conceal, or distract consumers' attention from, the underlying ingredients and additives and the processing techniques used in the production of margarine.

The pharmaceutical company Pitman-Moore released the first polyunsaturated-rich margarine in 1958, called Emdee, and initially marketed it as a medicinal product.[39] The same year, Fleischmann's launched its margarine made from corn oil with advertisements that proclaimed its heart-health benefits, although only a year later the U.S. Food and Drug Administration (FDA) ruled that such heart-health claims were "false and misleading."[40] Then, in 1960, immediately after the AHA's new policy statement endorsing the diet-heart hypothesis, producers of polyunsaturated-rich vegetable oils such as Mazola Corn Oil and Wesson Oil took out full-page newspaper ads echoing the AHA's statement regarding the benefits of polyunsaturated fats.[41] A *Business Week* article at the time noted that "some of the margarine makers think they have discovered in recent medical findings a weapon that will enable them to lop off a fat slice of butter's share of the market."[42]

Not until 1971 did the FDA begin allowing producers of margarine and other processed foods to advertise the types of fats contained in food products.[43] While margarine and oil producers could not make explicit health claims for their products, the knowledge of the claimed relationship among polyunsaturated fats, blood cholesterol, and heart disease had already been sufficiently popularized, so the lay public was able to make the connection between the nutrient-content claims and the implied health benefits of these new foods.[44]

In response to developments in nutrition science and dietary advice, food scientists continued to nutritionally reengineer margarine. By the mid-1970s, nutrition experts were differentiating between LDL (low-density lipoprotein, the so-called bad cholesterol) and HDL (low-density lipoprotein, the "good" cholesterol), leading to a reordering of the fat hierarchy.[45] They continued to classify saturated fatty acids as bad fats, because they increased both HDL and LDL cholesterol levels, whereas in their view, polyunsaturated fats remained good fats because they lowered LDL cholesterol levels. In the 1980s, scientists recategorized monounsaturated fats as potentially the best fats of all, since they lowered LDL cholesterol levels but seemed also to raise HDL cholesterol levels. Margarine manufacturers responded to these shifts in scientific classification by using oils high in monounsaturated fats, particularly canola oil and olive oil blends, in some of their margarine brands.

The 1980s marked the beginning of the low-fat era, with nutrition experts and public health institutions recommending that people reduce their consumption of fat, and saturated fats in particular. Margarine producers responded with a range of reduced-fat and low-fat products. They renamed these low-fat margarines *spreads*, since the term *margarine* requires the product to contain at least 80 percent fat. To produce these low-fat spreads, manufacturers replaced some of the vegetable oils present in margarine with water. They also used new formulations of emulsifiers to better blend the oil with the water, as well as other ingredients and additives to imitate the texture, mouthfeel, and taste of regular, high-fat margarines.

The food manufacturing and food service industries were increasingly using hydrogenated vegetable oils in a range of other food products, including in deep-frying oils for restaurants and fast-food outlets. However, by the 1980s many fast-food chains, such as McDonald's and Burger King, were still frying many of their foods in beef fat, or in saturated fat–rich tropical oils such as palm oil and coconut oil.[46] Beginning in 1984, the prominent public health advocacy group Center for Science in the Public Interest (CSPI) played a pivotal role in pressuring restaurant chains to switch from using animal fats and vegetable oils high in saturated fats, to hydrogenated vegetable oils. The CSPI also stigmatized what they called "those troublesome tropical oils" due to their high saturated fat content, particularly palm oil (51 percent saturated fat) and coconut oil (92 percent). In their 1988 report *Saturated Fat Attack*, the CSPI defended the food industry's use of hydrogenated oils and dismissed any health concerns the public may already have harbored: "Hydrogenated (or partially hydrogenated) fats are widely used in foods and cause untold consternation among consumers. . . . Overall, hydrogenated fats don't pose a significant risk. The exceptions are hydrogenated coconut, palm, or palm kernel oils, which are bad to start with, but even worse after hydrogenation."[47] The CSPI was stretching credibility here by suggesting that hydrogenation was only a problem when applied to tropical oils such as palm and coconut oils. These tropical oils were in fact the least likely to be hydrogenated, due to their naturally high saturated fat content. In 1986, McDonald's succumbed to the damaging publicity and switched its deep-frying oils from beef fat to hydrogenated vegetable oil. By 1990, most fast-food chains had followed suit.[48]

In this era of good-and-bad nutritionism from the early 1960s to about 1990, nutrition experts promoted margarine as a healthier spread than butter exclusively on the basis of their respective fatty acid profiles. The assumption that margarine is healthier than butter was to become an *everyday nutritionism*—that is, an everyday nutritional expression, formulated within the logic of nutritionism, and that has been embraced and repeated by nutrition experts and the lay public alike. Margarine had shifted from attempting to merely imitate butter to being portrayed in advertisements as superior to butter in terms of its health benefits, as well as in terms of its other enhanced features, such as its spreadability, shelf life, and cheaper price. A 1970s food technology book, *Fabricated Foods*, acknowledged margarine's successful transformation from a poor imitation to a "sophisticated fabricated food": "A well-known example of a fabricated food is margarine. Despite the long legal, marketing, scientific, and technological hurdles, margarine has become a respectable, highly regarded, and useful food. Many foods are now undergoing a transition from a poor imitation of an existing food to a sophisticated fabricated food."[49]

In the 1970s, the Italian cultural theorist Umberto Eco referred to "hyperreality" as the cultural space in which the distinction between the original and the copy begins to blur, such that the copy takes on an aura of being more real than the original. Eco referred to Disneyland, for example, as a "fantasy space more real than reality," in which reconstructions of real streetscapes, animals, and objects are not merely reproduced as replicas. Rather, Disneyland produces fantasies, or fantastic reconstructions, with qualities that surpass the merely real objects and the experiences upon which they were initially modeled.[50] Reflecting on the use of technologies to create these hyperreal experiences, Eco noted that "Disneyland tells us that technology gives us more reality than nature can."[51]

So it was with margarine, one of the first hyperreal foods that came to be considered better—more real—than the merely real and original product. Even the artificially colored, rich, golden luster of margarine made the pale yellow of butter look drab by comparison. The philosopher of technology Albert Borgmann has pointed to the hyperreal character of food products such as calorie-reduced, artificial whipped cream and other artificial fats and sugars: "Chemistry has been employed to disburden us of the calories that are the unwelcome extension of the real foods we love. Cool Whip is hyperreal whipped cream, cheaper, more durable, and far less caloric than the real thing."[52] The promotion of margarine and other hyperreal foods demonstrated that the level of nutrients was in the process of becoming the dominant level at which we engage with and understand food, undermining our concerns with the quality of the ingredients and the processing techniques used to manufacture them.

TRANS-FATS AS BAD FATS:
THE TAMING OF THE TRANS-FATS CONTROVERSY

The publication of the 1990 Mensink and Katan study demonstrating the adverse effects of *trans*-fats on blood cholesterol level posed a threat to the reputation of margarine. It could also have opened up nutrition science and its dominant paradigms to close scrutiny by the public, or prompted greater self-reflection on the part of nutrition experts. Instead, this new understanding of the dangers of *trans*-fats has since become the new nutritional certainty, and the reversal in dietary advice on *trans*-fats has been treated as little more than an embarrassing mistake. The *trans*-fat fiasco has, in fact, been used by many nutrition experts and food manufacturers to reinforce, rather than challenge, a number of aspects of the nutritionism paradigm. The addition of *trans*-fats to the bad fats category reinforced and extended the good- and bad-fats discourse, which had itself been partially displaced by the more simplified low-fat message during the 1980s. The expression "*trans*-fats are bad fats" has in fact become yet another everyday nutritionism in the contemporary nutriscape.

Scientists' framing of both *trans*-fats and saturated fats as "bad fats" undermines the distinction between an unmodified, naturally occurring nutrient, on the one hand, and an artificial, chemically reconstituted food component, on the other. The 2010 *Dietary Guidelines for Americans*, for example, reinforces this conflation of *trans*-fats and saturated fats by referring to them collectively as "solid fats."[53] The categorization of *trans*-fats as bad fats has also had the consequence of directing attention away from the hydrogenation process and other oil and margarine processing techniques and additives, and toward just one product of the manufacturing process—the *trans*-fats. An alternative to this good- and bad-fats discourse would be to categorize these chemically reconstituted oils as *bad oils*—a designation not likely to please the powerful vegetable oil industry.

Many nutrition experts and public health authorities have been quick to point out that under no circumstances should *trans*-fats simply be replaced with saturated fats—in the form of animal fats or palm and coconut oils—but instead should be substituted with *trans*-fat-free polyunsaturated- or monounsaturated-rich vegetable oils, such as canola, soybean, or

144   MARGARINE, BUTTER, AND THE *TRANS*-FATS FIASCO

olive oil. The proceedings of a 2006 AHA conference on *trans*-fats warned: "The unintended consequence of greatest concern is that fats and oils high in saturated fats, instead of the healthier unsaturated fats, might be used to replace fats and oils with *trans* fatty acids."[54] The AHA has thereby used the *trans*-fats controversy as an opportunity to renew their long-running anti-saturated fats campaign.

In 2007 the AHA launched an online campaign called "Meet the Fats." It features the Bad Fats Brothers—two sleazy cartoon characters called Sat and Trans who "clog arteries and break hearts." On the Meet the Fats website, mention is made that *trans*-fats are a component of partially hydrogenated vegetable oils. However, the emphasis is on identifying the types of foods in which both *trans*-fats and saturated fats are typically found:

> Go easy on bakery goodies like doughnuts and pastries and fried foods like French fries. And eat less fatty meat, chicken with skin, butter and full-fat dairy products. . . . Saturated and *trans*-fats can often be replaced with better alternatives, like monounsaturated and polyunsaturated fats. For example, use tub margarine instead of traditional stick margarine or liquid vegetable oil instead of butter. . . . Just because a label says "*trans*-fat-free" doesn't mean the food is healthy. It might still be high in the other bad fat—saturated—or have lots of empty calories.[55]

The assumption of this advice is that all of these foods contain significant quantities of *trans*-fats as well as saturated fats, even though some *trans*-fats were already in the process of being removed from many of these products. Whole categories of foods are stigmatized on the basis of their presumed *trans*-fat content, rather than distinguishing between good-quality and poor-quality varieties of these foods, with the latter more likely to contain *trans*-fats. Croissants, for example, are stigmatized as containing *trans*-fats, even though a traditionally prepared and good-quality croissant is typically made with butter. Nor is information given on what ingredients are now being used to replace these partially hydrogenated oils.

More important, at every point the Meet the Fats campaign equates the dangers of *trans*-fats and saturated fats, as well as the types of foods that contain both of these fats. The AHA also continues to advise consumers to "use soft margarine as a substitute for butter," as long as they are labeled *trans*-fat free.[56] The AHA is reported to have opposed the introduction of New York City's ban on *trans*-fats in its restaurants out of fear that this would lead to a shift back to the use of oils high in saturated fats.[57] Having been instrumental in promoting the switch to *trans*-fat laden foods, the AHA now only seems interested in criticizing *trans*-fats and hydrogenated oils to the extent that these can be linked to saturated fats. This is a continuation of the AHA's heavy promotion since the 1960s of polyunsaturated-rich vegetable oils.

The *trans*-fats controversy could also have been an opportunity to question nutrition experts' reductive focus on the LDL and HDL blood cholesterol biomarkers as the basis for evaluating the effects of foods on heart health. Instead, their focus on these biomarkers has been reaffirmed, and the *trans*-fat controversy has provided another opportunity for nutrition experts to disseminate the "HDL equals good, LDL equals bad" message. The dominant *trans*-fats discourse has also tended to reinforce rather than challenge the myth of nutritional precision, and particularly the claimed precision with which the association between fats and the incidence of chronic diseases is understood and can be quantified. Scientists have come to measure and quantify the detrimental health effects of *trans*-fats and saturated fats in much the same way. For example, an epidemiological study led by Walter Willett published in 2006 estimated that every year in the United States *trans*-fats directly contribute to 30,000 deaths from heart disease.[58]

Food regulatory agencies in most countries have been very slow to enact legislation to either regulate the levels of *trans*-fats in food products or to require *trans*-fat labeling. In 2004, the Dutch government was the first country to begin regulating *trans*-fat content, introducing legislation specifying a maximum of 2 percent *trans*-fats in all food products. The U.S. FDA, on the other hand, merely introduced *trans*-fat labeling on the Nutrition Facts label of packaged foods in 2006. However, the new labeling regulations in the United States still allow manufacturers to claim that foods containing up to 0.5 gram of *trans*-fats per serving are "*trans*-fat-free." So *trans*-fat-free in some cases may just mean low *trans*-fats. A person could therefore unwittingly consume several grams of *trans*-fats per day from eating foods labeled *trans*-fat free. In 2006, New York became the first city in the United States to "ban" the presence of *trans*-fats in foods sold in its restaurants. However, the terms of this so-called ban meant that these foods could still contain up to 0.5 gram of *trans*-fats per serving.[59] The FDA's *trans*-fat food labeling regulations require that the total *trans*-fats listed on the label include not only industrial *trans*-fats, but also some kinds of ruminant *trans*-fats, thereby collapsing the distinction between them.[60]

The food industry has also been allowed to transform what could have been a marketing and commercial liability into a new marketing opportunity to promote the health benefits of their reformulated low-*trans*-fat and *trans*-fat-free products. In terms of nutrient-content claims, the labeling of foods as "*trans*-fat free" and "0 grams *trans*-fats" can give these food products a health halo, perhaps on a par with low-fat or no-fat nutrient claims.[61] In November 2006, the FDA went even further by approving the following disease prevention health claim for food products that contain less than 1 gram of fat and 0.5 gram of *trans*-fats: "Diets low in saturated fat and cholesterol, and as low as possible in *trans*-fat, may reduce the risk of heart disease."[62] This health claim suggests that the practice of *not* adding artificial or industrially manufactured *trans*-fats to a food product will somehow enhance its nutritional value and reduce heart disease risk.

Walter Willett seems to have been one of the few nutrition experts to confess to having previously promoted *trans*-fats consumption: "There was a lot of resistance from the scientific community [to the detrimental health effects of *trans*-fats] because a lot of people had made their careers telling people to eat margarine instead of butter. When I was a physician in the 1980s, that's what I was telling people to do and unfortunately we were often sending them to their graves prematurely."[63] Few other nutrition experts and public health institutions have publicly acknowledged and accepted responsibility for this reversal in dietary advice. Yet even though Willett admits that the initial recommendation to switch from butter to margarine was not based on solid evidence to begin with, he maintains that at the time "this recommendation made sense" based on scientists' understanding of the dangers of saturated fat.[64] It was simply overturned by new studies demonstrating the opposite. He defends this turn of events as an acceptable part of the onward march of "scientific progress": "To a scientist, this is the normal path of scientific progress—a recommendation based on a good guess is tested and toppled by one based on good science. To the rest of the world, though, it is a frustrating contradiction."[65] There is no suggestion here that scientists should have waited for more solid evidence, or that they should have erred on the side of promoting whole foods rather than a processed-reconstituted food such as margarine.

In the early 1990s, the CSPI also changed its tune and began vigorously campaigning against *trans*-fats, but without acknowledging its earlier role in coercing food companies to switch to hydrogenated vegetable oils in the 1980s, or its earlier exoneration of the health threats of these oils.[66] Even though the CSPI had played a major role in facilitating McDonald's initial switch to hydrogenated vegetable oils for deep-frying, in 2006 the CSPI successfully sued McDonald's for failing to change back to a low-*trans*-fat cooking oil as it had publicly announced it would do in 2003.

The court ordered McDonald's to pay $7 million of its settlement fee to the AHA, and these funds were subsequently used to fund the AHA's Meet the Fats campaign.[67]

There has also been a tendency among nutrition experts to gloss over this reversal in dietary advice regarding *trans*-fats and margarine. For example, in her 2006 book *What to Eat* Marion Nestle claims that there has been no significant shift in expert advice regarding margarine and hydrogenated oils since the 1960s, and defends the AHA's position on margarine and *trans*-fats:

> I often hear margarine used as a prime example of how nutrition advice changes all the time. First it was supposed to be good for you, then bad, and now it is supposed to be good for you again. But a careful reading of cardiologists' advice over the years gives a more consistent story. For more than forty years, the American Heart Association (AHA) has issued cautious and nuanced advice about margarine. It has always put hard margarines in the same category as butter.... In 1968, the American Heart Association noted that heavily hydrogenated margarines "are ineffective in lowering the serum cholesterol" and the next year suggested replacing butter with polyunsaturated margarines (these are the softer ones that come in tubs; they have less saturated fat and also less *trans*-fat).[68]

As noted earlier, there was a shift in the AHA advice during the 1960s, from acknowledging the cholesterol-raising effects of all hydrogenated oils, to only warning against hard (i.e., heavily hydrogenated) margarines and recommending soft margarines. Yet even these softer margarines contained significant quantities of *trans*-fats. The AHA explanation for their preference for soft margarines was that they contained more polyunsaturated fats and less saturated fats than hard margarines, but without explaining that the fats in both products had been chemically transformed and contained *trans*-fats. The AHA's nuanced distinction between hard and soft margarine was also probably overwhelmed by the more simplified nutritional mantra to replace butter with margarine.[69]

The lack of serious reflection on the lessons of the *trans*-fat fiasco is evidence of a failure to interrogate the broader paradigm and assumptions that continue to inform scientific research and dietary advice. Most nutrition and public health experts have simply adjusted their dietary messages and joined the campaign against *trans*-fats. Going against this trend, epidemiologist Paul Marantz and his colleagues have warned of the public health *risks* of the campaign to stigmatize and regulate *trans*-fats without sufficient reflection or evidence of the consequences of doing so. For example, they suggest that the marketing of foods as *trans*-fat free may "affect dietary behavior in unpredictable ways," such as fostering people's belief that more *trans*-fat-free foods can be consumed.[70] It is also unclear what the *trans*-fats would be replaced with, and what the health consequences of these changes might be. They therefore warn against any repeat of other ill-considered and ill-fated dietary campaigns, such as the low-fat campaign and the promotion of margarine over butter.

On the basis of the principles of food processing quality and precaution, however, there are good grounds for immediately removing hydrogenated oils from the food supply. Hydrogenation fundamentally transforms the chemical structure of fats, and these chemically reconstituted oils should not have been permitted to enter the food supply in the first place—particularly in such quantities—until they had been proven safe and nutritious. But the question of what they might now be replaced with is equally important.

FROM *TRANS*-FATS TO *I*-FATS: REENGINEERING MARGARINE IN THE "VIRTUALLY *TRANS*-FAT-FREE" ERA

Nutrition experts, by focusing only on the presence of *trans*-fats in food products, have framed the solution to the *trans*-fat problem in terms of the need to eliminate or even just to minimize levels of artificial *trans*-fats in margarine and other foods. This allows for not only the continued use of fully and partially hydrogenated oils by food manufacturers and restaurants but also the use of other processing techniques for chemically transforming oils to obtain novel fats with similar end-product characteristics as the partially hydrogenated oils.[71]

While nutrition experts and public health institutions have welcomed the gradual removal of *trans*-fats and partially hydrogenated oils from the food supply, they have largely been silent on the issue of their replacements.[72] Just as prior to the 1990s the public was not properly informed that the oils used in margarine production and other foods had been hydrogenated and contained *trans*-fats, it would seem this denial of information is being repeated in this virtually *trans*-fat-free era. While some food manufacturers and restaurants are simply returning to the use of unprocessed and non-chemically engineered vegetable oils, this is just one of the many available options being pursued within these industries.

Partially hydrogenated oils have been a cheap, all-purpose ingredient for a range of food products and applications across the food manufacturing, restaurant, and fast-food industries. The challenge for many food companies since the 1990s has been to develop a range of alternative processing techniques and ingredients to meet the specific requirements of these various products and applications. In many cases, these companies have opted for a combination of fully hydrogenated, partially hydrogenated, and unhydrogenated oils, often using improved processing techniques for chemically transforming liquid oils.[73] Another parallel strategy has been for these companies to switch to using varieties of vegetable oils with more favorable fat profiles, often through breeding and genetically engineering plants to yield seed oils with selected characteristics, such as high-oleic canola oil (an oil with a high monounsaturated fat content). Alternatively, they may use new additives—including emulsifiers, enzymes, and modified starches—to create the required texture, consistency, and taste in processed foods.[74]

The processing techniques that margarine manufacturers have started using to produce hardened vegetable oils typically involve a combination of fractionation, interesterification, and full hydrogenation.[75] Fractionation is a process for physically separating the solid and liquid fractions of oils. Because of its highly saturated character, palm oil is the one manufacturers use most often in this process.[76] Margarines can be rendered harder or softer by varying the ratio of these solid and liquid fractions. Interesterification involves the use of a chemical catalyst (e.g., sodium methoxide) or enzymes to modify the physical properties of an oil or fat blend.[77] As with partially hydrogenated oils, the interesterified oil may then be washed, bleached, and deodorized—although the deodorization process is also known to produce small quantities of *trans*-fats. The end product may also contain other chemical residues.[78]

Manufacturers can use interesterification to blend liquid oils with hard fats to produce a modified oil with the desired properties, such as a higher melting point. The hard fats used in this process may be fully or partially hydrogenated oils, or else the hard fractions of vegetable oils such as palm oil. The interesterification process itself does not produce *trans*-fatty acids, nor does it modify the existing fatty acids, but it does rearrange the constituent fatty acids within the larger fat molecules.[79] In this sense, these interesterified fats—or what I call *i*-fats for short—have a chemically transformed molecular structure and, like *trans*-fats, are a novel kind of fat not otherwise found in nature.[80] The interesterification process produces not one but a number of different types of rearranged fatty acid molecules.[81] Each of these novel fatty acid sequences can be expected to be metabolized differently, and some may have adverse health effects.

Many table margarines are now labeled as virtually *trans*-fat free, meaning that they contain 1 percent or less of *trans*-fats. A common margarine manufacturing practice is to combine fully hydrogenated and unhydrogenated vegetable oils, modifying the composition of incorporated fats through the use of interesterification and fractionation techniques.[82] Unilever's popular Flora brand, for example, is manufactured using this combination of full hydrogenation, fractionation, and interesterification techniques applied to a blend of sunflower, canola, and palm oils.[83] Unilever has been one of the pioneers in margarine innovation and has quickly responded to shifts in the nutriscape over the past fifty years, leading the development of polyunsaturated margarines in the 1960s, low-fat spreads in the late 1970s and 1980s, and virtually *trans*-fat-free and cholesterol-lowering margarines from the mid-1990s.[84]

Food manufacturers' development of virtually *trans*-fat-free alternatives to other food products and applications has involved choosing the right combination of techniques and oils for the task.[85] For instance, interesterified and fully hydrogenated oils can be used as shortening agents for baked food products. For deep-frying applications, one option is to blend lightly hydrogenated oils with unhydrogenated oils to achieve a low-*trans*-fat end-product.[86] However, food companies have tended to favor new varieties and blends of nonhydrogenated vegetable oils to lower the *trans*-fat content, such as low-linolenic soybean oil and high-oleic canola oil varieties. These new oil varieties are more stable and less prone to oxidation, in part due to their lower levels of highly unsaturated omega-3 fats. These oils are therefore better suited than conventional unhydrogenated oils to repeated frying and other exposures to high temperatures.[87] Some of these new oil varieties have been genetically engineered, such as Monsanto's herbicide-tolerant, low-linolenic soybean oil.[88]

Despite food companies' rush to remove and replace *trans*-fats, scientists have conducted few studies on the health effects of these individual or combined processing techniques and ingredients being used to replace them, such as fully hydrogenated, low-*trans*-fat partially hydrogenated, fractionated, and interesterified oils. A couple of studies of *i*-fats have claimed that they do not have adverse effects on LDL and HDL cholesterol levels, while other preliminary studies have suggested that they do.[89] One study has also reported that interesterification may increase the susceptibility of oils to oxidation, which is now considered to be a possible cause of inflammation in the body (and therefore as promoting cardiovascular disease).[90] Other studies have not found adverse effects of reformulated margarines on biomarkers of cardiovascular disease and inflammation.[91] It may be some time before the health impacts of interesterification and *i*-fats are adequately tested. It is therefore appropriate to invoke the precautionary principle here and to remove these chemically reconstituted oils from the food supply until they can be shown to be safe and healthful.

In 2004 the FDA introduced new regulations allowing interesterified fats (at least those with a stearate content of more than 20 percent) to be labeled as "interesterified oils," or even as "high-stearate" or "stearate-rich" oils—even those that had been hydrogenated before being interesterified.[92] This enabled food companies to avoid making reference on labels to hydrogenated oils—a term that has become tainted in the minds of many consumers. At the same time, there is no obligation on food companies to state whether an oil has been interesterified. These labeling regulations not only conceal from consumers the presence of hydrogenated or interesterified oils but also reduce the ability of nutrition and public health experts to monitor and evaluate the possible health effects of these modified fats.[93] So far, however, nutrition experts have done little to alert the public to the presence of these reconstituted *i*-fats in the food supply.

CHOLESTEROL-LOWERING FUNCTIONAL MARGARINES: PURE SIMULATION IN THE NUTRISCAPE

As the *trans*-fat controversy was unfolding in the 1990s, margarine manufacturers such as Unilever had already begun quietly reformulating their products to minimize their *trans*-fat content below the 1 percent level. While this modification of the underlying production techniques was taking place, margarine's nutritional facade also continued to be redesigned in response to the changing nutritional trends and consumer expectations in the era of functional nutritionism. With the development of cholesterol-lowering and omega-3-enriched varieties, margarine has managed to not only retain but also to enhance its healthful image to nutricentric consumers.

Beginning in the mid-1990s in Europe, and then in the United States, food companies introduced margarine varieties that contained high concentrations of cholesterol-lowering plant sterols and stanols.[94] Johnson & Johnson's Benecol, for example, was introduced in Europe in 1995 and proved especially popular in Finland, a country with high rates of heart disease.[95] In 2000 Unilever introduced its Pro Activ sterol-enriched margarine in Europe.[96] Plant sterols and stanols are naturally occurring components of plants, fruits, and vegetables and are chemically similar to cholesterol. They thereby block the absorption of cholesterol in the body and have been shown to lower blood cholesterol levels.[97] However, the sterols and stanols added to margarine and other food products have been extracted from a range of food and nonfood sources—such as wood pulp or vegetable oils—which may then undergo further processing.[98] The sterols and stanols in Benecol, for example, are primarily sourced from tall oil derived from the pulping of pinewood. The crude tall oil is first fractionated into its component parts, with the plant sterols hydrogenated to form stanols and then esterified with monounsaturated and polyunsaturated fats.[99]

Manufacturers now add these extracted and reconstituted sterols and stanols to a range of foods and drinks, including orange juice and milk. In order to achieve significant blood cholesterol–lowering effects, these stanols and sterols are added in greater quantities than typically found in single whole foods. However, while many studies have demonstrated the ability of sterol- and stanol-enriched food products to reduce LDL cholesterol levels, there are as yet no human studies that demonstrate that the plant sterols and stanols added to food directly reduce the incidence of heart disease. Instead, this causal connection is assumed on the basis that other cholesterol-lowering therapies—particularly those involving statin drugs—have been associated with a reduced risk of coronary heart disease.[100]

Choosing margarine as the first vehicle for these cholesterol-lowering food additives was a clever marketing decision by food companies, given that the claimed link between margarine and blood cholesterol levels was already well established in the public mind. Yet the communication of the claimed health benefits of cholesterol-lowering margarines could not rely on the type of nutrient-content claims that had previously been effective for marketing standard margarines. The low level of public awareness of plant sterols, and of their effects on blood cholesterol, meant that simply promoting a margarine's sterol content —such as the claim "high in plant sterols"—would be largely meaningless to the lay public. Instead, a more explicit health claim stating that this product actively lowered blood cholesterol levels was required. In 1999, the FDA gave approval for two margarine brands—Johnson & Johnson's Benecol and Lipton's Take Control—to be advertised with explicit health claims that these foods were able to lower cholesterol levels.[101] In the FDA's terminology, these are technically known as *structure/function claims* because they refer to particular bodily functions or processes, in contrast with disease prevention type of health claims, which require a higher level of scientific substantiation.[102]

These plant-sterol enriched margarines can be described as transnutric foods, since they involve the addition of a nutrient or food component that is not otherwise associated with margarine, butter, or other spreads. The claim that the direct modification of blood cholesterol levels leads to a reduction in heart disease risk is also a form of biomarker reductionism and, more specifically, of biomarker determinism, because it assumes that there is a direct causal relationship between blood cholesterol levels and heart disease.

One of the known side effects of consuming plant sterols in the concentrated quantities being added to these margarine products is that they have been shown to block the absorption of beta-carotene and therefore to lower vitamin A levels in the body. In this sense, sterol-enriched margarines produce a nutrient-level contradiction, whereby the addition of a particular nutrient or food component inadvertently reduces the availability to the body of another beneficial nutrient. Consumers of sterol-enriched foods are therefore encouraged to compensate for this nutrient-level contradiction by eating more fruits and vegetables to increase their vitamin A levels.[103] Recent studies have also raised questions about other possible detrimental health effects of increased plant sterol intake, with some studies ironically suggesting that sterol and stanol esters may increase the risk of atherosclerosis.[104]

The introduction and commercial success of cholesterol-lowering margarines and spreads signal the rise to dominance of the functional nutritionism paradigm since the 1990s. Functional nutritionism is characterized by a heightened emphasis on the relationship between individual foods and nutrients, on the one hand, and specific internal bodily functions, biomarkers, and health conditions, on the other. Cholesterol-lowering margarines appeal to this focus on particular biomarkers of bodily health. The production and marketing of cholesterol-lowering spreads also represent a further shift in the relationship among margarine, butter, and the nutriscape. In the era of good-and-bad nutritionism, hyperreal margarine's primary reference point was butter, with margarine's claimed health benefits justified by reference to the nutrient profiles of these two products. In the functional era, however, margarine now inhabits a surreal world of spreads with diverse features designed to meet a range of consumer demands. In terms of its claimed health benefits, margarine's primary reference point is no longer just butter, for it is designed to simulate the nutritional characteristics and health benefits of a range of foods, including plant foods (plant sterols), fish (omega-3 fats), and vegetable oils (polyunsaturated and monounsaturated fats). Margarine's primary reference points are in fact no longer foods at all but nutrients. These margarines and other functional food products inhabit a world of nutrients and nutritional concepts, having floated free of any engagement with actual foods.[105]

Butter has also succumbed to this logic of the nutritional code and has been reengineered and remarketed since the 1990s in response to the success of margarine and to the changing nutriscape. In some respects, the relationship between butter and margarine has been turned on its head, with butter now attempting to simulate some of margarine's nutritional characteristics and other features.[106] For example, more spreadable varieties of butter blended with vegetable oils were released in the late 1980s and early 1990s and were packaged for convenience in margarine-like plastic tubs. These butter-oil blends also produce what many nutrition experts would view as a more favorable fat profile compared with plain butter. Another type of spreadable butter is whipped butter that has been aerated with nitrogen gas. Food manufacturers have also developed reduced-fat and low-fat varieties of butter that replace with water some of the milk fat found in butter, which then require other additives such gelatins and starter cultures to maintain a butterlike texture.[107]

In 1992 the Belgium company Balade introduced a low-cholesterol product in Europe named Light Butter. This butterish product had 90 percent of the cholesterol in its milk fat removed by the addition of crystalline beta-cyclodextrin, an enzyme-modified starch derivative that binds to the cholesterol and enables it to be easily removed.[108] This is another case of a more highly processed food being promoted as a healthy alternative to the original product. Many other dairy products have also been nutritionally engineered, from reduced-fat milk and cheeses to sterol-enriched yogurts, yogurt drinks, cheeses, and milk products.[109]

The history of margarine, butter, and the *trans*-fats controversy reveals the extent to which a reductive understanding of nutrients and biomarkers has in some cases been used by nutrition experts and the food industry to promote highly processed and reconstituted foods as nutritionally superior products. Those nutrition experts who now proclaim the benefits of sterol-enriched margarine varieties continue to prioritize the claimed health benefits of specific nutrients and food components over the types of processing and additives used in their production. Not even the acknowledged mistakes associated with the *trans*-fat controversy seem to have given the nutrition profession much pause for reflection on the dominant nutritionism paradigm. On the contrary, the celebration of cholesterol-lowering spreads by many nutrition experts demonstrates the continued dominance of this paradigm, and its ability to adapt to and absorb any potential threats to its legitimacy in the functional era.

CHAPTER SEVEN

The Era of Functional Nutritionism

Functional Nutrients, Superfoods, and Optimal Dietary Patterns

It is just a matter of time until a person's omega-3 status will replace serum cholesterol, LDL to HDL ratio, and even C-reactive protein . . . to assess that person's risk for sudden cardiac death and other diseases.
—SUSAN ALPORT, *THE QUEEN OF FATS*, 2007

The omega-3 fats are one of the wonder nutrients of the present era of functional nutritionism. Many studies over the past decade have reported that an inadequate intake of omega-3 fats is associated with higher incidences of heart disease, cancer, arthritis, and dementia. More positively, many nutrition experts suggest that increasing your omega-3 intake can actively decrease your risk of suffering these diseases, improve your brain function, and enhance your overall health and longevity. This emphasis by nutrition experts on the importance of raising omega-3 intake has created a new anxiety about the perceived scarcity of omega-3 fats in the food supply and in many people's diets, while also encouraging people to think they can reap a range of health benefits and enhancements if they increase or optimize their intake of these fats.

The food industry has stoked these fears of an omega-3 scarcity, not just by promoting foods that naturally contain high levels of omega-3 fats, such as fish, but also by fortifying and reengineering a range of foods with omega-3 fats, such as orange juice, dairy products, and margarine. PepsiCo, for example, produces Tropicana Healthy Heart Orange Juice laced with microencapsulated fish oils. The marketing director of Tropicana recognizes the obvious consumer appeal of this fortified juice: "People just aren't eating salmon or sardines twice a day. But they will drink two glasses of orange juice, if it has no fishy taste and all the benefits."[1]

The celebration of omega-3 fats encapsulates the zeitgeist of the present era of functional nutritionism that began around the mid-1990s. Functional nutritionism is characterized by a greater emphasis on the more positive, beneficial, and health-enhancing role of nutrients, rather than the earlier focus on the harmful properties of so-called bad nutrients. A new set of beneficial nutrients and other food components are now valued for their "functional" attributes—that is, their ability to target and enhance particular bodily functions—such as omega-3s for enhanced brain functioning, plant sterols for lowering blood cholesterol, and probiotics for gut health. These functional nutrients are also attributed with the ability to reduce the risk of chronic diseases, while the inadequate intake of these beneficial nutrients is now blamed for increasing chronic disease risk.

The rise of functional nutritionism has in part been driven by scientific developments that enable experts to develop a more precise understanding of nutrients and bodies at the molecular level, as well as the development of new techniques for reengineering the nutritional profile of foods. But this paradigm shift has also been precipitated by some of the perceived limitations and controversies of the earlier era of good-and-bad nutritionism, such as the discrediting of the low-fat campaign, the backflip on *trans*-fats and margarine, the overemphasis on bad nutrients and negative dietary messages, and the limitations of single-nutrient studies. The shift to functional nutritionism has also been facilitated by the introduction of new health claims regulations in the United States and elsewhere since the mid-1990s that allow food companies to directly advertise the precise health benefits they claim for their products.

While nutrition research and dietary guidelines continue to be framed in terms of nutrients, there has also been a belated interest since the early 2000s in research addressing foods and dietary patterns in their own right. Researchers have more actively studied the health effects of foods and food groups, such as whole grains, milk, meat, nuts, sweetened beverages, as well as nutritionally engineered foods such as cholesterol-lowering margarine and probiotic yogurts. Some of these foods have been elevated by nutrition experts and popular commentators to the status of "superfoods" or "functional foods" capable of enhancing and optimizing health and specific bodily functions. Dietary patterns such as the Mediterranean, Japanese, and vegetarian diets have also been studied and celebrated, while the paleolithic diet has become an enormously popular counternutritional dietary approach.

This chapter explores the characteristics of this now dominant functional understanding of nutrients, foods, and the body, through an examination of omega-3 fats, nutrigenomics, nutritional supplements, superfoods, dietary pattern analysis, vegetarian and paleo diets, and the new emphasis on hormones and other internal biochemical processes.

FUNCTIONAL NUTRIENTS

The era of good-and-bad nutritionism was dominated by a narrow range of nutrients and food components (fats, carbs, cholesterol, fiber, vitamins, calcium), with the aim primarily being to minimize the consumption of bad nutrients in order to lower the risk of chronic diseases. In the functional era, by contrast, there has been a proliferation of categories and subcategories of nutrients, but with each nutrient now more precisely targeted to particular bodily functions and health outcomes. Within mainstream nutritional discourses, there is now a much greater emphasis on the beneficial and health-enhancing nutrients and food components and on their ability to target and enhance specific bodily functions and to optimize bodily health.

Experts continue to speak the language of "good and bad nutrients," incorporating a broader range of more differentiated and nuanced distinctions. Following the decline of the low-fat campaign, they have returned to the familiar good- and bad-fats distinction but with *trans*-fats joining saturated fats in the bad fats category and omega-3 fats added to the good fats category. The polyunsaturated fats that have been celebrated since the 1960s are now primarily differentiated into the very good omega-3 fats, on the one hand, and the not quite as good omega-6 fatty acids. Nutrition scientists have also valued differently the subtypes of omega-3 fats, with the long-chain DHA (docosahexaenoic acid) and EPA (eicosapentaenoic acid) varieties found in fish the most highly prized, compared with the ALA (alpha-linolenic acid) omega-3 fats commonly found in plant foods. As noted in chapter 4, the various subgroups of saturated fatty acids have also been shown to have variable effects on blood cholesterol levels, such that—even within the terms of the diet-heart hypothesis—these saturated fats are not considered so bad after all. The American Heart Association continues to openly promote the good- and bad-fat discourse and has published its own updated interpretation of this fat hierarchy:

1. Very beneficial: omega-3 polyunsaturated fats
2. Beneficial: omega-6 polyunsaturated fats

3. Good: monounsaturated fats
4. Avoid/limit: saturated fat (to 7 percent of calories)
5. Avoid/limit: *trans*-fat (to 1 percent of calories)[2]

Nutrition experts have also increasingly differentiated carbs into "good carbs" and "bad carbs," based either on levels of processing or on glycemic response. The old distinction between complex carbs (i.e., starches) and simple carbs (i.e., sugars) has largely been abandoned, displaced by the distinction between whole carbs (i.e., whole grains, starchy vegetables) and so-called refined carbs (i.e., refined cereals and sugars). A growing number of experts have identified the rise in consumption of refined carbs since the 1970s as a major contributor to the rise in obesity and diabetes levels in the United States, particularly because of their role in raising blood sugar and insulin levels. The other nutritional concept for distinguishing between good and bad carbs is the glycemic index (GI), which, as discussed in chapter 5, essentially undermines the clear distinction between whole foods and refined-processed foods.

One "bad carb" that some experts now implicate in rising rates of obesity and diabetes is sugar, particularly in the form of the sucrose and high-fructose corn syrup added to sweets and beverages or found in fruit juices. Throughout the good-and-bad era, most nutrition experts considered sugar a source of "empty calories" and as just another "refined" or "simple" carb that should not be consumed in excess. In this spirit, some promoters of the GI concept have continued to exonerate sugar because of its moderate GI score. However, while the high intake of glucose from added sugars has been known to stimulate blood glucose and insulin levels, the role of fructose has come under greater scrutiny in recent years for its various deleterious effects in the body.[3] Pediatric and obesity expert Robert Lustig, for example, describes fructose as the "smoking gun" at the scene of the obesity epidemic.[4] He also argues that sugar induces all of the diseases associated with the metabolic syndrome, including hypertension, cardiovascular disease, and fatty liver disease.[5]

Despite this renewal of the good- and bad-nutrient discourse, in the functional era the emphasis within mainstream dietary guidelines and food marketing practices has shifted from avoiding bad nutrients to harnessing the more positive and beneficial attributes of good nutrients and other food components. A range of new "wonder nutrients" such as omega-3 fats, vitamin D, phytochemicals, antioxidants, plant sterols, and probiotics now commands the attention of nutrition experts and the food industry. Many nutrition experts consider these nutrients and food components not just good but "functional." They now promote these functional nutrients—and the functional foods in which they are contained—as having almost medicinal or therapeutic qualities and the capacity to minimize the risk of specific chronic diseases and to enhance specific bodily functions, rather than just meeting our "basic" nutritional requirements. Within the functional nutritionism paradigm, these good, beneficial, or functional nutrients are valued for their specific and targeted effects on particular bodily functions and health states. In order to manage one's weight, for example, rather than just eating less food—or fewer calories—we can also select high-protein or low-GI foods that target satiety and so decrease hunger.[6]

Nutrition researchers have also become more interested in nonnutrient components thought to offer health benefits, and food manufacturers have not hesitated to add these prized food components to processed foods. These include plant sterols and stanols for reducing blood cholesterol levels, and probiotic cultures of microorganisms claimed to improve gut health. The many types of antioxidants found in plant foods are now valued for their role in preventing oxidation and inflammation in the body. The ginkgo biloba nut—which some experts believe may improve cognitive performance and memory, though there is little scientific evidence for such claims—is being added to energy drinks and breakfast cereals, together with claims that they enhance "mental alertness" and "sharp thinking."[7]

The most celebrated vitamin in the present era is vitamin D. Many vitamin D experts now attribute a range of diseases and conditions—including cancers, cardiovascular disease, diabetes, autoimmune diseases, bone fractures, and arthritis—to low levels of vitamin D in the body and therefore recommend very high doses of vitamin D in supplements or from fortified foods, particularly in cases where a person's exposure to adequate sunlight is limited.[8] Such high doses go beyond what has previously been considered necessary to prevent obvious nutrient deficiency diseases and to maintain everyday "good health" and instead become part of the pursuit of an "optimal" or "enhanced" state of health. As Tufts University vitamin D expert Susan Harris puts it: "We're no longer talking about avoiding frank deficiencies. We're talking about maintaining optimum health, and reducing our risks in more subtle ways."[9]

In the functional era it is the underconsumption of beneficial nutrients—such as omega-3 fats, vitamin D, resistant starch, folate, and antioxidants—that carries a fair portion of the blame for people's poor health, alongside the overconsumption of bad nutrients. In some cases, such as with omega-3 fats, until the 1980s nutrition scientists were ignorant about or barely studied these nutrients and food components, yet they are now suddenly represented as vital food components. Some experts also suggest that micronutrient deficiencies over a more prolonged period of time may be implicated in a range of chronic diseases. Nutrition scientist Robert Heaney, for example, has argued that the "minimum daily requirements" that continue to define the setting of dietary guidelines are based on an outdated emphasis on avoiding absolute nutrient deficiency diseases. He instead recommends considerably larger doses of some nutrients, such as vitamin D, in order to reduce chronic disease risk and to actively enhance health.[10]

The nutritional anxiety that we are just not getting enough of these functional nutrients from "ordinary" or "conventional" foods and dietary patterns has intensified the perception of nutrient scarcity that first emerged in the era of quantifying nutritionism. This perception, combined with the new assumptions and imperatives of the functional era, now drives consumer demands for "nutrient-dense" whole foods, nutritionally engineered functional foods, and dietary supplements. The food and supplement industries are more than willing to commodify these expanding nutritional requirements and fetishes. For example, Dannon's Activia brand blueberry-flavored yogurt contains not only 19 grams of sugar per 113-gram tub but also added calcium, vitamin A, and what they call "Bifidus Regularis," a friendly bacterium that can help to "regulate your digestive system."[11] Cargill's new Smart Balance, Heart Right, Fat Free Milk has cholesterol-lowering plant sterols, DHA and EPA omega-3 fats, vitamin D, and 25 percent more protein and calcium per serve than whole milk.[12]

In the era of functional nutritionism, there has also been a shift in nutritional messaging from a focus on the quantity of single nutrients to more nuanced multinutrient advice for optimizing health outcomes. From being told to *eat more* of the protective and growth-promoting nutrients in the quantifying era and to *eat less* of the bad and fattening nutrients in the good-and-bad era, we are now being urged by nutrition experts and popular commentators to *eat smarter*. An article in *Men's Health* magazine begins, for instance, with the helpful tip that "you don't have to go on a diet to lose those extra pounds. Just eat smart."[13] Rather than simply seeking to maximize or minimize the consumption of particular nutrients, the new imperative is for people to optimize the quantities and ratios of nutrients they consume and to identify nutrient components and nutrient combinations that target particular bodily functions. For example, many nutrition experts recommend not simply increasing the consumption of omega-3 fats but also lowering the ratio of omega-6 to omega-3 fats in order to restore the balance of these fats to a more optimal level.[14] The marketing of multinutrient supplements also taps into a new recognition that single nutrients may work better in combination with other nutrients.

While the concept of "nutrient density" has been in circulation since at least the 1970s, it has come to the fore in nutritional discourses over the past decade.[15] The term *nutrient density* originally referred to the nutrient content per gram of food but is now used by many nutrition experts to refer to both the quantity and "quality" of nutrients contained in a food.[16] While definitions of nutrient density emphasize the presence of positive, health-enhancing components, at the same time the presence of what these experts consider to be bad nutrients—such as saturated fats—can seriously reduce a food's nutrient density score. As the U.S. Department of Agriculture (USDA) 2010 *Dietary Guidelines for Americans* defines the term,

> Nutrient-dense foods and beverages provide vitamins, minerals, and other substances that may have positive health effects with relatively few calories. The term "nutrient dense" indicates that the nutrients and other beneficial substances in a food have not been "diluted" by the addition of calories from added solid fats, added sugars, or added refined starches, or by the solid fats naturally present in the food.[17]

Full-fat cuts of meat and baked chicken with the skin on fare poorly in terms of nutrient density according to the USDA's criteria, despite the fact that these foods are a concentrated source of many valuable nutrients. The concept of nutrient density at least has the virtue of shifting the focus away from single nutrients and onto the overall nutrient profile of a food. It nevertheless maintains the focus on nutrients and largely involves adding up the relative benefits of a number of single nutrients.

BIOMARKERS, HORMONES, AND OPTIMAL HEALTH

The functional era has seen a shift not only in the way nutrients are understood but also in the way the body and bodily health are interpreted, represented, and personally experienced. The earlier concern with preventing and minimizing the risks of chronic diseases has been extended and intensified, with the focus of nutrition scientists shifting from heart disease and cancer to diabetes and obesity.

On top of this intensified concern with minimizing disease risks, many nutrition experts now superimpose the new goal of people achieving an enhanced or optimal state of health and of optimizing bodily functioning and performance. This includes brain health, stomach health, sports performance, and longevity. To achieve this enhanced state of health in turn requires the maximization or optimization of the consumption of functional nutrients. Within this ideology of functional nutritionism, simply eating a diverse and balanced whole foods diet appears inadequate to the task of obtaining these nutrients in the right quantities, thereby creating a demand for superfoods, nutritionally engineered foods, and dietary supplements.

This more precise and targeted approach to nutrients and the body has been enabled by nutrition and medical scientists' deeper understanding of internal biochemical processes and their identification of a new range of disease biomarkers and other quantifiable measures of bodily functioning and disease risk.[18] Hormones such as insulin, leptin, and glucagon have become the new target biomarkers to be measured, monitored, and directly manipulated. The former obsession with blood cholesterol levels remains and has intensified with the ability to measure not only levels and ratios of triglycerides and low- and high-density lipoproteins but also the size and density of the particles. C-reactive protein has been identified as a marker of inflammation.[19] For diabetes management, insulin, blood sugar, and hemoglobin A1c levels have become important biomarkers to measure and control. The GI is a type of biomarker of blood sugar levels, but it is used to measure individual foods rather than individual bodies. Health professionals also use the body mass index (BMI)—a simple external measure of body size and weight—as a biomarker of risk for a range of diseases. As discussed in chapter 2, these biomarkers are themselves often interpreted in a reductive manner.

The functional era has seen a proliferation of dietary risk factors and biomarkers of disease and health, with risk factors further extended to the cellular, molecular, and genetic levels. The science of nutrigenomics, for example, promises to extend our understanding of risk factors to the genetic level, such as by identifying "at-risk" genes that predispose us to poor nutritional health.[20] This expansion of at-risk biomarkers, and of people's susceptibilities to diseases, may transform yet more healthy people into patients requiring monitoring, testing, and proactive treatment.[21]

Functional nutritionism is characterized by not only a more extensive understanding of the relationship between nutrients and biochemical processes but also the attempt by scientists and food technologists to more directly target, control, and manipulate these internal bodily processes, functions, and biomarkers. This more direct intervention within the body can to some extent be achieved by dietary changes in whole food consumption. However, this interventionist logic increasingly demands the use of nutritionally engineered foods, dietary supplements, and pharmaceuticals that claim to directly target biochemical processes and biomarkers, as well as other direct medical interventions such as surgery.

The medical advice to aggressively lower blood cholesterol levels, for example, is difficult to achieve by simply eating or avoiding particular types of whole foods. For this reason, many nutrition experts promote plant sterol–enhanced foods, such as cholesterol-lowering margarines, as suitable means for lowering blood cholesterol levels. However, the drive to lower blood cholesterol levels has mostly been met through the prescription of statin drugs first developed in the 1990s. These drugs have become the largest class of pharmaceuticals in the world, with global sales now exceeding $25 billion.[22] A broad range of pharmaceuticals is now also available for suppressing hunger or for managing blood sugar and A1c levels in people with diabetes. For obesity management, bariatric surgery that reduces the size of the stomach is offered to patients as a means of reducing their BMI.

THE FUNCTIONAL BODY

Functional nutritionism has brought to the fore a new way of representing and experiencing the body, the functional body.[23] The notion of the functional body describes a heightened appreciation by individuals of the internal workings and functioning of the body and their relation to specific nutrients and foods. The nutritional focus of both scientists and the lay public increasingly penetrates the body, making "the invisible visible"[24] and further opening up the body's internal functioning to direct research, monitoring, regulation, and intervention.

Nutricentric persons directly experience this functional body, in the sense that they identify with and internalize a functional approach to nutrients, foods, and bodily functions. As consumers, we would not respond so favorably to the marketing of functional foods—the foods that are supposed to target and benefit specific bodily functions and health outcomes—if we did not already inhabit functional bodies. The marketing and consumer acceptance of functional foods presuppose a corresponding view and experience of our own bodies in these functional terms. This functional body is also represented more specifically as a nutritionally enhanced body, in the sense that these functional foods and nutrients are claimed to enhance and optimize particular bodily functions.

This opening up of the functional body to the nutritional and medical gaze has been a defining feature of the discourses and practices of nutrition science and medicine for more than two centuries. However, nutrition education campaigns and commercial marketing strategies in recent years have had an even greater focus on, and made more explicit references to, our internal bodily processes.[25] Rosalind Coward has referred to the way the alternative health and whole foods movements in the 1980s had also begun to open up "a whole inner geography of the body":

> Instead of the previous simple notion of food in our bellies, we now have a whole complex and detailed vision of the food broken down by various organs into chemicals and enzymes. . . . In this scenario, the interior of the body—its chemical interactions, its nutritional needs and the operations of ingestion, digestion and expulsion—can be known in highly individual ways. A new conception of the body and the person has opened up, an interior world of highly charged biochemical interactions.[26]

Sociologist Deborah Lupton has also highlighted how this new way of engaging with the body had been popularized in the late twentieth century: "The technicolour image of the 'diseased' artery 'clogged' with layers of cholesterol has moved from medical textbooks to posters in chemist shops and pamphlets on coronary heart disease."[27] While the science and discourse of "artery-clogging fats" has been in circulation since the 1960s, this scientific understanding and way of representing the body has increasingly become a lived, embodied reality. Popular Australian diet doctor John Tickell articulated the functional experience of his own body when he explained in a magazine interview why he could not bring himself to eat more than a mouthful of rich chocolate cake at his own birthday party: "I imagined it clogging up my arteries."[28]

Current nutritional concepts and marketing campaigns similarly appeal to and promote this functional body. Some advertisements for cholesterol-lowering margarines, for instance, provide explicit descriptions of how plant sterols enter the intestines and block cholesterol being absorbed into the blood. In the promotion of probiotic yogurts, consumers are encouraged to imagine the "good" and "bad" microorganisms competing for dominance in their stomachs so that this image may come to mind when people purchase or eat these foods. The concept of the glycemic index similarly invites the lay public to imagine the speed at which sugars are released into the bloodstream and the effects this has on hunger and energy levels.

In some recent weight-loss diet books, such as Byron Richards's *Mastering Leptin* and Natasha Turner's *The Hormone Diet*, the popular focus on internal bodily processes and the new fascination with hormones and hormonal regulation play a major role.[29] In *The Perfect 10 Diet*, diet doctor Michael Aziz cleverly exploits this growing familiarity with hormones by explaining the role of the ten key hormones that he claims mediate weight management, including insulin, glucagon, and leptin: "It's not your fault! Nobody has taught you how to balance your hormones. And other diets do not work because they wreak havoc on your hormones. The Perfect 10 Diet is the breakthrough diet that does not rely on trying to trick your body. This is real-world weight loss that balances your body's natural hormones to do the work for you."[30]

The functional/nutritionally enhanced body of the functional era coexists with and incorporates the overnourished/at-risk body and the nutrient-deficient/quantified body of earlier eras. With the development of new tools for measuring and monitoring internal biomarkers, the functional body is an intensely quantified body. The functional body also remains a body "at risk"—in fact, the dietary risks have multiplied and extended, as have the biomarkers of disease risk. A whole new world of nutritional and health anxieties has been opened up focusing on the inadequate intake of functional nutrients. Are we getting enough omega-3 fats and vitamin D? How are our blood glucose, insulin, and cholesterol markers holding up?

These internal bodily functions and biomarkers become more amenable to—and targets of—direct nutritional and therapeutic intervention by nutrition and medical experts. Many food and pharmaceutical companies have rushed in to colonize, commodify, and control the body's inner geography, offering products that claim to target and directly manipulate blood sugar levels, blood cholesterol, insulin, and satiety. These products include cholesterol-lowering margarine, low-GI breakfast cereals, and high-protein appetite-quenching shakes.

Could it be that the problem with the Western diet is a gross deficiency in this essential nutrient?
—MICHAEL POLLAN, *IN DEFENSE OF FOOD*, 2008

The most celebrated macronutrients of the functional era are the omega-3 polyunsaturated fatty acids. Omega-3 and omega-6 are the two major categories of polyunsaturated fats. They are also "essential fatty acids" because the body requires them but does not produce them, so they must be consumed in the diet.[31] Omega-3 fats are also divided into three main subcategories—ALA (alpha-linolenic acid), EPA (eicosapentaenoic acid), and DHA (docosahexaenoic acid). ALA is abundant in the leaves of plants and is converted in the body of humans and animals into smaller quantities of EPA. DHA and EPA are most readily found in fish and grass-fed animals, and a number of studies have identified these two omega-3 fats as the most beneficial.[32]

It was not until the late 1970s and early 1980s that nutrition scientists began to study and acknowledge the potentially beneficial functions of the omega-3 fats. Danish physicians Jørn Dyerberg and Hans Olaf Bang—who studied the fat intake of Americans, Danes, and Greenland Inuits—attributed Inuits' extremely low mortality from coronary heart disease to their omega-3-rich diet of whale blubber, seal fat, and fish.[33] Many studies have since reported that omega-3 fats may be beneficial for brain and visual development and functioning and for combating inflammatory reactions, coronary heart disease, arthritis, certain kinds of cancers, diabetes, obesity, and diseases of the brain such as dementia and obesity.[34] Omega-3 fats may deliver these various health benefits via a number of metabolic pathways, such as their beneficial effects on blood cholesterol levels, inflammation, and insulin sensitivity.[35]

Many of these studies have found an association only between omega-3 consumption and improved health outcomes, and some studies failed to show any measurable benefits.[36] A 2006 systematic review of eighty-nine trials, for example, concluded that omega-3 fats "do not have a clear effect on total mortality, combined cardiovascular events, or cancer."[37] By contrast, a 2009 epidemiological study examining the association between a number of dietary and lifestyle risk factors, led by researchers from the Harvard School of Public Health, boldly concluded that between 72,000 and 96,000 American deaths per year could be attributed to omega-3 deficiency.[38] Regardless of the credibility of such figures, the reporting of these and countless other studies pointing to the benefits of omega-3 intake continues to build the hype around this macronutrient. Strengthening these trends, in 2003 the U.S. Food and Drug Administration (FDA) approved a qualified health claim on food labels stating that "supportive but not conclusive research shows that consumption of EPA and DHA omega-3 fatty acids may reduce the risk of coronary heart disease."[39] In 2012 the European Food Safety Authority approved a new food labeling health claim stating that DHA omega-3 fats "contribute to the optimal brain development of infants and young children."[40]

Many nutrition experts endorse the view that contemporary foods and "Western" diets are generally deficient in omega-3 fats due to changes in food production methods and consumption patterns. Industrially produced meat and eggs contain lower levels of omega-3 fats than their free-range or pastured counterparts, and refined vegetable oils are generally low in omega-3 fats but very high in omega-6 fats. Some food processing techniques, such as the hydrogenation process applied to vegetable oils, also remove omega-3 from foods, which has the commercial benefit of improving the stability and shelf life of oils and foods.[41]

Based largely on laboratory and animal experiments, many scientists argue that omega-3 and omega-6 fats compete for certain enzymes in the body and that a high intake of omega-6 fats may reduce the body's ability to transform the available omega-3 fats into a more beneficial form that is anti-inflammatory.[42] If that is the case, then omega-3 dietary recommendations may be meaningful only in relation to an individual's existing as well as past omega-6 intake. It has been estimated that lowering omega-6 intake may significantly decrease an individual's requirements for omega-3 fats and that this is therefore an alternative strategy to increasing omega-3 intake.[43] Many experts recommend a significant reduction from the present omega-6/omega-3 ratio of about 20-to-1 down to a ratio 5-to-1 or even 1-to-1, although there is much disagreement and debate on the level and the significance of this ratio.[44] Some experts also believe that a high intake of omega-6 fat is pro-inflammatory and therefore potentially harmful.[45]

National dietary guidelines, public health institutions, and nutrition experts almost universally promote an increase in omega-3 consumption, especially in the form of DHA-rich fish and fish oil supplements. The 2010 *Dietary Guidelines for Americans*, for example, recommends regular fish intake largely on the basis of its omega-3 fat content.[46] However, the more nuanced message to simultaneously decrease omega-6 consumption is less widely endorsed.[47] The recommendations by many omega-3 experts to reduce the ratio of omega-6 to omega-3 are somewhat in tension with mainstream dietary guidelines that since the 1960s have promoted the increased consumption of grains and oils that are typically high in omega-6 fats. The American Heart Association remains a vigorous promoter of vegetable oils high in polyunsaturated fats. It recommends an increase in omega-3 consumption but not a reduction in omega-6 consumption, and it denies that the currently high omega-6:omega-3 ratio poses any health risks with respect to cardiovascular disease.[48] Leading nutritional epidemiologists Dariush Mozaffarian and Walter Willett also claim there is inadequate scientific evidence of the harmful effects of high omega-6 fat intake, with Willett continuing to promote the benefits of omega-6-rich vegetable oils.[49]

The new scientific insights into the biological functions of omega-3 and omega-6 fats in the body have certainly broadened our understanding of foods and food constituents and provide a more complex picture of how various types of fats interact in the body. This research has also illuminated some of the ways modern agricultural and breeding practices and food processing techniques have altered the nutritional composition of foods, and it seems to provide further support for diets based on minimally processed and traditionally farmed foods. It also brings into question the health consequences of the decades-long promotion of polyunsaturated fats in the form of omega-6-rich vegetable oils. However, some proponents of omega-3 fats avoid any blanket criticism of refined vegetable oils by promoting omega-3-rich oils such as canola.[50] Similarly, omega-3 depletion in the products of factory-farmed meat and eggs can also be partially addressed through the addition of omega-3 fats to the feed of confined animals, rather than by having farmers revert to free-range, pasture-fed, and less cruel animal-rearing practices.

The high omega-3 fat requirements claimed by some nutrition experts and the deficiency of most foods in the DHA forms of omega-3s found in oily fish have created a strong demand and perceived need for omega-3-fortified foods and nutritional supplements. While increased fish intake is strongly encouraged, the *Dietary Guidelines* recommendation of two servings per week is considered difficult to achieve due to cost, availability, and taste constraints, and therefore many experts promote fortified foods and supplements as suitable alternative sources of EPA and DHA omega-3 fats.[51] This demand for omega-3 fats and fish oils has thereby been commodified and transformed into a range of convenient and accessible products. A number of foods are now fortified with omega-3 or fish oils, such as orange juice and yogurt, with these fish oils usually enclosed in microcapsules that mask the fishy taste and reduce the oxidation of the fats. Plant crops are also being genetically engineered for enhanced omega-3 content, including a canola plant containing DHA forms of omega-3 fats.[52]

Despite changes in the availability of omega-3 fats in industrially grown and processed foods, the claims of many experts of the prevalence of omega-3 deficiencies in the population seem exaggerated. The minimum requirements for these essential fatty acids—and even the quantities required for so-called optimal health—may turn out to be relatively low and to therefore be easily obtainable from a range of readily available whole foods. The widespread promotion of fish and fish oil as a necessary component of a healthy or an optimal diet—primarily due to their high DHA omega-3 content—is also questionable given the good health of many populations around the world who eat little seafood, including vegetarians and land-locked communities.[53]

At the same time, nutrition experts rarely acknowledge, let alone publicize, the potential hazards of omega-3 fat consumption. Like all polyunsaturated fats, omega-3 fats are susceptible to oxidation—particularly when extracted, refined, processed into fish oil and omega-3 supplements, or subject to high-temperature heating or deep-frying. Omega-3 fats that have become oxidized may well promote, rather than prevent, inflammation in the body, which is now believed to play an important role in cardiovascular disease.[54] High intake of omega-3 fats in supplements has also been associated with excessive bleeding.[55] Once again, this suggests that the quality of the food in which this nutrient is contained may be the best guide to its relative beneficial or detrimental effects. Whole food sources—such as fresh whole fish, unrefined plant foods, and pasture-fed animals—provide omega-3 fats in what may be the safest and most beneficial form. On the other hand, refined-extracted and deep-fried food sources of omega-3—such as the omega-3 fats naturally occurring in refined vegetable oils that have been repeatedly heated for frying—are prone to oxidative damage. The fish oils and omega-3 supplements added to many processed foods are also more susceptible to oxidation.[56]

SUPERFOODS, FUNCTIONAL FOODS, AND NUTRITIONAL SUPPLEMENTS

Despite the continued focus of nutrition experts on single nutrients in scientific research and dietary guidelines, many experts have increasingly emphasized the importance of the interactions between nutrients within foods, food combinations, and dietary patterns. A still small but rapidly growing number of studies have evaluated the health benefits of single foods or food groups in their own right, independent of their specific nutrient profile.[57] Nevertheless, the understanding and promotion of foods continue to be framed by the nutritionism paradigm, and within the terms of functional nutritionism in particular. Foods are increasingly being understood, described, engineered, and marketed in these functional terms.

Determining the precise health effects of single foods or food groups is no less difficult and complex a scientific exercise than it is for single nutrients. Observational studies may use highly inaccurate consumer questionnaires to determine the relative health status of individuals within populations who eat a certain number of servings of a food per week, such as meat or whole grains. The dietary component of the Nurses' Health Study that was established in 1980 is an example of a very large, long-term study of this kind. Given the complexity of dietary and other confounding health-related behaviors, the best that such studies can offer are associations between foods and health outcomes. Yet the researchers on these studies continue to publish papers claiming causal relations between them.[58] Alternatively, more controlled experiments may involve placing groups of people on diets that include or exclude particular foods or food groups and monitoring their biomarkers and health outcomes. Because of the difficulties and high financial costs of conducting such trials, these studies usually have a relatively small number of participants and are of short duration, therefore limiting the conclusions that can be drawn from them.

One of the difficulties of drawing conclusions about single foods from any of these types of studies is that a food may be strongly correlated with other foods and broader dietary patterns. For example, a recent study in Finland found that people with the highest fish consumption—a food often associated with beneficial health effects—also had the highest consumption of vegetables, fruit, berries, potatoes, and wine.[59] Similarly, a paper published in 2012 based on a statistical analysis of the Nurses' Health Study and the Health Professionals Follow-up Study showed that among study participants, as red meat consumption increased, so too did smoking rates, BMI, diabetes rates, and alcohol and overall calorie intake, while physical activity and fruit and vegetable consumption progressively declined.[60] Despite all of these correlations between meat intake and this host of unhealthy dietary and lifestyle behaviors, the authors of this report still claimed that most of the excess deaths in the high meat-consumption groups could be attributed to the meat.

The use of biomarkers as measures of disease risk and health status means that these food-based studies are also dependent upon, and subject to, the limitations of the often reductive understanding of the role of these biomarkers. Studies of egg consumption, for example, may be designed to measure their effects on LDL levels, and from this their assumed impact on heart disease risk is calculated, rather than through directly measuring the association between egg consumption and heart disease incidence. Despite these complexities, these direct and indirect associations between foods and health outcomes have in some instances been interpreted by nutrition experts as cause-and-effect relationships or have been used to exaggerate the health benefits or dangers of these single foods. Such reductive interpretations of the role of single foods in bodily health can be described as a form of *food-level* reductionism or single-food reductionism.

Nutrition experts have for many years promoted fruit and vegetable consumption as protective against cancer and other chronic diseases, in part due to their antioxidant content. The beneficial effects of fruit and vegetable consumption on cancer risk have been the basis for the "5-a-Day"-style fruit-and-vegetable campaigns promoted in the United States, the United Kingdom, Germany, and many other countries. "It would seem that one of the few, if not only, non-controversial issues in nutrition," noted one nutrition scientist in 2008, "is that fruit and vegetables are good for health, and generally the more, the better (with the possible exception of fruit juice and potatoes)."[61] However, evidence for such claims is far from conclusive, at least in the case of cancer risk. The results of the very large European Prospective Investigation into Cancer and Nutrition study involving nearly half a million subjects were published in 2010, and the authors reported that they were able to detect only a "very small" decrease in cancer risk among those subjects consuming higher levels of fruits and vegetables.[62] Other researchers nevertheless claim that there is stronger evidence for the role of fruits and vegetables in reducing cardiovascular disease risk.[63]

Nutritional epidemiologist David Jacobs has argued that a number of observational studies of whole grain intake show a consistent association with good health outcomes and reduced risk of various diseases. Yet he acknowledges that high whole grain intake is also correlated with many other beneficial dietary components and lifestyle factors. For example, individuals who eat more whole grain foods tend to lead healthier lifestyles and choose healthier foods in general, including a high intake of fruit, vegetables, and fish and a minimal intake of highly processed foods.[64] Jacobs, writing with nutritional epidemiologist Nicola McKeown, therefore concedes that "it is impossible to declare unequivocally that the observed benefits of whole grains are due to the whole grains per se, and not due to 'the company they keep'."[65] A recent review of studies on the relationship between refined grains and health outcomes in fact concluded that consumption of up to 50 percent of all grain food in the form of refined grains is not associated with any increase in disease risk. However, less than 15 percent of total grain consumption in the United States is in the form of whole grain at present.[66]

Another way single foods are being evaluated is in terms of their "nutrient density"—a multinutrient rather than single-nutrient approach that nevertheless focuses on the relative quantities of good and bad nutrients. Within the terms of this nutricentric focus on nutrient density, whole foods—such as fruits, vegetables, nuts, whole grains, soy, and fish—are now celebrated for being "naturally nutrient rich." Eggs, for example, have been largely exonerated following the waning of the cholesterol scare and are now celebrated for their good-quality protein and (if from free-range hens) for their omega-3 content. On the other hand, many experts seem reluctant to categorize red meat as a nutrient-dense food rich in protein, iron, and zinc, because of its saturated fat content (as well as lingering concerns regarding its connection with colorectal and other forms of cancer). Yet much of the saturated fat in the American diet comes in the form of mixed grain dishes, dairy products, and processed meats, rather than from consumption of whole red meat.[67]

Functional nutritionism's goal of optimizing diets in order to enhance bodily functioning, and to control risky biomarkers, encourages the consumption of larger doses, or precise ratios and combinations, of functional nutrients. It implicitly—if not explicitly—promotes the idea that it is not enough to just eat a broadly balanced diet of whole foods in order to achieve an adequate intake of nutrients. Instead, the imperative is to seek out "nutrient-dense" foods to attain the functional nutrients required for optimal health. This has translated into a growing fetishism for "superfoods," which can be defined as ordinary whole foods with especially high concentrations of functionally beneficial nutrients, as well as the demand for nutritionally engineered processed foods and dietary supplements.

Many popular books are devoted to the superfoods theme, such as David Wolf's *Superfoods: The Food and Medicine of the Future*, Tonia Reinhard's *Superfoods: The Healthiest Food on the Planet*, and Steven Pratt and Kathy Matthews's *SuperFoods Rx: Fourteen Foods That Will Change Your Life*.[68] Top-ten lists of superfoods in books and popular weekend magazine articles commonly include broccoli, blueberries, oats, spinach, walnuts, and oily fish species such as sardines that are high in omega-3 fats. While playing down the notion of superfoods, physician and talk show host Mehmet Oz conveys much the same idea when he writes: "There is probably not some elusive superfood out in a distant rain forest waiting to be discovered. That said, we do know of some extraordinary foods that are already available in abundance."[69] The "extraordinary foods" he refers to include berries for their antioxidant and anti-inflammatory properties and broccoli for its high fiber and sulfur compounds.

While more sober nutrition experts shy away from the sensational term *superfoods*, the idea that some foods are especially health enhancing is indirectly supported by the FDA's granting of official "health claim" or "qualified health claim" status to some whole foods, including approved claims for fruit, vegetables, grains, and soy. For example, any grain products, fruits, and vegetables that contain fiber are permitted to use the claim that "diets low in fat and high in fiber-containing grain products, fruits, and vegetables may reduce the risk of some cancers."[70]

While dietary guidelines and most nutrition experts primarily promote the consumption of whole foods as the best means for a nutritionally optimal diet and optimal health, the logic of functional nutritionism places a question mark over the ability of many people to obtain the optimal level of functional nutrients from unmodified whole foods alone. Concerns over the nutritional quality of whole foods due to industrial farming and breeding practices have been a feature of the debate over the need for vitamins and dietary supplements since the early twentieth century. These same concerns have been heightened by the scientific debate in recent years over the relative nutrient concentrations of organic and conventional (i.e., chemical-industrial) produce, or between free-range (i.e., pastured) and intensively reared animals.[71] Such debates contribute to people's anxieties over the nutritional adequacy of the food supply.

The new emphasis within the functional nutritionism paradigm on an increased or optimized intake of functional nutrients accentuates this perception of nutrient scarcity, even among individuals and socioeconomic groups that otherwise have access to an abundance of diverse foods. In this context, nutritionally modified or nutritionally enhanced whole foods or processed foods, as well as dietary supplements, are able to be marketed to consumers as alternative and necessary sources of these supposedly scarce nutrients.

Nutritionally engineered foods may take the form of relatively unprocessed whole foods that have simply had a few nutrients added to them, such as plant sterol–enriched milk, or orange juice with omega-3 fats. But they also take the form of highly processed foods with added nutrients or carefully chosen ingredients, such as margarine, breakfast cereals, and snack bars. Food crops have also been genetically engineered to have higher levels of particular nutrients, such as omega-3-enhanced canola seeds. All these nutritionally engineered foods fall broadly under the banner of so-called functional foods. Many nutrition experts and institutions, such as the Academy of Nutrition and Dietetics (formerly the American Dietetic Association)—the body representing America's registered dieticians—endorse the functional foods concept and the consumption of at least some of these nutritionally engineered foods.[72] These functional food products and their associated health claims are examined in more detail in chapter 8.

This functional nutritional paradigm has also fueled the continued rise in consumer demand for dietary supplements. Surveys suggest that more than half of the U.S. population regularly uses some type of dietary supplements, with multivitamin and mineral supplements being among the most common forms.[73] As medical anthropologists Mark Nichter and Jennifer Thompson observe, "Supplement use appears to have become a common means by which Americans engage in wellness, protect themselves from illness, and treat disease."[74] The multinutrient supplement is still typically taken as a form of "nutrition insurance" to protect against the threat of nutrient deficiencies. However, the goals of supplementation in the functional era have increasingly been oriented toward enhancing health, reducing chronic disease risks, and undoing the damage of an unhealthy diet or lifestyle. Supplements are also part of a personal strategy through which individuals proactively take greater control of their health, in the face of a proliferation of risks, hazards, and health threats.

Mainstream nutrition organizations, such as the Academy of Nutrition and Dietetics, continue to argue that the "wise selection of nutrient-rich foods is generally the best strategy for meeting nutrient needs."[75] They also highlight the "dietary gaps" that exist in many people's diets, indicating that "additional nutrients from supplements can help some people meet their nutrition needs as specified by science-based nutrition standards."[76] Taking a multivitamin or multinutrient supplement has become more or less standard nutritional and medical advice.[77] For example, in *Eat, Drink, and Be Healthy*, Walter Willett of the Harvard School of Public Health adopts the standard view of multivitamin supplements as a nutritional insurance policy: "A multivitamin can't in any way replace healthy eating. It gives you barely a scintilla of the vast array of healthful nutrients found in food. It doesn't deliver any fiber. Or taste. Or enjoyment. The only thing it can do is offer a nutritional backup or fill in the nutrient holes that can plague even the most conscientious eaters."[78] Willett admits that there is far from scientific consensus or strong evidence for the health benefits of vitamin supplements or their optimal intake levels. But he figures that the likely harm is minimal as long as doses are "reasonable." Other mainstream and alternative health experts recommend much higher doses of specific nutrients and promise more substantial health benefits, such as actively reducing the risk of chronic diseases or enhancing physical and mental functions.

Despite this general endorsement of dietary supplement use, large trials of single-nutrient and multinutrient supplements continue to disappoint, with many showing no significant benefits. For example, a 2007 study found that calcium derived from food seemed to be more effective than calcium supplements for increasing bone density.[79] In some cases, supplement use has been found to correlate with detrimental health outcomes, rather than beneficial effects, such as in trials of beta-carotene and vitamin E.[80] Other health risks are also associated with dietary supplementation, such as the dangers from poor-quality preparations and of the excessive intake of specific nutrients.[81] On the other hand, taking dietary supplements may at least be a more transparent means of consuming added nutrients and food components, and of monitoring one's intake, than receiving them in randomly fortified foods.[82]

THE SEARCH FOR THE OPTIMAL DIETARY PATTERN

Over the past decade, there has been growing interest among nutrition scientists and epidemiologists in the study of dietary patterns that are defined in terms of the combination of foods and food groups that make up those diets. This is in part motivated by a belated recognition by many nutrition experts of the limits of trying to understand dietary health in terms of single nutrients or even single foods. While this new emphasis on food combinations and dietary patterns is a welcome relief from both single-nutrient and single-food reductionism, a number of elements of the dominant nutritional paradigm are reproduced in the studies and advice related to dietary patterns. This includes the continued vilification or celebration of particular nutrients and foods and the blurring of important distinctions among types of foods.

As late as 2002, dietary pattern analysis could still be described by Frank Hu of the Harvard School of Public Health as "a new direction in nutritional epidemiology."[83] Hu identified some of the limitations of the traditional focus on a single or a few nutrients or foods:

> People do not eat isolated nutrients. Instead they eat meals consisting of a variety of foods with complex combinations of nutrients that are likely to be interactive or synergistic. . . . An examination of dietary patterns would parallel more closely the real world in which nutrients and foods are consumed in combination, and their joint effects may best be investigated by considering the entire eating pattern.[84]

Dietary pattern analysis may thereby overcome other limitations of nutrient-level approaches, such as that many nutrients may be closely correlated with each other, making it difficult to examine their separate effects.[85] Hu also argued that studying dietary patterns could be used as a kind of last resort when nutrient-level approaches had failed, such that "the dietary pattern approach may be more useful when traditional nutrient analyses have identified few dietary associations for the disease (e.g., breast cancer)."[86]

Some of the dietary patterns that have been formally studied have been consumed by geographically or culturally specific populations, such as the Cretan diet or the Japanese Okinawa diet, and tend to be characterized as being especially healthful. However, a new approach pioneered over the past decade has identified specific dietary patterns within contemporary societies using sophisticated statistical modeling techniques.[87] Few people may actually be following these specific dietary patterns. Instead, people who tend to eat particular combinations of foods, and who therefore approximate these dietary patterns, will effectively be counted as representing this pattern. In this sense, these dietary patterns may be more of a statistical construct of researchers rather than a cultural reality.

The three dietary patterns most extensively studied have been the Mediterranean diet, the Dietary Approaches to Stop Hypertension (DASH) diet, and the so-called prudent diet.[88] These diets tend to closely resemble mainstream dietary guidelines in that they are defined as high in plant-based foods and low in red meat.[89] Importantly, they are largely based on whole foods and limit the consumption of highly refined and processed foods and beverages. In these respects, they are defined in contrast to the so-called Western diet, or the standard American diet, which is defined as being high in red meat and highly refined and processed foods.

The Mediterranean diet is the most celebrated of these dietary patterns, no doubt partly due to its gastronomic appeal. Nutrition scientist

Ancel Keys first celebrated the claimed benefits of the Mediterranean diet in the early 1960s when he coined this term to refer to the diet of poor Cretan peasants immediately following World War II. Despite the broad range of foods and dietary patterns in the countries of the Mediterranean, and even within Greece, proponents of this dietary concept have primarily defined it in terms of a "high intake of vegetables, fruits and nuts, legumes, fish and seafood, and cereals; low intake of meat and meat products, and dairy products; a high ratio of monounsaturated to saturated lipids; and moderate intake of ethanol (alcohol)."[90] Various Mediterranean scoring systems have been developed to measure the adherence to a Mediterranean-style dietary pattern in countries otherwise following diverse dietary patterns.[91] Numerous studies of populations within and outside of Mediterranean countries following this dietary pattern claim to have demonstrated its many health benefits, such as for reducing overall mortality and the risk of cardiovascular disease, cancer, and diabetes.[92]

Another celebrated dietary pattern is the so-called prudent diet first identified by researchers in 1998, which is defined in direct opposition to the stigmatized Western dietary pattern.[93] The prudent diet is, as one researcher has defined it, "characterized by higher intakes of fruits, vegetables, legumes, fish, poultry, and whole grains, while the Western pattern by higher intakes of red and processed meats, sweets and desserts, French fries, and refined grains."[94] The Dietary Approaches to Stop Hypertension (DASH) diet is somewhat similar, designed to reduce blood pressure and the risk of cardiovascular disease.[95] The DASH diet is low in fat, saturated fat, and salt; emphasizes fruits, vegetables, whole grains, fish, poultry, and low-fat dairy products; and restricts the consumption of red meat, sweets, and sugar. True to its name, several studies have shown the DASH diet to be effective in lowering blood pressure, as well as in improving blood cholesterol profiles.[96]

While these three dietary patterns are no doubt healthful, it is not exactly clear what is being tested or what conclusions can be drawn from these scientific studies. First, the main premise of these studies is that it is a particular combination of foods in these dietary patterns that brings about these health benefits, such as white versus red meat, or olive oil versus butter. However, every one of the recommended dietary patterns is primarily a whole foods diet made up of good-quality foods; that is, they are largely devoid of refined grains, added sugars, or highly processed foods. These diets are invariably compared against the standard American diet rather than against other good-quality, whole food dietary patterns.[97] The health benefits of these celebrated dietary patterns in comparison with standard diets could therefore be largely attributed to their whole food character and to the absence of highly processed and refined foods rather than the particular mix of whole foods they contain or their macronutrient profiles. For example, could adherence to a Mediterranean-style diet by individuals in the United States simply be a dietary marker of an overall good-quality diet, defined here in terms of the consumption of good-quality, minimally processed foods? As with most nutrient-level and food-level studies, researchers have shown little interest in examining or emphasizing the quality of the foods themselves in these dietary pattern studies, particularly in terms of the levels of processing they have undergone.

One of the ways the issue of food quality has been obscured is the tendency in many of these studies to treat red meat as being as unhealthy as the highly processed foods in the Western dietary pattern. But if both high meat consumption and processed food consumption define the standard Western diet, and this dietary pattern is also associated with poor health outcomes, then might meat simply be guilty by association—a product of the poor quality of the food company it keeps? Those who eat a good-quality diet may choose to eat less red meat and to instead consume a more diverse range of quality foods. Some studies that have independently assessed each food category in these dietary patterns have failed to find an association between meat and poor health outcomes.[98] At the same time, insufficient attention is paid to the quality of meat consumed in these studies, such as whether it is in the form of steak, fatty hamburger meat, or reconstituted sausage. When the quality of the meat has been included as a factor, it is usually the highly processed meats that are associated with poorer health outcomes.[99]

Moreover, the term *Western diet* has been used to describe dietary patterns in North America and Europe over the past century, despite the enormous changes in foods and typical dietary patterns over this period. Before World War II, the typical American diet was—in comparison with other countries at the time—relatively high in meat and dairy products but with few of the highly processed, preprepared, fast, and snack foods and beverages that have proliferated since the 1960s. Given these enormous changes, how meaningful is it to describe "typical" dietary patterns at both the beginning and the end of the twentieth century as "Western"?

While a diet high in meat and processed foods certainly describes the dominant dietary pattern in America in the 1980s, there are also countertrends in diet in the same period. One could equally describe a Western diet—a diet enjoyed by a good portion of the population in North America and Europe over the past century—as one characterized by the year-round abundance of good-quality meat, fish, and fresh fruits and vegetables. Long-distance transportation, refrigeration, and other technological innovations have made good food available to anyone with the money to afford an abundance of fresh, preserved, and out-of-season fruits and vegetables. A highly processed diet is more likely to describe the eating pattern of low-income communities in the West, rather than of the higher socioeconomic classes in these countries.

VEGETARIAN DIETS

Vegetarian diets have also attracted greater interest and expert endorsement over the past decade, particularly because they are broadly compatible with the plant-based emphasis of current dietary guidelines. From the 1960s to the 1980s, much of the nutrition literature focused on the nutritional inadequacy of vegetarian diets and the potential for nutritional deficiencies among vegetarians.[100] Since the 1990s, however, a number of studies have reported the overall good health of vegetarians living in affluent countries.[101] Vegetarian diets receive explicit acknowledgment as healthful dietary patterns in the 2010 *Dietary Guidelines for Americans*. The Academy for Nutrition and Dietetics also now concludes that "appropriately planned vegetarian diets, including total vegetarian and vegan diets, are healthful, nutritionally adequate, and may provide health benefits in the prevention and treatment of certain diseases."[102]

Compared with the general population, the benefits of a vegetarian diet reported in some studies include lower rates of obesity, coronary diseases, diabetes, and some cancers, as well as increased longevity.[103] Such evidence has largely been derived from epidemiological studies measuring associations between vegetarian and nonvegetarian dietary patterns.[104] However, the health of vegetarians has also been found in these studies to be comparable with health-conscious nonvegetarians with a similar socioeconomic background and lifestyle.[105] There is some debate and uncertainty as to whether any observed benefits of a vegetarian diet are related to the absence of meat or to the consumption of a diverse diet rich in fruits, vegetables, legumes, and whole grains. It could also be due to the tendency for vegetarians to be more mindful eaters and more health conscious compared with the general population, including eating less highly processed foods and having lower smoking rates.[106] A good-quality vegetarian diet may therefore be no more or less healthful than a good-quality nonvegetarian diet, particularly when the latter is rich in a diversity of plant-based foods.[107] There are many types of vegetarian diets—such as those that include or exclude fish, eggs, or dairy products—making generalizations about the health consequences of vegetarianism difficult.[108]

It is also possible to eat a poor-quality vegetarian diet, particularly one based on a poor combination of whole foods or an overreliance on highly processed and refined foods. People on low incomes need to exercise special care to achieve a nutritionally adequate vegetarian diet, because meat and other animal products can in some cases be a very economical source of nourishment. Nevertheless, the apparent good health of many vegetarians—at least those eating a good-quality vegetarian diet—demonstrates that there are indeed a variety of possible healthful dietary patterns and that meat is not essential for everyone. Vegetarian diets also tend to be higher in carbs and lower in fat than are nonvegetarian diets, so the apparent good health of many vegetarians runs counter to the arguments of low-carb proponents of the inherent dangers of a high-carb diet.[109]

A prominent advocate of vegetarian and vegan diets is retired nutritional epidemiologist Colin Campbell. His popular 2005 book *The China Study* presents evidence based on his and other studies for the all-around benefits of a "plant-based diet."[110] However, Campbell goes further to argue that animal-based foods in any quantity—including all types of meat and dairy foods—contribute to a host of chronic diseases and should ideally be eliminated from the diet. Campbell identifies a range of components in animal-based foods that promote these diseases, such as animal protein, cholesterol, and high calcium levels, rather than just the saturated fat vilified by most nutrition experts. But "animal protein" bears the brunt of the responsibility in Campbell's book. Even though there are many types of proteins found in animal foods (and even though the studies he cites in support of his hypothesis mostly relate to casein, a protein found in milk), Campbell is bold enough to generalize to all types of animal protein.

The China Study is only loosely based on the large epidemiological study of the same name, which is described in the book as "the most comprehensive study of nutrition ever conducted." He notes that this study "produced more than 8,000 statistically significant associations between various dietary factors and disease," but from these thousands of associations Campbell has distilled one simple and definitive dietary lesson: "People who ate the most animal-based foods got the most chronic disease. Even relatively small intakes of animal-based food were associated with adverse effects. People who ate the most plant-based foods were the healthiest and tended to avoid chronic disease."[111] Such interpretations and sweeping generalizations seem more the product of his own ideological bias against animal foods. He has no hesitation indicting dietary cholesterol and arguing that "eating foods that contain any cholesterol above 0 mg is unhealthy."[112] Campbell's arguments have been taken up by many vegetarian groups as scientific justification of the healthfulness of their dietary choices, and his work is celebrated in the anti-meat documentaries *Forks over Knives* and *Planeat.*

Interestingly, Campbell is explicitly critical of "scientific reductionism" and of attempts to explain the health effects of foods on single nutrients:

> This mistake of characterizing whole foods by the health effects of specific nutrients is what I call reductionism. For example, the health effect of a hamburger cannot be simply attributed to the effect of a few grams of saturated fat in the meat. . . . Even if you change the level of saturated fat in the meat, all of the other nutrients are still present and may still have harmful effects on health. It's the case of the whole (the hamburger) being greater than the sum of its parts (the saturated fat, the cholesterol, etc.).[113]

Campbell uses the Nurses' Health Study as an example of this form of reductionism. This study analyzed—but failed to find—any substantial reduction in breast cancer rates for nurses who followed a low-fat diet. Campbell argues that while the nurses in the study reduced their fat consumption, they did not reduce their intake of animal foods and merely switched to lower-fat animal products. For Campbell, the continued consumption of animal products explains why there was no substantial reduction in cancer rates and demonstrates that "tinkering with one nutrient at a time, while maintaining the same overall dietary pattern, does not lead to better health or to better health information."[114]

While Campbell's point about the reductive interventions of the Nurses' Health Study is valid, he is willing to engage in an equally reductive interpretation of nutrition studies to prove his point about the health dangers from consumption of animal-based food. This includes drawing definitive and questionable conclusions from food-based epidemiological studies that he claims link animal-food consumption to higher rates of chronic disease, as well as providing simplified and exaggerated interpretations of single nutrient studies of animal protein, calcium, and dietary cholesterol. In this sense, Campbell himself engages in dietary-level, food-level, and nutrient-level forms of reductionism.

The functional era has also seen a growing interest in the diets of the longest living populations in the world, such as the Okinawans in Japan, the Abkhazians in Russia, and the Hunzans in Pakistan.[115] These are explored in popular diet books such as John Robbins's *Healthy at 100*, Dan Buettner's *The Blue Zones*, and Bradley Willcox and colleagues' *The Okinawa Program*.[116] The premise of much of this literature is that some traditional dietary patterns may be more healthful than others. The aim is to search for the super dietary pattern that gives people optimal health and longevity. Many commentators on traditional diets suggest that there are some common features of these diets from which general lessons can be drawn, such as their emphasis on the consumption of fruit, vegetables, and legumes but only a little meat. Some of the foods that contribute to these superdiets are invariably categorized as superfoods or functional foods. Craig Willcox and Bradley Willcox, promoters of the Okinawan diet, identify a number of low-GI functional foods that they consider to be important factors in the health and longevity of Okinawans, such as tofu, shitake mushrooms, and seaweeds.[117] In nutricentric terms, they describe the Okinawan diet as "a low-calorie, nutrient-dense, antioxidant-rich dietary pattern low in glycemic load."[118] As with the Mediterranean diet and the prudent diet, the favored interpretation of these traditional diets tends to reflect current dietary guidelines. Yet some traditional dietary patterns also contradict current guidelines, such as the Alaskan Eskimo and American Samoan diets that are relatively high in meat.[119]

A celebration of traditional diets is found in the 1939 book *Nutrition and Physical Degeneration*, in which dentist and health researcher Weston A. Price documented the extremely good physical and dental health of many communities around the world living on their traditional, indigenous foods.[120] He found that their diets were rich in vitamins and other nutrients and included many foods high in vitamins A and D, such as organ meats and butter from grass-fed cattle. Price also observed the deterioration in health of communities around the world when exposed to what were often the cheapest and poorest-quality "Western foods," particularly white flour and sugar. But he went further to describe the "progressive decline of modern civilization" in Western countries as well, due to the overconsumption of modern foods such as white flour, sugar, polished rice, vegetable fats, and canned goods.[121]

Price's research is now celebrated and promoted by the Weston A. Price Foundation, a U.S.-based organization with a thriving international network that promotes traditional foods and forms of food preparation.[122] The foundation is very critical of refined and highly processed foods, emphasizing the importance of the traditional preparation of whole foods, such as soaking and fermenting whole grains and legumes, and the consumption of raw milk, animal organs, and tropical oils. The Weston A. Price Foundation is also critical of mainstream nutrition science and dietary guidelines that have stigmatized fat, saturated fat, and animal foods. While the foundation recognizes the diversity of healthy dietary patterns studied by Weston Price, it strongly promotes animal foods as the best source of beneficial nutrients and is rather disdainful of vegetarian and vegan diets, as well as of the plant-based focus of recent American dietary guidelines.[123] Like the low-carb movement, the foundation portrays contemporary health problems as partly due to the overconsumption of "refined carbs" (refined flour and sugar) and to a lack of good-quality meat and animal foods in the American diet—despite the fact that the per capita meat intake of Americans is among the highest in the world.[124]

Since the 1990s there has also been growing scientific interest in paleolithic or "ancestral" diets that characterized preagricultural societies. These paleo diets have now gained an enormous popular following around the world. Best-selling paleo diet books in the United States include Loren Cordain's *The Paleo Diet*, Robb Wolf's *The Paleo Solution*, and Mark Sisson's *The Primal Blueprint*.[125] These proponents of paleo diets take a much longer view of what constitutes a traditional eating pattern, and they date the decline in human health to the rise of agriculture 10,000 years ago. This approach celebrates the types of foods thought to have been eaten by our ancestors and to which they claim humans are biologically best adapted. The apparent absence of chronic diseases in paleolithic people is taken as proof of the healthfulness of their diets, rather than, say, a consequence of their shorter life spans (they were more likely to die from accident or infectious disease). Consequently, its advocates present the paleo diet as the solution to our diet-related health problems.

Paleo diets generally promote meat (particularly free-range meat), fish, fruits, vegetables, nuts, and seeds, while disparaging the "neolithic foods" of the postagricultural era, particularly grains (including whole grains), beans, refined vegetable oils, refined sugar, and any products of modern food processing and engineering.[126] Some paleo researchers claim that most hunter-gatherer societies derived more than half of their dietary energy from animal foods.[127] There are, however, differing positions among advocates of paleo diets on some food groups, such as the appropriateness of consuming milk and dairy products, given that they are a product of the domestication of animals. On the other hand, critics challenge a number of components of the paleo diet story. There is still considerable scientific uncertainty and debate as to what paleolithic people actually ate. The diversity of paleolithic diets has also been noted, as well as the possibility that humans had already adapted to a diversity of foods and patterns in paleolithic times.[128]

Rather than celebrating the way diverse postagricultural human cultures have constructed a range of healthful dietary patterns over the past 10,000 years, proponents of paleo diets appeal to the supposedly immutable character of human biology, and particularly of our genetic constitution. As leading paleo diet advocate Loren Cordain puts it in his popular diet book *The Paleo Diet*:

> The Paleo Diet is the one and only diet that ideally fits our genetic makeup. Just 333 generations ago—and for 2.5 million years before that—every human being on Earth ate this way. It is the diet to which all of us are ideally suited and the lifetime nutritional plan that will normalize your weight and improve your health. I didn't design this diet—nature did. This diet has been built into our genes.[129]

Cordain here encapsulates the kind of biological or genetic determinism that pervades the paleo literature. He suggests that "our genes were shaped by the selective pressures of our Paleolithic environment, including the foods our ancient ancestors ate." In turn, "our genes determine our nutritional needs." Since "many modern foods are at odds with our genetic constitution," we must return to eating the foods eaten by our hunter-gatherer ancestors.[130] We are, apparently, still poorly adapted to "neolithic" foods such as grains, beans, and dairy, since our bodies have not managed over the last 10,000 years to adapt to this new diet.

Such arguments are based on a classical form of genetic determinism, which views the human genome as largely static and unchanging and as a fixed set of genes that supposedly code for—and determine in a one-to-one fashion—very specific nutrient and foods requirements. This very long view of what constitutes a traditional human diet skips over and denigrates millennia of apparently healthy agricultural diets. The last 10,000 years of agricultural and food production innovations, of culinary development and food preparation techniques, and of dietary health experimentation and wisdom are dismissed as being entirely detrimental to human health.

The paleo diet is largely defined and justified in terms of the choice of foods available in the paleolithic period, rather than in terms of nutrients.

However, Boyd Eaton, pioneer researcher of ancestral diets, has estimated that the macronutrient profile of these diets was high protein (19–35 percent), high fat (22–58 percent), and low carb (20–40 percent).[131] Eaton argues that mainstream dietary recommendations have, in fact, been gradually shifting toward the ancestral nutritional profile. This convergence might be accelerated, he suggests, if the research community were to embrace the ancestral paradigm as a guide for the research and design of dietary guidelines.

Despite the limitations of this paleo paradigm, it does provide a useful standpoint from which to critically assess the consumption of refined and processed foods, and even of some whole foods, that characterize contemporary "Western" diets. In practice, following a paleo diet often involves eating good-quality foods, in terms of both agricultural practices and food processing methods. The exclusion of products containing refined grains and flours automatically excludes a large portion of the processed and packaged foods and beverages on the market. Paleo proponents question the consumption of extracted and refined vegetable oils, which have been consumed in enormous quantities only in the twentieth century. They also tend to promote free-range and organically raised animals in order to more closely approximate the nutritional profile of the meat consumed before the domestication of animals. While they frame their approach as a contrast to agricultural diets, in some respects they have more in common with traditional agricultural and peasant foods and eating patterns than with the processed food diets of the late twentieth and early twenty-first centuries.[132]

NUTRIGENOMICS AND PERSONALIZED DIETS

Alongside nutrition experts' interest in identifying functional nutrients, superfoods, and optimal dietary patterns, there has been a shift in nutrition research and dietary guidelines toward a recognition of the need for more "personalized" diets for individual bodies. The targeting of specific bodily functions and conditions that characterizes functional nutritionism has enabled a shift away from the idea of a universal, one-size-fits-all, standardized healthy diet that meets the nutritional requirements of a universal and standardized body. In the good-and-bad era, this universal and standardized approach was typified by the low-fat/high-carb diet and the *Food Guide Pyramid*. In the functional era, by contrast, there has been a greater emphasis on diets tailored to individuals and their "unique" bodily requirements and health concerns.

To advocate personalized diets does not necessarily entail the abandonment of the idea of there being *an* optimal diet but requires at least that it be tweaked and tailored to the bodies, needs, and tastes of individuals or subgroups of the population. The USDA's *MyPyramid*, introduced in 2005, demonstrated a fairly modest shift to "personalized eating plans." Whereas the old *Food Guide Pyramid* gave a simple and universal plan of types and quantities of foods to eat in a simple graphic, *MyPyramid* required you to visit the website and enter your biographical information (age, sex, weight, height) before you received your tailored—yet still standardized—dietary recommendations.[133] In 2011 the USDA replaced *MyPyramid* with *MyPlate*, which involves a similar level of personalized dietary advice.

We can now choose from a wider range of nutritional concepts, and indeed, from a range of packaged food products, to address our specific needs for heart health, diabetes, sporting performance, or weight loss. Individual bodies can be more precisely differentiated with respect to age, weight, sex, and existing diseases and for different stages of the life course, such as pregnancy, youth, and old age. More sophisticated personalization may involve measuring a person's internal biomarkers of nutritional status and disease risk to build up a picture of their "unique" biochemical profile or their "biochemical individuality."[134]

The language of "personalization" and "individualization" indicates a departure from one-size-fits-all dietary guidance and a move toward greater appreciation of individual or collective differences. A personalized diet could mean one based on a person's individual and cultural experiences and experimentations with food, or one in which a nutrition expert carefully assesses the particular body, dietary needs, and life situation of an individual. However, within the functional nutritionism paradigm, individual bodies tend to be reduced to a number of easily measurable biomarkers and nutritional indicators. Personalized nutrition thereby takes the form of a more differentiated range of otherwise standardized nutritional concepts and products. In the broader field of medical care, this type of differentiated health care has been referred to by sociologist Steven Epstein as "niche standardization," in which medical practices are standardized for particular social groups.[135]

One strand of this discourse of personalized nutrition is the new science of nutritional genomics, or nutrigenomics—the science of understanding the interactions between genes and nutrients. One of the applications of nutrigenomics is to understand how people's responses to particular nutrients, foods, and dietary patterns are influenced by their genetic profiles. For example, it could be used to explain why some people appear to do well on either a low-fat or a low-carb diet.[136] By examining the interactions between nutrients and genes, nutrigenomics may also help to unravel some of the complexities of food-body interactions that have eluded nutrition scientists to date.[137]

Proponents of nutrigenomics hold out the promise of extending our understanding of the relationship between food and nutrients to the genetic level of the body, with claims that we may soon be able to tailor diets to each individual's "unique" genetic profile. In 2003 FDA Commissioner Mark McClennan evoked such a future of genetically determined diets: "Nutrigenomics envisions a future in which personalized genetic profiling takes the guesswork out of deciding what you should eat. By adjusting nutrient composition in a person's diet according to genetic profiles, gene-based nutrition planning could one day play a significant role in preventing chronic disease."[138] These claims of a new level of precision and control, and the prospect of overcoming the imprecisions (and "guesswork") of the prenutrigenomic era, are key features of nutrigenomic discourses.

The notion that we each have our own unique genetic profile, for which a personalized diet for optimal health can be determined, suggests the ultimate in individualization. However only those genetic differences that can be easily quantified, categorized, and translated into dietary recommendations are likely to be utilized. This genetic level of health assessment and dietary advice may take the form of another set of standardized biomarkers—in this case genetic biomarkers—that are used to categorize individuals into subgroups of the population that carry a particular gene.[139] Based on this categorization, an individual might be issued with a targeted set of "niche standardized" dietary guidelines.

To the extent that the genetic reductionism that has characterized research in the biological sciences is combined with the nutritional and biomarker reductionism of nutrition science, nutrigenomics may simply take the form of genetic nutritionism.[140] As with nutrition science in general, it is not simply the study of nutrients or genes, but the paradigms within which this research and knowledge is interpreted and applied, that will shape whether or not nutrigenomics perpetuates the decontextualized, simplified, fragmented, exaggerated, and deterministic character of much nutrition science research and dietary advice. The promises of genetic and nutritional precision that define this ideology of nutrigenomics is yet another claim by scientists that they have discovered the "truth" about food and health—this time at the deeper molecular and genetic levels of our bodies.

While nutrition experts have for many years talked about the potential of nutrigenomics, concrete progress in the science has been slow, and it is likely to be many years before it develops sufficiently to be translated into scientifically credible dietary guidance. But this has not stopped a number of enterprising companies selling nutrigenomic tests directly to the public that claim to be able to offer personalized advice to optimize an individual's health.[141] The food manufacturing and supplement industries are also standing by, ready to design and market foods and pills that target and commodify these newly constructed needs. These products may take the form of nutrigenomically engineered and nutrigenomically marketed functional foods that claim to target and perform best on people who possess a particular gene or genetic profile.[142] Nutrigenomics may in these ways add to the many new possibilities that have emerged in the functional era for food companies to personalize and target their nutritional marketing strategies.

The era of functional nutritionism has, above all, created a number of new opportunities for food companies. The range of nutrients and food components and the range of health or functional benefits have multiplied, thereby supplying the industry with ever more opportunities to differentiate and market their products. The corresponding range of nutritional requirements, anxieties, and aspirations of nutricentric consumers has also proliferated, which food and supplement companies, drug companies, and the weight-loss industry are ready and willing to commodify. Nutrition experts have moved to providing ever more nuanced, qualified, targeted, precise, and personalized nutritional knowledge. But the food industry is now in such a position of power over government regulators, consumers, and the research agenda that they are poised to appropriate and exploit any new scientific research or dietary advice that can be used to inform the design and marketing of their products. Chapter 8 looks more closely at the food industry's nutritional engineering and nutritional marketing practices.

CHAPTER EIGHT

Functional Foods

Nutritional Engineering, Nutritional Marketing, and Corporate Nutritionism

Functional foods move beyond necessity to provide additional health benefits that may reduce disease risk and/or promote optimal health.
—ACADEMY OF NUTRITION AND DIETETICS,
"FUNCTIONAL FOODS," 2009

Food Technology is an industry journal that showcases the latest technologically modified and nutritionally engineered foods, offering an array of claimed health benefits and marketed with a proliferating range of nutritional buzzwords. Probiotic ice cream, heart-healthy chocolate chip muffins, satiety smoothies, calorie-burning green teas, fiber-rich snack bars, omega-3-fortified baby foods for brain and eye development, and low-glycemic-index meal replacements are part of a new generation of so-called functional food products. Other health-enhancing products include fat-free yogurts with three grams of fiber per cup; heart-healthy chocolate bars with high concentrations of flavonols to reduce blood pressure; a Women's Wonder Bar chocolate bar with soy, cranberry seed oil, and flax for "easing symptoms of premenstrual syndrome and menopause"; and candy and chews with echinacea for "boosting immunity."[1]

Alongside these premium-positioned food products are much more conventional processed foods, sweets, and beverages that have had some nutrients added to or subtracted from them. These are the standard fare of the supermarket shelves, including vitamin-enhanced breakfast cereals, low-fat reconstituted chicken nuggets, calcium-fortified orange juice, caffeinated and sugar-dense "energy" drinks, and processed/refined white sliced breads with invisible added fiber. Even confectionery and soft drinks are being nutritionally enhanced, such as Diet Coke Plus with added vitamins B_6 and B_{12}, zinc, and magnesium and Diet Pepsi Max with added ginseng and increased caffeine. Some of these products fit into the category of "lesser evil" foods—foods of poor nutritional quality that have been nutritionally improved by reducing the quantity of some of their "bad" nutrients and food components.[2]

Within the food industry and among nutrition experts, the code phrase for all of these types of foods marketed with nutrient-content and health-related claims is *functional foods*, foods they claim can target and enhance particular bodily functions and overall health. The functional foods term is, however, so poorly and broadly defined that virtually any food with added nutrients, or carrying some type of health claim, seems to qualify. Through their ability to overwhelm consumers with nutritional and health claims on food packaging and in advertisements, food corporations have become the primary disseminators of the most simplified and reductive understanding of food and nutrients in the present era of functional nutritionism.

This chapter examines food companies' various nutritional engineering strategies, and their use of nutrient-content and health claims, to create a demand for their products (summarized in appendix table A.6). I also consider how the food industry and governments have proposed or implemented other front-of-pack labeling schemes, such as nutrition scoring and traffic-light labeling systems, in order to inform or influence consumers' understanding of the nutritional quality of food products.

FROM RESTORING NUTRIENT BALANCE TO HEALTH-ENHANCING FOODS

In *Food Politics: How the Food Industry Influences Nutrition and Health*, Marion Nestle characterizes functional foods—or "techno-foods," as she refers to them—as "flatly reductionist; the value of a food is reduced to its single functional ingredient. . . . This logic is flawed in that it fails to consider the complexity of food composition and the interactions amongst food components."[3] Nestle portrays the food industry's reductive rationale for the design and marketing of these functional foods as a deliberate misuse and distortion of the otherwise sound and rigorous scientific knowledge that she claims underpins mainstream dietary guidelines.

However, while the food industry has certainly exploited nutrition science for its own commercial interests, the types of reductionism that Nestle identifies are also a key feature of the nutritionism paradigm that nutrition scientists and experts have themselves adopted and promoted over the past century. The focus on single, isolated, decontextualized nutrients has been a long-standing feature of scientific research since the mid-nineteenth century and of dietary guidelines since the 1970s. The idea that these isolated nutrients can impart their full benefits when added as a supplement to foods is also supported by the nutrient fortification programs promoted by governments and public health institutions, as well as the health claims approved for use by food regulatory agencies. The single-nutrient and multinutrient supplements that many nutrition experts endorse are similarly underpinned by these kinds of reductionist assumptions.

The food industry's nutritional engineering and marketing strategies have reflected the broader changes in nutritional paradigms over the past fifty years. As discussed in chapter 4, throughout the era of good-and-bad nutritionism, mainstream dietary guidelines were dominated by negative dietary advice regarding the dangers of consuming too much of the wrong types of foods and nutrients.[4] Nutrition experts branded highly processed foods, as well as some animal foods, as containing too many "bad" nutrients and ingredients. Food manufacturers responded to these negative nutritional messages by designing food products and marketing strategies that focused on lesser evil messages, such as those accompanying reduced-fat and reduced-calorie foods, as well as vitamin-fortified and fiber-fortified processed foods.

The aim of much of this nutritional engineering and marketing was to restore the appropriate "nutrient balance" to one's diet, either by reducing the bad nutrients and calories or by adding good nutrients considered to be lacking in modern foods and dietary patterns. In some cases food manufacturers achieved these nutritional reductions by incorporating processed-reconstituted ingredients, such as artificial sugars and fats. Consumers themselves might consume these nutritionally engineered food products in order to compensate for perceived imbalances, deficiencies, or excesses in their overall diets.[5] In the early 1990s, journalist Michelle Stacey noted the tendency for consumers to trade the perceived health benefits of one food for the consumption of less healthy fare: "A prime reason for having diet soda in existence at all is to compensate for other indulgences—it's an equation, a numerical trade-off, and perhaps a little game we play with ourselves. Thanks to Atwater we know that a one-calorie soda leaves a hole that a 500-calorie piece of pie could fill."[6] This nutritional trade-off is a game many of us still seem to play, by selectively responding to nutritional guidelines and food marketing claims.

Since the 1990s, a range of novel food products carrying more positive health messages have taken center stage. As discussed in chapter 7, a new and broader set of nutrients and food components such as omega-3 fats, plant sterols, probiotics, and antioxidants now compete for attention on food labels. Rather than just compensating for the perceived nutritional deficiencies or excesses in one's diet, such as of vitamin C or calcium, some of these nutritionally engineered foods aim to provide nutrients and other food and nonfood components that are meant to provide additional and targeted health benefits. Sports drinks such as Red Bull, for example, contain added taurine, which the company claims is "involved in neurological processes and positively influences the performance of the heart,"[7] while probiotic yogurt drinks are laden with specific "good bacteria" that target gut health. Food companies also market their foods not merely as restoring and maintaining good health but as enhancing health, optimizing bodily functioning and performance, and delivering a broad range of targeted health benefits relating to such issues as weight management, joint and bone health, immunity, digestive health, cardiovascular health, mental performance, and physical energy.

The commercial success of some of these foods marketed for their health benefits is illustrated by the popularity of probiotic yogurt drinks, such as Yakult and Dannon's DanActive. The specific live microorganisms in these foods are intended to add "good bacteria" to your stomach, much like traditional yogurts. Yakult contains the bacterial strain *Lactobacillus casei Shirota*, named after the Japanese scientist who identified this strain and invented the product. Dannon's DanActive is powered by the strategically named *Lactobacillus casei Defensis* bacteria, which Dannon claims can "help strengthen the body's natural defenses."[8] Manufacturers make a wide range of health claims about their probiotic products, from how they can alleviate indigestion and diarrhea to how they can strengthen the immune system and reduce the severity of colds and flu. However, unlike regular yogurts, these yogurt drinks are not conventional foods that you eat as a snack or as a part of a meal; instead, they are sold in small packages containing a daily medicinal dose of beneficial bacteria. Consumers have therefore been convinced to purchase these products entirely for their claimed health benefits.

Another trend in food companies' marketing practices in the functional era has been their more explicit reference to internal bodily processes in their food marketing campaigns. This form of marketing plays upon and promotes the way nutricentric individuals have developed a functional view or experience of their own bodies, in which they visualize the way these foods directly act upon particular parts of the body or bodily functions. Advertisements for cholesterol-lowering margarines, for example, provide explicit descriptions of how plant sterols enter the intestines and block the absorption of cholesterol into the blood, while probiotic yogurts are advertised with reference to "good microorganisms" in the stomach. Advertisements for Yakult explain to consumers that their product "contains billions of live and active 'good bacteria.' . . . When you drink Yakult daily, it makes it difficult for the bad bacteria to take over. Yakult also gives you more of the good bacteria that may help balance your digestive system."[9]

Defining Functional Foods

Many of these nutritionally engineered and nutritionally marketed foods are now referred to by food and nutrition experts as functional foods. The functional foods concept was first introduced in Japan in the 1980s, a country that has led the development of modified foods targeting good health. The world's first product identified as a functional food was a soft drink containing added dietary fiber, Fibre Mini, launched in Japan in 1988.[10] Yet despite the widespread use of the term, functional foods have been notoriously hard to define.

Some definitions emphasize the marketing dimension of functional foods. For example, leading Dutch nutrition scientist Martijn Katan defines functional foods simply as "a branded food that claims explicitly or implicitly to improve health and wellbeing."[11] Marion Nestle has similarly defined functional foods as "products created just so that they can be marketed using health claims."[12] These definitions are the most straightforward, and I believe the most accurate, since they identify the marketing of a food product with either a nutrient-content claim or a health claim as the essential characteristic of a functional food. For this reason, the term *functionally marketed foods*—defined as foods marketed as having specific and targeted health or functional benefits—may be a more accurate and less presumptive term for these products than *functional foods*.[13] However, the way most nutrition experts and food scientists define functional foods goes further than Katan's and Nestle's descriptions by asserting that such foods not only *claim* to deliver but actually *do* deliver precisely targeted and enhanced health benefits.

Most definitions of functional foods suggest that these products provide health benefits "beyond" the "basic nutrients" contained in conventional foods, and that they provide "targeted health benefits" that either reduce the risk of chronic diseases or deliver an enhanced state of health. The widely quoted European "Consensus Document" prepared by the International Life Sciences Institute states: "A food can be regarded as 'functional' if it is satisfactorily demonstrated to affect beneficially one or more target functions in the body, beyond adequate nutritional effects, in a way that is relevant to either an improved state of health and well-being and/or reduction of risk of disease."[14] The American Academy of Nutrition and Dietetics (AND) position paper on functional foods categorizes "all foods as functional at some physiological level because they provide nutrients or other substances that furnish energy, sustain growth, or maintain/repair vital processes. However, functional foods move *beyond necessity* to provide *additional health benefits* that may reduce disease risk and/or promote optimal health."[15] The AND begins by admitting that all foods are functional in some way yet still goes on to suggest that functional foods are a separate class of especially healthful foods! They claim that these foods go "beyond necessity" and provide more than just the nutrients necessary for energy and growth, for they supposedly also provide "additional health benefits."

In terms of "conventional" functional foods (or whole foods), most fruits, vegetables, and nuts seem to qualify. The AND identifies the beneficial properties of citrus fruits for protection against stomach cancer, tree nuts such as almonds to counter heart disease, cruciferous vegetables such as broccoli and cabbage and tomatoes (lycopene) for preventing various cancers, and fermented dairy products to deal with irritable bowel syndrome. The "modified foods" the AND identifies include calcium-fortified orange juice, folate-enriched breads, plant sterol–enriched margarines, "energy-promoting" beverages "enhanced" with ginseng and guarana, and genetically engineered oil seeds that have been "enhanced" with omega-3 or that are *trans*-fat free.

The meanings of the terms *basic nutrients* and *beyond basic nutrients* in these definitions of functional foods are particularly vague. Many so-called functional foods have been fortified with nutrients and food components that are readily available in ample quantities in other foods or in a generally well-balanced diet, such as omega-3 fats, fiber, folate, and calcium—so it is unclear how they provide more than the "basic nutrients" found in conventional foods or well-balanced diets. Moreover, the claimed benefits of any larger doses of particular nutrients in these foods seem, at the very least, to be greatly exaggerated. These nutritionally engineered foods may well partially compensate for some specific nutrient deficiencies in those individuals consuming inadequate diets. But there is, arguably, little evidence that such fortified foods in themselves provide a more optimal range of nutrients, or additional health benefits, from those you can get from good-quality, minimally processed foods.

The claim that these foods are able to target and enhance particular bodily functions gives functional foods—and the scientific knowledge on which they are based—an aura of precision. Virtually all foods have at least one nutrient that scientific evidence suggests plays some role in normal bodily functioning. However, particular bodily functions, not to mention chronic diseases, are mediated and affected by multiple food and nonfood factors. To single out one food or food component and claim it enhances particular bodily functions, or prevents the incidence of chronic diseases, invariably exaggerates both the health effects and the precision of the scientific knowledge underpinning these health claims.

Public health nutritionists have been critical of the way the functional foods concept blurs the boundary between food and medicine.[16] As with the terms *nutraceuticals* and *pharmafoods*, companies market functional foods as having medicinal or druglike qualities.[17] This medicalization of food is hardly new or confined to these newly developed functional foods. Since the nineteenth century, the nutritionism paradigm has essentially promoted a pharmaceutical model in which direct and precise effects on particular bodily functions are attributed to single, isolated nutrients and food components. In the functional era, what is novel within this already medicalized view of food is the extent to which foods are being technologically reengineered to reflect this medicalized understanding, and also that companies are permitted to advertise some of these claimed health benefits.

Despite attempts by many nutrition experts and food scientists to define and position functional foods as a distinct category of especially healthful foods, I suggest that there are no distinguishing compositional criteria or health benefits that set these foods apart from other conventional foods. It is not—as these experts would have us believe—that a new class of especially healthful foods has emerged due to advances in nutrition science and food engineering. Rather, there has been a change in the types of foods being nutritionally engineered and the ways in which they are being marketed in the functional era. What is new is that these foods are being marketed in functional terms, with the benefit of labeling regulations permitting direct health claims to be attributed to these foods.

Foods identified as functional may be conventional, whole, or minimally processed foods, such as oats or yogurt, and these are sometimes referred to as "naturally functional foods."[18] But functional foods are more commonly identified as foods that have been nutritionally engineered. Nutritionally engineered foods can be defined as foods that have had their nutrient profile deliberately modified in some way, usually through the addition or removal of particular nutrients or the ingredients in which they are contained. These engineered foods may be whole foods that have been bred or farmed in a way that modifies their nutrient profile, such as genetically engineered Golden Rice with enhanced beta-carotene levels, or omega-3-enhanced eggs produced by manipulating the feed of confined chickens. Nutritionally engineered foods may also be minimally processed foods that have been nutritionally modified during processing, such as fat-reduced milk, probiotic yogurts produced with specific cultures, or calcium-enhanced orange juice.

Some nutritionally engineered foods, however, are highly processed and reconstituted foods, produced using refined and poor-quality ingredients, a range of chemical additives, and plenty of added salt and sugar. Kellogg's Cocoa Krispies is an example of such a highly processed, high-sugar food marketed for its health benefits on the basis of a few added nutrients. In 2009, during the H1N1 influenza epidemic, Kellogg's emblazoned the claim "Now helps support your child's immunity" in very large type across the front of Cocoa Krispies packaging. This claim for targeted immunity protection was made on the basis that the vitamins A, C, and E added to the product are assumed to play a role in boosting immunity. A Kellogg's spokeswoman responded to critics of this marketing strategy by claiming that "Kellogg's developed this product in response to consumers expressing a need for more positive nutrition."[19]

Nutritionally engineered foods are often the product of an arbitrary and novel mixing of different types and quantities of nutrients not found in whole foods. Nutritional engineering may involve the addition of nutrients already present in a particular food in its unprocessed form. This includes vitamin C–enhanced orange juice or white flour fortified with the vitamins and minerals that are removed from the whole grain during the refining process. However, nutritional engineering often entails the introduction of nutrients not otherwise found in significant quantities in a particular food and not commonly associated with that food, such as the addition of plant sterols to margarine, calcium to orange juice, fiber to drinks, fish oil to bread, and vitamins to water.[20] I refer to some of these forms of nutritionally engineered products as trans-nutric foods because they involve the transfer of nutrients across recognized food categories and boundaries.

This transfer of food components from one food to another enables food manufacturers to claim that the trans-nutric product provides the health benefits of *both* foods, thereby delivering multifunctional health benefits.[21] Orange juice with added calcium, for example, carries the nutritional aura of both oranges (vitamin C) and milk (calcium), while milk enhanced with plant sterols suggests the benefits of both dairy and plant foods. Trans-nutric foods are thus based on and promote a logic of nutritional interchangeability, in which foods come to be viewed as interchangeable sources of a set of standardized and generic nutrients.[22] In crossing food group boundaries, trans-nutric foods also tend to blur the distinction between types of foods and food categories, and this can undermine dietary advice based on traditional distinctions between food groups, such as those represented in the *Food Guide Pyramid* or *MyPlate*.[23]

The nutritional engineering of a food often involves the translation of nutritionally reductive scientific knowledge into nutritionally reductive technological products. In many cases, the claimed health benefits of these foods not only rely on the accuracy of the scientific knowledge upon which these nutritional modifications are based (e.g., the claimed benefits of omega-3 fats in the case of omega-3-fortified foods). They also assume that these single nutrients will directly improve human health regardless of the particular types of foods or the food "matrix" in which they are embedded.[24] Nutritionally engineered foods will deliver to their consumers a substantial dose of an extracted or synthesized nutrient or food component. However, it is only a simplified and narrow range of valued, popularly recognized, easily attainable, and isolated nutrients that tend to be added to food products, rather than the much wider range of known and unknown food components and combinations. The ways in which the body absorbs and metabolizes these nutrients may also be compromised if they are not consumed together with the nutrients and food components with which they are otherwise combined in whole foods. Importantly, these foods rarely undergo independent testing to assess their claimed benefits or potential risks. Instead, their benefits are simply extrapolated from those attributed to the isolated nutrients.[25]

These nutritional modifications may involve replacing some minimally processed ingredients with more highly processed ones. The production of reduced-fat foods, for example, has often involved replacing vegetable oils or butter with ingredients such as sugar, refined flours, or chemically modified starches. A range of engineered fat substitutes have been developed that are designed to replace the bulk, body, and mouthfeel of fats, while also at times having a lower calorie count. Some of these caloric and noncaloric fat substitutes include maltodextrin, beta-glucan, pectin, guar gum, and xanthan gum.[26]

The nutritional engineering of foods can create nutrient-level contradictions, whereby the enhancement or removal of a particular nutrient by food manufacturers interferes with the quantities or absorption of other desirable nutrients. For instance, studies have shown that the concentrated quantities of plant sterols in cholesterol-lowering margarines block the absorption of beta-carotene and therefore lower vitamin A levels in the body.[27] Consumers of sterol-enriched foods are therefore encouraged to compensate for this nutrient-level contradiction by eating more fruits and vegetables to increase their vitamin A levels.[28] Similarly, excessive calcium intake is known to interfere with iron absorption.[29] In this sense, such nutrient-level contradictions may involve a certain nutritional trade-off between nutrients or between particular health outcomes. These types of contradictions highlight some of the limitations of attempting to directly manipulate the quantities of particular nutrients in foods and diets, particularly where our knowledge of the complexity of nutrient interactions within foods and within the body is inadequate.

One of the problems associated with the random "nutrification" of the food supply is that it is very difficult for members of the lay public to monitor the concentrated doses of nutrients they receive from eating a range of fortified foods.[30] Nutrition scientists David Jacobs and Linda Tapsell have suggested that isolating and adding nutrients and food components to foods should instead be thought of as "drugs delivered via a food."[31] Indeed, consumers of these products may be better served by consuming these added nutrients in the form of dietary supplements, because it would at least enable them to estimate the doses of supplemental nutrients they are consuming.

NUTRITIONAL TECHNO-FIXES: FROM GM FOODS TO NANOFOODS

The nutritional engineering of foods is essentially a narrowly framed technological solution—or nutritional techno-fix—to the perceived limitations of particular foods or dietary patterns. If the problem is that highly processed foods have been stripped of beneficial nutrients, then engineering them back into foods is a way of convincing consumers to continue eating these products. Similarly, if impoverished populations have inadequate access to good-quality foods and diets, then specific nutrient deficiencies can be addressed through the nutrient fortification of their staple foods, rather than by tackling the broader socioeconomic inequalities that deny people an adequate income to afford better quality diets.

Food scientists have developed sophisticated processing techniques to add and subtract nutrients and ingredients from foods while retaining the desired taste, texture, appearance, and durability of food products. A range of novel technologies are being developed and applied by food and agricultural scientists for these purposes, such as the breeding of genetically engineered crops with modified nutrient profiles, and new processing techniques for manipulating or adding nutrients and other components to foods and drink products. For example, food companies adding small quantities of fish oil to products—in order to claim the health benefits of their long-chain omega-3 fats—have had to meet the significant technological challenge of trying to overcome the "fishy" taste of these oils. So food scientists developed microscopic capsules containing the fish oil that are intended to dissolve and release the fish oil in a person's stomach rather than in the mouth.[32]

While genetically engineered crops with modified nutrient profiles have been promised for many years, none of these modified crops have yet reached the stage of commercial release. The most celebrated of these genetically modified crops has been the rice variety dubbed Golden Rice that scientists have engineered with enhanced levels of pro-vitamin A. The promoters of Golden Rice have touted it as a technological solution to vitamin A deficiency for the world's poor, since vitamin A is a major cause of blindness and of increased susceptibility to infection, particularly in children.[33] Plant breeders have also genetically modified canola seeds to produce the type of long-chain omega-3 fats (DHA) found in fish.[34] Another genetically modified functional food crop under development is a variety of wheat with enhanced levels of resistant starch. When incorporated into food products, this modified wheat may enable these products to be marketed as having a low glycemic index.[35]

The new nanotechnologies represent the next wave of technological innovation across the food system, including developments in agricultural production and breeding, and in food processing and packaging. Nanotechnology is a set of tools and techniques for directly manipulating, transforming, and mass-producing materials, living organisms, and products at the level of atoms and molecules, or at the nanometer scale (one-billionth of a meter). Food manufacturers are already using nanotechnology to develop new processing techniques and additives with novel or improved properties. These new techniques and materials may simply enable the more efficient production of cheap, palatable, and durable convenience foods. But nanotechnology is also being used to nutritionally engineer foods through the addition of nanoscale nutrients and food components. These nanonutrients may in some cases be more easily absorbed than the larger-scale equivalent nutrients and could therefore be added to foods in smaller quantities. Scientists are also developing nanoscale encapsulation techniques for the addition of nutrients and food components to foods, such as nanoencapsulated fish oil, that may provide greater stability than existing microsized capsules, enabling them to better withstand cooking, refrigeration or long-term storage.[36]

It is primarily the larger food manufacturing corporations that have the resources necessary to develop, test, seek regulatory approval for, and market these various forms of functional food technologies and products. So the trend toward functional food development is likely to accelerate the trends toward the corporate concentration and control of the food manufacturing sector.[37] The world's largest food and beverage corporation, Nestlé, launched its Nestlé Health Science venture in 2011. The new center draws on cutting-edge science to develop new products with "enhanced" health benefits. It will also be capable of generating the scientific data that governments increasingly require to substantiate new health claims.[38] One of the first products to roll out of the lab was a new version of its BOOST Drink containing twenty-six essential vitamins and minerals and ten grams of protein per bottle. Nestlé is targeting this drink at "older adults" who can, according to the company's marketing blurb, use it as "a convenient way . . . to accomplish their daily nutritional goals while maintaining their busy lifestyle."[39]

In 2012 the Quaker Oats Company, a division of PepsiCo, announced the creation of the Quaker Oats Center of Excellence, described by the company as a "cross functional entity focused on elevating the relevance and benefits of oats through science, agriculture and innovation." The center will conduct research intended to build on the already positive public image of oats based on studies and health claims for the heart-heath benefits of oats in the 1990s. In a press release the director of the center, Marianne O'Shea, states, "Oat science has already revealed important benefits such as heart health and satiety, but we've only scratched the surface when it comes to the power of the oat and all it can do."[40]

NUTRITIONAL MARKETING AND
THE NUTRITIONAL FACADE

In her annual summary of the "Top 10 Functional Food Trends" in the *Food Technology* journal, food scientist and industry consultant Elizabeth Sloan identifies the shifting trends among food manufacturers and health-conscious consumers.[41] Some of these recent trends include what she calls "Retro Health," a return to "traditional" strategies focusing on "avoidance foods," such as reduced fat, calories, and sodium in foods. Another trend—"Prime Timers"—targets the health concerns of the over-fifties age group, who might be more interested in functional foods that claim to address problems of cholesterol levels, bone health, memory, and digestion. The more active consumers are covered under the market segment she calls "Daily Dynamics": foods and beverages that "boost" energy, improve sports performance, enhance memory, or reduce stress. Of the successful new food products launched in 2006–2007, for example, Sloan reports that 30 percent carried an added-nutrient claim, such as added calcium or soy; 23 percent carried a reduced-calorie claim; and 22 percent a high-fiber/whole-grain claim.[42]

One of the aims of nutritional marketing is to create what I refer to as a *nutritional facade* around a food product—an image of the food's nutritional characteristics and benefits. This nutritional facade then becomes the focus of food marketing campaigns. The other purpose of a nutritional facade is to cover up or distract attention from the underlying ingredients and processing techniques used to manufacture a food. Nutritional marketing typically focuses on the presence or absence of one or two nutrient components of a food—such as the presence of vitamin C, calcium, and omega-3 fats, or reduced quantities of fat, cholesterol, or calories. A 2010 survey of selected supermarkets in the United States found that half of all products stocked carried a nutrient-content claim and that, of these, half were processed foods high in added salt, sugar, and fat.[43] In *Appetite for Profit*, public health attorney Michele Simon refers to the nutritional marketing of such foods as "nutri-washing," another variation of the corporate strategies of white-washing and green-washing.[44]

These nutritional marketing practices reproduce and promote both nutrient-level and single-nutrient reductionism. The reductive focus on nutrient composition conceals the quality of a food and its ingredients, as well as its overall nutrient profile. This is particularly the case with highly processed breakfast cereals targeted at children and that typically contain highly refined grains, sugars, and chemical additives yet are marketed on the basis of the extensive list of added vitamins and minerals. Kellogg's Froot Loops Marshmallow cereal, for example, has the nutrient-content claim "Good Source of Vitamin D" emblazoned at the top of the cereal box even though it contains a whopping 48 percent sugar.[45] A 2006 study of breakfast cereals marketed to children revealed that those marketed with "low-fat" claims had, on average, no less sugar, salt, or calories than other breakfast cereals.[46] The nutrient content claims on the front of the pack, as well as the nutrition information on the Nutrition Facts label, also fail to distinguish between nutrients intrinsic to a food or its ingredients, on the one hand, and those added to a food product during processing, on the other.[47]

The enormous commercial success of Vitaminwater products also suggests that cutting-edge nutrition science is not always required when appealing to the nutricentric consumer. Simply adding a few vitamins and minerals to water is enough to add an aura of health, even when that water also contains added flavorings and 32 grams of sugar per bottle. Instead of esoteric ingredients backed by rigorous scientific studies and government-endorsed health claims, the manufacturers of Vitaminwater—now owned by the Coca-Cola corporation—just sprinkle a few nutrients into the mix and use suggestive names for each variety, such as "Revive," "Energy," "Focus," and "Defense." The Vitaminwater labels also carry the nutritional claim that this product is a "nutrient enhanced water beverage." However both the suggestive names ("Defense") and the accompanying commentaries ("Help support your immune system with the zinc and vitamin C in this bottle") stray beyond nutrient claims and into the more highly regulated territory of direct health claims.[48]

HEALTH CLAIMS AND FUNCTIONALLY MARKETED FOODS

For much of the twentieth century, the U.S. Food and Drug Administration (FDA) prohibited the use of health claims on food labels advertising a link between foods, nutrients, or other food components, on the one hand, and specific diseases, bodily functions, and health conditions, on the other. In 1984 the Kellogg company began advertising its All-Bran breakfast cereal with the claim that high-fiber foods might help prevent cancer, in defiance of FDA regulations. The FDA initially attempted to stop Kellogg's marketing campaign but backed down under pressure from within its own oversight department.[49] In the following years, the FDA tolerated the proliferation of health claims on food labels while it developed new labeling guidelines. The Nutrition Labeling and Education Act that was finally introduced in 1990 allowed companies to seek approval for health claims by submitting evidence for the claims to the FDA.[50]

The first authorized health claim under the new legislation was issued in 1997—linking the beta-glucan soluble fiber from whole oats to the lowering of blood cholesterol levels—following evidence submitted by the Quaker Oats Company. Quaker had assembled scientific studies supporting its claim—including a meta-analysis of previous studies published in 1992 that it had cosponsored—reporting that bran had a modest lowering effect on blood cholesterol levels.[51] To scientifically substantiate health claims, the FDA required evidence of the specific nutrient or active ingredient in oats that was responsible for the claimed health effects. In this case, the FDA accepted Quaker's claim that the active ingredient in oats imparting its health benefits is the beta-glucan soluble fiber. Quaker was even able to quantify the precise effect, claiming that three grams of beta-glucan would reduce cholesterol by 5 percent in most people. The wording approved by the FDA for this health claim was as follows: "Soluble fiber from oatmeal, as part of a low saturated fat, low cholesterol diet, may reduce the risk of heart disease." Quaker quickly capitalized on this approved health claim by heavily advertising the health benefits of its oat products, which translated into impressive annual sales growth in the following years.[52]

The FDA currently distinguishes three types of health-related claims on food labels—health claims, qualified health claims, and structure/function claims—for which it requires different levels of scientific substantiation.[53] Health claims—or scientifically substantiated health claims—refer to a direct relationship between a food component and the risk of disease and require the highest level of scientific substantiation for regulatory approval. The current FDA-approved health claims include the link between calcium and osteoporosis; soy protein and the risk of coronary heart disease; saturated fats, *trans*-fats, and dietary cholesterol and heart disease risk; and folic acid and neural tube defects. Some whole foods or whole food extracts have also received approval for substantiated and qualified health claims, such as whole oats and oat flour, nuts, tomatoes and tomato sauce, and green tea. Qualified health claims are claims that have not yet met all of the FDA's scientific substantiation criteria required for authorized health claims.[54] Nevertheless, they are permitted to carry similar types of claimed health benefits (e.g., the link between omega-3 fats and the reduction of heart disease risk), provided they also carry the statement that "conclusive" evidence does not exist for such claims. The FDA introduced this category of qualified health claims in 2003 after a dietary supplement manufacturer legally challenged the FDA's claims approval process.[55]

Structure/function claims generally link single nutrients or foods to normal bodily functioning and growth, such as "calcium builds strong bones" and "fiber maintains bowel regularity." General Mills' Cheerios breakfast cereal, for example, carries the front-of-pack structure/function claim "Clinically Proven to Help Reduce Cholesterol," on the basis that it contains one gram of soluble fiber per serving. The fine print on the pack reveals that "3 grams of soluble fiber daily from whole grain oat foods, like Cheerios and Honey Nut Cheerios, in a diet low in saturated fat and cholesterol, may reduce the risk of heart disease."[56] Structure/function claims are relatively unregulated in the sense that they do not require preapproval by the FDA.[57] Yet these structure/function claims should be classified as fully fledged "health claims" and require the same level of scientific substantiation as disease prevention claims since they may be interpreted by consumers in much the same way.[58] A report by the U.S. General Accounting Office confirms that "consumers find it difficult to understand the differences between qualified health claims and health claims ... Consumers have similar difficulties understanding the differences among health, structure/function, and other health- and nutrient-related claims."[59]

Claims about nutrient content in food advertisements rely on consumers making their own connections between a nutrient and its perceived health benefits and are therefore limited to commonly recognizable nutrient-health associations. Direct health claims, on the other hand, open up a wider range of marketing possibilities for the food industry. Cholesterol-lowering foods such as sterol-enriched margarine may not have been introduced without the regulatory approval to make explicit cholesterol-lowering claims on the pack, since the nutrient-content claim "contains plant sterols" would be meaningless to most consumers. By highlighting the presence of an unfamiliar additive, such as plant sterols, these foods may even be looked upon suspiciously by consumers who prefer minimally processed foods. Making direct health claims may therefore be effective for reaching and influencing consumers unfamiliar with the latest nutritional trends and scientific developments.[60]

Health claims invariably exaggerate and decontextualize the health benefits of particular foods. All nutrients and whole foods probably have multiple health benefits, many of which scientists are either unaware of or are unable to substantiate. To pick out any of these claimed health effects, and to allow them to be used on food packaging and in advertisements, is flawed in at least two respects. First, it exaggerates the scientific certainty of such an association. Second, it exaggerates and decontextualizes the significance of the particular food/nutrient and its related health benefits, in relation to the plethora of other such food-health relationships.

Studies examining consumers' understanding and interpretation of health claims have identified a number of ways in which the healthfulness of functionally marketed foods may be exaggerated in the minds of consumers. A seminal study published in 1999 by food researchers Brian Roe, Alan Levy, and Brenda Derby has identified a number of possible effects of health claims, such as the so-called "halo effect," in which "the presence of a health claim induces a consumer to rate the product higher on other attributes not mentioned in the claim."[61] Another is the "magic-bullet effect" that leads consumers to attribute inappropriate and exaggerated health benefits to a food product.[62] They also observed how health claims on the front of food packaging are prioritized over the information on the Nutrition Facts label and may discourage consumers from searching for further information on the package.[63] For example, you could pick up a box of Cocoa Krispies that carries the front-of-pack claim that it is "a good source of 5 vitamins including folate" and "now helps support your child's immunity" while overlooking the Nutrition Facts label that shows it contains 36.5 percent sugar.

NATURALLY MARKETED FOODS

While the direct or implied health claims on food labels and in advertisements usually relate to nutrients, an increasingly common marketing strategy is to draw attention to the presence of "whole" and "natural" ingredients in food products.[64] These can be referred to as *naturally marketed foods* and include products in which minimally processed whole foods make up the bulk of the food or food ingredients, such as a box of oats or an ice cream made primarily from whole food ingredients (e.g., cream, eggs, sugar, and fruit). But they also include highly processed foods containing small quantities of whole foods, such as processed white breads with a few whole grains added.

Like low-fat label claims, whole grain and natural claims create a health halo effect around a product, such that they may exaggerate the quality or healthful properties of a food in the eyes of consumers. Consumer surveys have shown that many people assume that foods advertised with whole grain claims are also high in fiber. However, one study of foods marketed with such whole grain claims found that a high proportion of them did not contain enough fiber to meet the FDA's definition of a "good source" of fiber.[65]

The use of "natural" and "whole" claims is hardly new. In *Appetite for Change*, Warren Belasco analyzes the ways in which the counterculture's celebration of natural and whole foods in the 1960s and 1970s was quickly appropriated by manufacturers of breakfast cereals and other convenience foods.[66] These products sometimes referred either to the absence of chemical additives or to the presence—however minor—of ingredients that conveyed wholesomeness, such as honey, nuts, or stone-ground wheat. However, there has been a resurgence of foods marketed with these claims—paralleling the rise of the "real food" movement—and they are beginning to outstrip foods marketed with nutrient claims. Almost half of the successful new products released in 2010–2011 reportedly carried either a natural/organic or a high-fiber/whole grain claim.[67]

Food companies have also responded to consumers' growing concerns with highly processed foods and ingredients by developing what industry analysts have started to call "clean label" foods.[68] These are foods that display a short list of ingredients and few highly processed or chemical-sounding ingredients. An example of a clean label is Häagen-Dazs Five ice cream that contains just five simple ingredients: milk, cream, sugar, eggs, and one other ingredient for flavor, such as cocoa or lemon. These new processing and marketing strategies are in response to the growing demand for good-quality foods, defined largely in terms of being minimally processed. It is perhaps also a sign that nutritional marketing is beginning to lose some of its selling power with some classes of consumers.

FRONT-OF-PACK LABELING SCHEMES AND PROMOTIONAL LOGOS

A range of front-of-pack and point-of-purchase labeling systems are already in place to convey to a shopper at a glance the relative healthfulness of a food.[69] The labeling schemes developed by food companies for their own products are largely intended to promote the healthier, "better for you," or lesser-evil products within their product range. The labeling schemes run independently of food companies, on the other hand, rank all foods on the supermarket shelf, whether of good or poor quality. Government-mandated labeling systems, such as calorie labeling and traffic-light labeling systems, are another source of guidance for consumers about the nutritional contents of foods. These labeling schemes are primarily focused on nutrients and are usually based on a specific nutrient profiling system to evaluate and rank foods.[70]

The more "positive" promotional logos introduced by food companies include Kraft's Sensible Solutions, PepsiCo's Smart Spot, and the controversial Smart Choices Program. Smart Choices was introduced in 2009 by a number of leading food companies in conjunction with nutrition experts and organizations, and administered by the American Society for Nutrition.[71] This scheme was voluntarily suspended in 2010 when its green logo began appearing on sugary breakfast cereals such as Froot Loops and Cocoa Puffs, drawing close media scrutiny and destroying the program's credibility. The Froot Loops fiasco highlighted the lenient criteria that food companies inevitably adopt to rank their own products.[72] Food manufacturers also use third-party health endorsements, such as the American Heart Association's Heart-Check symbol and the Whole Grains Council's Whole Grain Stamp. Most of these schemes are based on meeting some minimum qualifying criteria, such as the quantities of salt, sugar, total fat, cholesterol, saturated fat, trans-fat, and selected vitamins and minerals contained in a product.

In 2011 the Grocery Manufacturers of America, representing all the major food manufacturers, introduced its own voluntary Facts Up Front front-of-pack nutrition labeling system under which companies can place an icon on food packaging that displays calories, saturated fat, salt, and sugar per serving. Critics of these voluntary initiatives argue that they are an attempt by the food industry to circumvent more stringent and mandatory government-regulated schemes, such as traffic light systems. But the Facts Up Front labeling system also suggests that the industry considers there to be little to fear from providing quantified, nutrient-by-nutrient information about their products.

Other types of nutritional scoring and ranking systems are displayed on the shelf or at the point of purchase rather than on the label. For instance, the NuVal system, developed by an independent panel of nutrition and medical experts led by Yale University researcher David Katz, ranks foods from 1 to 100 and is currently being used in a number of supermarket chains across the United States. The Guiding Stars program developed by one supermarket chain allocates between 0 and 4 stars to each item within a food and beverage category. These schemes intend to offer a single indicator of the nutritional quality of a food and are a means of ranking foods within each product category.[73]

Another type of front-of-pack labeling is the traffic light scheme developed by the U.K. Food Standards Agency that retailers and manufacturers can voluntarily use on the front of packages.[74] The U.K. traffic light system lists only the quantities of total fat, saturated fat, sodium, and sugar and color-codes each of these red, amber, or green depending on the quantities of each food component in a product. Salt and sugar are key ingredients in highly processed foods and may be reliable indicators of the overall quality of a food. But this labeling system maintains the long-standing focus on and stigmatization of fat and saturated fat. Even within the terms of nutricentric food labeling, the omission of calories from the U.K. traffic light system seems odd. Some studies have demonstrated that consumers prefer and find easier to comprehend such simple color-coded labeling systems, and this may be precisely why they are so vigorously opposed by the food industry.[75] The industry is reported to have spent around one billion euros successfully lobbying the European Food Safety Authority to reject a proposal for the introduction of a mandatory traffic-light labeling system across Europe.[76]

These front-of-pack labeling schemes are usually underpinned by nutrient profiling systems that have been developed by independent nutrition experts, government institutions, or food or retailing companies. Nutrient profiling has been defined as the science of ranking foods based on their nutrient composition.[77] It involves evaluating foods based on a range of constituent nutrients and weighting the various beneficial and detrimental (i.e., good and bad) nutrients in order to produce a single nutrient-density score or nutritional classification. These profiling systems use varying methods for evaluating and classifying foods.[78] Nevertheless, in most schemes, the bad nutrients are the usual suspects, saturated fats, *trans*-fats, calories, sugar, and salt; the good nutrients usually include protein, fiber, polyunsaturated fats, vitamins A and C, calcium, and iron.[79] Most profiling schemes focus on nutrients, although some combine nutrient and food ingredient criteria. While maintaining our attention on nutrients, nutrient profiling systems at least move us beyond the reductive focus on single nutrients. Nevertheless, this multinutrient evaluation of foods is largely based on the simple addition and weighting of the single nutrients in a food and therefore reproduces—and possibly even magnifies—some of the limitations and biases of single-nutrient reductionism.

CORPORATE NUTRITIONISM

In the present era of functional nutritionism, there is now a deep complicity between nutritionism and food corporations. In many respects, we can refer to this as the era of corporate nutritionism, as food corporations become the primary promoters and beneficiaries of this reductive understanding of nutrients, foods, and the body. While a level of corporate influence, and of government appeasement of food industry interests, is not new, it is since the 1980s that food corporations have come to control the nutritional agenda, and have become the dominant promoters of the nutritionism paradigm. It matters less and less what nutrition experts or the government's dietary guidelines advocate, for their advice will invariably be appropriated and reinterpreted by the research, development, and marketing departments of food corporations and overwhelmed by a barrage of nutritional and health claims.

The marketing of foods with nutrient-content and health claims has become the primary means through which the public now encounters nutritional information. Beyond its role in selling products, nutritional marketing now also shapes and disseminates the functional nutritionism paradigm itself. Through these nutritionally engineered products and nutritional marketing practices, the food industry promotes the most simplified, decontextualized, deterministic, and exaggerated ways of understanding nutrients, foods, and the body. The food industry has also capitalized on, and accentuated the shift to, a more positive and functional view of foods and nutrients that target internal bodily functions. It also exacerbates the anxieties surrounding the perceived lack of these nutrients in conventional foods and dietary patterns.

The sheer volume of nutritional advertising has maintained the focus of many consumers on nutrients and other functional components of foods, rather than on the quality of food products and their ingredients. The marketing budgets of some food corporations now run into the hundreds of millions of dollars, easily overwhelming government agencies' modest nutrition education and health promotion efforts. Many of these food companies are transnational corporations that are able to invest significant resources in the development of new products, in new technologies for designing nutritionally engineered foods, and in scientific research to support the claimed health benefits of their products.

The ability of food companies to promote their products and cultivate consumer demand, unhindered by restrictive regulations, has been facilitated by compliant and cooperative governments and nutrition experts and institutions. Government agencies such as the U.S. Department of Agriculture and the FDA have seemed more intent on enabling these food marketing possibilities than restricting them. The introduction of new food labeling regulations in the United States in the mid-1990s permitting a range of direct health claims on food packaging and in advertisements has allowed food companies to capitalize on a broader range of nutritional concerns and functional nutrients. At the same time, food companies' use of these nutrient and health claims has been poorly regulated and monitored by these agencies.

Government agencies have also formulated national dietary guidelines for the public in ways that further, or at least protect, the interests of food producers or manufacturers, as discussed in previous chapters. The earliest American food guides, such as the *Basic Four* food guide, gave a prominent place to meat and dairy foods. The *Food Guide Pyramid* and the latest *MyPlate* food guide have similarly given prominent place and ample recommended servings of dairy products. As Marion Nestle has argued, the *Dietary Guidelines for Americans* has typically been worded so as not to advise eating less of any specific foods. "Eat less" recommendations have been translated into nutrient-level language, such as eat less saturated fats or less sugar, rather than naming the foods in which these food components are typically consumed.[80]

The food industry spends millions of dollars each year lobbying politicians as a means of more directly influencing government food policies and regulations.[81] The defeat of the proposed traffic-light labeling scheme in Europe, described earlier, following intense industry lobbying demonstrates the power of food corporations to undermine what many public health institutions consider to be a powerful and effective labeling system. Another documented example is the sugar industry's lobbying of the World Health Organization to remove its proposed recommendation that added sugars should be limited to 10 percent of daily caloric intake in its 2004 *Global Strategy on Diet, Physical Activity and Health* report.[82] While resisting direct government regulation, the food industry has instead undertaken to self-regulate its actions, such as through pledges to reduce children's food advertising or to reformulate its products by selectively reducing their sugar or salt content.[83]

Food companies have become increasingly active in directly funding scientific studies into particular foods or nutrients conducted by university-based researchers.[84] Some reviews of these industry-funded studies have found that they are, on average, more likely to publish favorable findings for the nutrient or food under investigation, thereby lending support for the industry sponsor's products.[85] These more favorable studies may have been used as scientific substantiation to support a food company's submission to regulatory agencies for approval for health claims, such as Quaker's funding of studies on the health benefits of oats described earlier. These studies may also be referred to directly in advertisements for food products. Food companies also seek to influence expert dietary advice in other ways, such as by funding nutrition and public health organizations or university departments. For example, the American Academy of Nutrition and Dietetics and the British Nutrition Foundation accept funding from food corporations.[86] Another strategy of food corporations has been to set up industry front groups that purport to offer an independent expert or consumer voice.[87] A recent example is Americans Against Food Taxes, which describes itself as "a coalition of concerned citizens— responsible individuals, financially strapped families, small and large businesses in communities across the country—opposed to the government tax hikes on food and beverages."[88]

In response to this growing corporate control of the nutriscape, there have been renewed attempts by public health experts and institutions, and in some cases government agencies, to impose more stringent regulations on food products and food marketing. Public health experts such as Kelly Brownell of Yale University and Marion Nestle have been vocal critics of the food industry's marketing campaigns and argue for stricter labeling and marketing regulations.[89] Despite its own role in promoting nutritionism, discussed in chapter 6, the advocacy group Center for Science in the Public Interest has been active in exposing the inadequacies of some food labeling and marketing regulations. It has lobbied governments for regulatory changes and litigated to pressure food companies to reformulate their products or to change their marketing practices. However, the center's campaigns seem rather selective and narrowly focused and are not anticorporate per se, given their support, for example, for genetically modified crops.[90]

Despite—or perhaps in response to—the food industry's colonization of the nutriscape, many people have also started to look beyond the nutri-centric focus of food marketing and dietary guidelines and are redefining and revaluing food quality in other terms. Chapter 9 considers some of these alternative approaches to food and the body.

CHAPTER NINE

The Food Quality Paradigm

Alternative Approaches to Food and the Body

*In an era when the laxative Metamucil has claimed it contains as much fiber as two bowls
of oatmeal, or the table sweetener Equal has tried to position itself "as a healthy alternative"
like "2% milk," nutrients alone cannot define a healthy food. What we mean by "nutritious"
is something more. We mean, I think, something like "wholesome."*
—JOAN DYE GUSSOW, "CAN AN ORGANIC TWINKIE BE CERTIFIED?," 1997

What do we mean when we say something is nutritious? The nutritionism
paradigm defines the nutritiousness and healthfulness of foods primarily
in terms of their nutrient composition. Low fat, high fiber, calcium,
omega-3, nutrient dense, low glycemic index—this is the kind of language
that permeates expert and lay dietary discourses around the health effects
of foods, since it is the only language that has so far been able to claim
scientific authority and legitimacy. But we also understand the nutritiousness and healthfulness of food in other ways. Joan Gussow has pointed to
wholesomeness as one such characteristic of nutritious foods, which she
contrasts with such highly processed products as Twinkie sponge cakes.[1]
She and many other food experts typically think of healthful foods as being minimally processed and as having few added chemically synthesized
compounds, as well as having been grown without the use of chemicals.

Virtually everyone interested in food and nutrition today promotes
and celebrates the production and consumption of good-quality food, or
what is now often simply called "real food." While "quality" is a contested
term, among contemporary food movements there is a fair degree of consensus about what constitutes good-quality or real food. The local food
movement, the international Slow Food movement, counternutritional
food advocacy groups such as the Weston A. Price Foundation, leading
chefs, and affluent foodies all generally celebrate fresh, minimally processed and traditionally, organically, and locally grown and prepared foods.

Most recommended dietary patterns, such as the Mediterranean, vegetarian, low-carb, low-fat, and paleo diets are also invariably based on good-quality, minimally processed, fresh foods.

Aside from the way in which a food has been produced and processed, a number of other approaches have been used to identify healthful foods and dietary patterns. Cultural and traditional knowledge and practices of food production and consumption continue to act as a guide for many people and communities around the world as to how to choose, prepare, and combine healthy and tasty foods. The sensual and practical experiences of growing, preparing, and eating food offer other ways of identifying healthful foods, as well as alternative ways of engaging with our own bodies.

The alternative paradigm I outline in this chapter shifts the focus from nutrients to foods and dietary patterns. But it also places food production and processing quality at the center of our understanding of food and health. The food quality paradigm ultimately involves integrating food production and processing quality, cultural-traditional knowledge, and sensual-practical experience, as well as the nutritional-scientific analysis of nutrients, foods, and dietary patterns (appendix table A.9). It also provides a way of contextualizing and qualifying nutritional-scientific knowledge. In discussing these other approaches, the aim here is not to replace one set of "truths" with another. Rather, it is to value a range of approaches to food and the body and to suggest that they can all contribute to a more integrated and less reductive understanding of the healthfulness of foods.

CATEGORIZING FOOD PRODUCTION AND PROCESSING QUALITY

The starting point for my critique of nutritionism was the way in which nutrition science and dietary advice have obscured food processing quality and blurred the qualitative distinction between minimally and highly processed foods. Nutritional knowledge can complement our understanding of the way different processing techniques may enhance, transform, or degrade the quality of a food. Nutrition science is at its best when it can reveal and elucidate some of the differences among them, but is at its worst when it conceals or blurs important distinctions among these levels of food quality. Much nutrition research supports the argument that minimally processed foods are healthier than highly processed foods, but this is not always the case, particularly because most research has focused on single nutrients or single ingredients. Even most food-level studies tend to evaluate and compare the health effects of various whole or minimally processed foods, rather than examining highly processed foods and the various processed ingredients, additives, and chemical residues they may contain.

Partly because of the dominance of the nutritionism paradigm, nutrition and food experts have had little interest in developing a language—that is, a set of terms, categories, and concepts—for identifying and distinguishing foods on the basis of processing quality. The exceptions are generic terms such as *processed* or *highly processed food* and more derogatory terms such as *junk food*. Claude Fischler's term for highly processed and technologically transformed foods is "unidentified edible objects"; Joan Gussow refers to "the objects once called food" and "edible substances"; and Michael Pollan paraphrases Gussow by calling these foods "edible food-like substances."[2] In the absence of schemes for categorizing foods according to levels and types of processing, some types of foods tend to be placed in either the "good food" or the "bad food" basket, regardless of the way in which they are produced. In some food guides, for example, foods such as bread, yogurt, and fruit are typically depicted as healthy, while pizza, hamburgers, and muffins are portrayed as unhealthy or junk food. But this categorization fails to acknowledge that there are both poor- and good-quality varieties of all of these types of foods.

One of the few nutrition experts in recent decades to have focused primarily on the nutritional effects of food processing, and to have developed a classification system based on types of processing, was the late Canadian biochemist Ross Hume Hall. In his book *The Unofficial Guide to Smart Nutrition* (2000), Hall proposed a 1-to-4 ranking system within each food group based on the method of agricultural production and the types of processing that foods have been subjected to. The three main criteria he used to rank foods were the degree of processing, the quantity of nonnutritional chemicals added to the food, and the amount of fiber contained in the end product. Hall ranked minimally processed, fresh, organic, and free-range products the highest, followed by increasingly refined, frozen, and preserved foods, and food products that have been subjected to various forms of chemical processing and industrial manufacture. In the fruit group, for example, Hall ranked fresh and raw produce the highest, followed by frozen, then dried, and then canned fruit. In the meat category, top-ranked are free-range meats, then cuts of fresh meat, then commercial hamburger and frozen meats, followed by bacon, sausages, and low-fat meats.[3] Hall's rankings mainly refer to individual ingredients rather than to final food products and mixed-ingredient foods. His ranking system also conflates the agricultural and processing aspects of food quality. Hall was clear that these rankings reflect the nutrient profile of these foods, with the highest-ranked foods having a more beneficial nutrient profile. In this sense he relied on conventional nutritional criteria to justify these rankings. Nevertheless, he prioritized the level of processing and the methods of agricultural production within his ranking system.

The food classification system I outline here distinguishes among three broad categories of food ingredients (table 9.1) and three corresponding

TABLE 9.1
Levels of Processing of Food Ingredients

Whole Food Ingredients (Minimally Processed and Beneficially Processed Ingredients)
- *Definition:* Whole foods; foods minimally processed or beneficially processed through fermentation, preservation, sprouting, and cooking
- *Techniques:* Manual, and in some cases mechanical, preparation (e.g., peeling, chopping, mixing); natural fermentation; canning, bottling
- *Examples:* Whole grains, particularly fermented and sprouted; fresh and fermented vegetables and fruits; whole meat, animal organs, and fish; unhomogenized, raw or fermented full-fat milk and dairy products (cream, butter, yogurt); nuts and seeds; fermented soy products; spices

Refined-Extracted Ingredients (Concentrated Ingredients)
- *Definition:* Extracted, refined, and concentrated ingredients and foods, often involving the removal of other beneficial food components from a whole food
- *Techniques:* Manual practices; mechanical technologies; grinding; some chemical, thermal, high-pressure, and biotechnological methods; fractionation techniques
- *Examples:* Refined and ground grains and flours; refined corn starch; extracted and refined sugar; extracted and refined vegetable oils; lard; reduced-fat and fractionated milk; milk powder; fruit juices; soy milk and other soy fractions; high-fat minced meat; some nutritional supplements and extracts, such as fish oils

Processed-Reconstituted Ingredients (Detrimentally Processed Ingredients)
- *Definition:* Ingredients and foods that are broken down into their constituent components, and transformed, reconstituted, or significantly degraded during processing, preparation, and cooking
- *Techniques:* Chemical technologies; cellular and genetic biotechnologies; nanotechnologies; high-pressure and heat extraction; irradiation; hydrogenation and interesterification
- *Examples:* Chemically reconstituted and chemically synthesized preservatives, colors, flavors, and other additives; hydrogenated and interesterified oils; artificial sweeteners; high-fructose corn syrup; chemically modified starch; textured vegetable or soy protein; nanoscale and nanoreconstituted ingredients and additives; continually reused deep-frying oils; chemically processed meats; mechanically extracted meat; some nutrient supplements and additives, such as plant sterols and stanols

TABLE 9.2

Levels of Processing of Foods and Food Products

Whole Foods (Minimally Processed and Beneficially Processed Foods)

- *Definition:* Foods and meals prepared primarily with good-quality whole and minimally or beneficially processed ingredients; beneficial combinations of ingredients and foods; may also include some quantities of refined-extracted ingredients

- *Examples:* Butter; sourdough (fermented) whole wheat bread; whole meat and home-minced meat; eggs; full-fat dairy products; mixed meals prepared with these foods; homemade cakes and muffins

Refined-Processed Foods

- *Definition:* Foods produced with a combination of whole and refined-extracted ingredients, and only small quantities of processed-reconstituted ingredients

- *Examples:* White yeasted bread; cake and muffins with large quantities of sugar; dairy products with added sugar; foods produced with larger quantities of oils, fat, salt, refined flours and fatty meats

Processed-Reconstituted Foods (Detrimentally Processed Foods)

- *Definition:* Highly processed foods that are constructed primarily out of processed-reconstituted and refined-extracted ingredients and additives

- *Examples:* Margarine; soft drinks and sweetened beverages; modern industrial bread (with added gluten, emulsifiers, and preservatives); commercially deep-fried fast foods; reconstituted fish sticks; chicken nuggets; commercial sausages, hamburgers and processed meat products; breakfast cereals made with highly refined grains and high in sugar; most commercial snack foods and confectionaries made primarily from refined and modified flour, starch, sugars and oils

---

types of final food products based on levels and intensity of technological processing (table 9.2).[4] Foods and ingredients are categorized as, first, whole, minimally processed or beneficially processed; second, refined-processed or refined-extracted; and third, processed-reconstituted or detrimentally processed. The choice of three categories is arbitrary—more could be included, and other, more accessible and evocative names could also be used. But three categories avoid the overly dichotomized and simplified choice when only two categories are used (e.g., whole foods vs. highly processed foods), while also accentuating the distinction between foods that may be less nutritious than whole foods but okay to eat in moderation, and those that are not just devoid of nutritiousness but may be more directly harmful in any quantity.[5]

The criteria for distinguishing these three categories of processing quality are based primarily on the type and intensity of technological intervention. Each successive category within this tripartite classification system generally involves a reduction or degradation in food quality, due to the removal of beneficial food components, the concentration of certain food components, or the further technological transformation and degradation of the foods and ingredients. However, the quality of foods, including their nutritional quality and their health effects, can also vary greatly within each category, depending, for example, on the type of processing they are subjected to, and the relative quantities of refined and reconstituted ingredients. I also make no claims regarding the *specific* health effects of any of these food categories; for example, I do not argue that all processed-reconstituted foods cause specific chronic diseases or lead to weight gain.

The first category is ingredients that are whole or have been minimally processed or beneficially processed. Unless eaten raw and whole, most foods are processed in some way, but the processing and transformation in this case typically occur at the level of the whole food—or what can be referred to as the organic level, that is, at the level of the whole food product or whole organism as we encounter them with our unaided senses. They include ingredients prepared using chopping, peeling, cooking, culturing, and fermentation techniques. All of this processing can be done with your own hands using simple equipment in a domestic kitchen, although mechanical technologies such as mechanical mixers can also be used to process foods at this level.

Importantly, some of these processing techniques may improve or enhance the quality of food by making them more palatable and nutritious, by removing or negating potentially harmful components, or by preserving them for year-round consumption.[6] Cooking foods, for example, can enhance the palatability, safety, and nutritional quality of a food, an often-cited example being how cooking tomatoes increases the bioavailability of lycopene.[7] The fermentation of foods using a range of traditional techniques may also provide a range of benefits. This includes fermented grains and flour, fermented dairy products such as yogurt and cheese, fermented vegetables and soy products, and dried and canned beans and vegetables. In examining the fermentation practices of various cultures, ethnopharmacologist Nina Etkin argues that fermentation has been used in quite specific ways to produce foods that are "more nutritious and otherwise healthful than their unprocessed counterparts."[8]:

Fermentations destroy some undesirable elements of the raw product; improve food digestibility and constituent availability and/or solubility; enrich substrates with vitamins and amino acids; preserve foods, some for months or even years; transform vegetable protein to products that have meatlike qualities; bring forth flavors, aromas, and textures; and are relatively inexpensive preparations that salvage wastes that otherwise would not be usable as food.[9]

The second processing category, refined-extracted ingredients, includes items that are produced through the extraction, refinement, and concentration of food components from a whole food, such as white flour, vegetable oil, lard, cane sugar, and fruit juice. This level of processing often entails the removal of what may be beneficial food components such as the outer shells of grains or the body of the fruit. The extraction and refinement of foods may involve the use of mechanical technologies for fine milling and oil extraction. In some cases this extraction also requires the use of chemical, high-temperature, and high-pressure technologies, as in the case of some vegetable oil and soy components. Some modern extraction and refinement techniques are potentially more damaging to the food and may degrade and transform the character of the food and its components. Refined-extracted ingredients may also be susceptible to further degradation from exposure to air or high-temperature cooking. For example, the process of refining and extracting vegetable oil from seeds and the continual reuse of these oils for deep-frying, place these oils both in the refined-extracted and processed-reconstituted categories. The extracted and synthesized nutrients and components added to foods and supplements, such as omega-3-rich fish oils, are also susceptible to oxidation and other forms of degradation.[10]

Refined-extracted ingredients can have an important role to play in preparing tasty and healthful meals, such as the use of oils for cooking or adding to salads. The process of refining and extracting foods is also a way of preserving and making these foods available all year round and enables ease of transportation and storage. While there is a long history of refining and grinding of grains and flour and of extracting vegetable oils, a range of modern technologies have enabled these ingredients to be extracted in greater volumes or to be more finely ground and refined. There is evidence that the overconsumption of large quantities of refined-extracted ingredients in concentrated forms, such as in the form of white flour and fruit juice, can have deleterious health effects, usually due to this level of concentration rather than because these ingredients are harmful in themselves. The enormous quantities of sugars now being consumed by Americans—in the form of cane sugar, high-fructose corn syrup, and fruit juices—is of particular concern, accounting for up to one-quarter of many children's calorie intake.[11] The consumption of isolated and concentrated doses of nutrients in the form of fortified foods and supplements may also pose health risks.[12]

The third processing category of processed-reconstituted ingredients typically involves the use of technologies for breaking down foods into their component parts, for transforming the molecular structure of foods and food components, and for synthesizing artificial ingredients and additives. These forms of processing may further remove or degrade otherwise beneficial food components, introduce novel components into foods, and transform food components into more harmful end-products. Processed-reconstituted ingredients can be manufactured using chemical technologies, biotechnologies, and nanotechnologies that reconstitute foods at the cellular and molecular level, such as the techniques of hydrogenation and interesterification, and high-pressure, thermal, and extrusion technologies. Food manufacturers' and fast-food restaurants' continual reuse of deep-frying oils can also oxidize and significantly degrade, and thereby transform, these oils. The deconstitution and chemical transformation of foods may also degrade or transform the way the body metabolizes these foods in ways yet to be studied or fully understood by nutrition scientists.

The reconstituted meat ingredient dubbed "pink slime" is an example of such a processed-reconstituted food. This mechanically separated and disinfected beef product is known in the meat industry as "lean finely textured beef" and "boneless beef trimmings." It is produced by heating beef trimmings to high temperatures to melt off the fat, and treated with ammonia to kill bacteria. Since 2001 this processed-reconstituted meat has been used widely by the food manufacturing and fast food industries, and in school lunch programs, as a filler in ground beef and processed meats, until it received widespread media coverage in 2012.[13]

The three categories of final food products—whole foods, refined-processed foods, and processed-reconstituted foods—can be defined in terms of the relative quantities of whole, refined-extracted, and processed-reconstituted ingredients they contain. Whole foods—or minimally processed and beneficially processed foods—are prepared primarily from whole food ingredients, though they may also include small quantities of refined-extracted ingredients. Refined-processed foods contain moderate quantities of refined-extracted ingredients, such as added sugar, salt, fat, and refined flour, but they may also contain small quantities of processed-reconstituted ingredients, such as chemical preservatives or flavors.

By contrast, I define processed-reconstituted foods as foods that have little if any direct relation to any particular whole foods but have instead been reconstructed, from the ground up, out of the deconstituted components of whole foods, refined-extracted ingredients, and other reconstituted and degraded ingredients and additives. These detrimentally processed products are often heavily adulterated with ingredients such as cane sugar, high-fructose corn syrup, artificial sweeteners, highly refined flours, chemically modified starches, soy fractions, mechanically extracted meat and animal fat, and refined and often chemically modified vegetable oils (e.g., hydrogenated and interesterified oils, *trans*-fats and *i*-fats). These food products might also then be subject to further processing, such as being deep fried in old/degraded vegetable oils, that thereby further degrade their quality. The health threats posed by processed-reconstituted foods has little if anything to do with the presence or absence of specific naturally occurring nutrients—such as fats, carbs, or vitamins—but rather with the combined effect on the body of high levels of reconstituted, degraded, and synthetic food components and additives.

Chicken nuggets and Twinkies are quintessential processed-reconstituted foods. A chicken nugget is typically manufactured out of mechanically extracted chicken, with a range of additives to hold it together and give it texture and flavor, such as textured vegetable protein, modified starch, and gum.[14] In *Twinkie, Deconstructed*, Steve Ettlinger meticulously describes the functions of twenty-five of the ingredients that go into the manufacturing of Twinkies, such as corn sweeteners, corn thickeners, polysorbate 60, and cellulose gum.[15] Other common examples of processed-reconstituted foods are children's breakfast cereals composed of highly refined flour and upward of 30 percent sugar, and much of the confectioneries and snack bars that line supermarket shelves.

A now largely discarded term for these processed-reconstituted foods is *fabricated foods*, a term once used openly by the food industry that immediately conveys the artificiality and highly constructed nature of these products. A 1975 food technology text titled *Fabricated Foods* defined them as "foods that have been taken apart and put together in a new form. Designed, engineered, or formulated from ingredients, they may or may not include additives, vitamins and minerals."[16] The authors of this textbook approvingly referred to margarine as an exemplary fabricated food. The terms *simulated foods*, *synthetic foods*, and *imitation foods* are other now rarely used food industry terms for fabricated foods.

A characteristic of many of these highly processed ingredients and final food products is that they are more quickly and easily consumed, and may be less satiating, relative to the same quantity of food consumed in the form of minimally processed foods.[17] The soft, almost premasticated meat in a fast-food chain's burger—filled with ground and reconstituted fatty animal off-cuts—is a case in point. The same quantity of meat in the form of a steak may take considerably more time to chew and digest. These processed-reconstituted foods also typically contain many "hidden ingredients" or, in nutricentric terms, "hidden calories," which can take the form of hidden carbs (e.g., flour), hidden fats (e.g., vegetable oil or extracted animal fats), or hidden protein (e.g., soy derivatives or milk powder).

A particular type of food may be represented in all three of these categories. For example, the best-quality breads are those made with whole wheat flour or a mixture of whole and white flour, contain no chemical additives, and are risen slowly, perhaps with a sourdough culture. Moderate-quality breads include those made from refined white flour and risen quickly with commercial yeast—perhaps in the form of a crunchy white Italian-style bread—and can be a tasty and filling accompaniment to other good-quality foods. The poorest-quality breads include the typical soft, sliced, supermarket loaf, manufactured using very highly refined flours and a range of additives, such as flour improvers, chemical preservatives, hardened fats, and added gluten. They may be "raised" using accelerated yeast-based or mechanical aeration techniques but without any significant fermentation of the dough.[18] The current denigration of refined (white) flour—both within mainstream dietary guidelines and by the low-carb movement—often fails to distinguish among the qualities of the food in which these refined flours are embedded. There is a qualitative difference between a good white sourdough bread and a soft white supermarket loaf, but these differences are blurred by the categories "refined grain," "refined carbs," or "high carb."

The question of food quality needs to be distinguished from that of *quantity*. It may be sensible to limit one's consumption of "rich" whole foods such as butter and bacon and of good-quality, homemade desserts high in sugar and refined flour. But this is not the same as calling butter, meat, or flour-based products "bad" or harmful foods. Refined-processed foods are more likely to become a health problem when overconsumed in one's overall diet, particularly when eaten in isolation and in the absence of other whole foods. However, these foods can form a healthful part of the diet when eaten in combination with whole foods. Processed-reconstituted foods, on the other hand, are not merely foods that one should not overconsume but foods one should really avoid altogether, because they contain a high level of potentially harmful constituents and are otherwise largely devoid of nourishment. Their production and availability should therefore be directly regulated, such as by mandating upper limits on the quantities of some refined-extracted and reconstituted ingredients that foods are permitted to contain. However, this characterization of processed-reconstituted foods as not so much bad foods, but nasty foods, runs counter to the Academy for Nutrition and Dietetics' claim that "there are no such thing as good and bad foods, only good and bad diets"—an expression also much-loved by food manufacturers.[19]

Nutrition researchers can use such a food categorization system to distinguish among types of foods in their dietary studies and to provide a way to understand and contextualize the health effects of nutrients, foods, and dietary patterns. Defining and categorizing food quality in terms of methods of primary production and processing, rather than in terms of nutrient composition, can be the basis of alternative dietary guidelines, nutrition education strategies, and food and nutrition policies and regulations. School food programs, for example, could be regulated on the basis of the production and processing quality of foods and food ingredients, rather than on nutrient-level criteria.[20] Similarly, the hurdle criteria for nutrient-content and health-claim regulations, as well as traffic light and other front-of-pack labeling schemes, could be based on food processing quality rather than on nutrient composition as is currently the case. A set of meaningful and accessible food categories and terms may also enable the lay public to more readily identify and describe the type and quality of foods on the supermarket shelf and on a fast-food menu.

To criticize the quality of highly processed foods is not to deny the many benefits that preprocessed, prepared, and packaged foods have brought to people over the past century. Processed foods of various kinds save time and labor in food preparation and have been important in easing the domestic burden of women in contexts where they have borne and continue to bear much of the responsibility for food preparation. These foods have also enabled a diversification of diets and have made new foods and tastes more accessible and more affordable to a broader population.[21] In making a wider range of foods available to people all year round and across geographical locations, they have most likely contributed to the improvement of many people's health. Even dedicated home cooks who largely cook from scratch use a wide range of prepared foods or ingredients—such as canned tomatoes, pasta, olives, and yogurt—as the basis of tasty and healthy meals.

It is not the convenience of processed or fast foods that is the issue here but rather their quality or level of processing.

PRIMARY PRODUCTION QUALITY

In terms of primary produce, the quality of foods can vary according to the types of agricultural technologies, production methods, breeding techniques, soil quality, and harvesting and transportation practices. We can use a series of dualistic criteria for distinguishing between good-quality and poorer-quality primary produce, such as organic, biodynamic, and wild-harvested versus chemical, industrially grown foods; free-range and pastured versus confined and grain-fed animal products; traditionally bred versus hybrid-industrial seed and animal varieties; and fresh, local produce versus those refrigerated and transported over long distances. The greatest concern here is the range of chemical pesticides, antibiotics, and growth hormones found in industrially produced foods and their possible effects on the body.[22] Aside from the toxicity of these chemicals at high levels of exposure, there has been little research on how these chemicals might affect bodily metabolism in other ways.

The nutrient profile of primary produce can vary considerably according to these methods of primary production. For example, grass-fed beef and free-range eggs generally have a higher omega-3 fat content than do products from confined and grain-fed animals. Modern cattle breeds and production methods also produce meat and milk with higher levels of saturated fats and hormones.[23] The health of the soils in which foods are grown may shape the nutritional content of foods, as can the breeds and the production methods used in animal production.

A number of studies have compared the nutrient composition of organic and conventionally grown foods, and some have measured the differences in health outcomes from their consumption.[24] Some studies have found that organic produce contains higher levels of particular micronutrients, while others have found little difference between them. However, this focus on nutrient content to evaluate the health benefits of organic produce distracts from the probably far more important benefits that come from the absence of chemical pesticides, fertilizers, antibiotics, and hormones used in their production, including how these chemical compounds may affect the body's metabolism of food and nutrients. The focus on the nutrient composition of organic foods may also accentuate the already widespread perceptions and fears of nutrient scarcity in the food supply and exaggerate the health implications of any nutrient-specific differences between organic and conventional foods. The consumers who can afford and are more inclined to purchase organic foods are probably the least likely to be consuming nutritionally deficient diets.

The Appeal to Culture and Tradition

Cuisine is to be understood as the art of manipulation and skillful combination, given that perfectly balanced foods do not exist in nature.
—MASSIMO MONTANARI, *FOOD IS CULTURE*, 2006

Culturally specific approaches to food offer another range of insights not only into how to identify healthful foods but also into how to prepare and combine them. Communities around the world—as well as within the United States—have developed culturally and geographically distinct dietary patterns and methods of food preparation. This accumulated knowledge is often embedded in the cuisines and recipes of cultures and communities, as well as in the traditional knowledge that links foods to particular health benefits and disease remedies.[25] These food cultures can also provide clues as to the quantities and ratios of types of foods to consume.

To the extent that traditional dietary patterns have evolved in a premodern or early modern context, they have primarily consisted of whole or minimally processed foods. Refined-extracted ingredients, such as oils and sugar, also have an important role to play in these traditional cuisines in making whole foods tasty and enjoyable to eat and as components of elaborate dishes. The particular combinations of whole foods that feature in these cuisines can bring out the health benefits of individual foods in ways that nutrition scientists do not yet fully understand or appreciate. How these whole foods are grown or sourced—such as using traditional agricultural practices, plant varieties and breeds of animals, or wild and freshly harvested plant foods—also contributes to their nutritiousness.

Traditional dietary patterns also provide a perspective from which to question the healthfulness of novel foods and food processing techniques, as well as changes in the form and quantity of foods consumed today. For example, refined vegetable oils and unfermented soy products are now being consumed in enormous quantities and are also advocated by many nutrition experts as promoting good health. Yet soy products have traditionally been eaten only in a fermented and carefully prepared form in Asian countries such as China, while the mass production of vegetable

oils has been enabled only by modern extraction and refining technologies developed over the past century.[26]

A number of recent popular food books celebrate the diversity and
healthfulness of traditional dietary patterns and the longevity of the people following these diets, such as the long-lived inhabitants on the Japanese island of Okinawa. These include Daphne Miller's *The Jungle Effect*,
Dan Buettner's *The Blue Zones*, Bradley Willcox et al.'s *The Okinawa Diet
Plan*, and John Robbins's *Healthy at 100*.[27] For the authors of many of these
books, it is not just the type of food but how the food is prepared and consumed that holds the key to the healthfulness of traditional diets. These
communities have developed ways of preparing foods that may enhance
the nutritional value of locally available foods while also mitigating the
potential harmful properties of some foods.

Communities around the world have thrived, and in many cases continue to thrive, on a broad range of dietary patterns. These include diets
that vary greatly in terms of the ratio of plant and animal foods and in
terms of the range of macronutrient ratios applicable.[28] In *The Jungle Effect*,
Miller identifies a number of common characteristics of many traditional
diets, including the use of spices and fermented foods, the use of meat
(including organ meats) in relatively small quantities, and communal eating practices. For Miller, it is not just the particular types of foods consumed but also the recipes that encapsulate the healthfulness of traditional diets, because of the way they often beneficially combine ingredients
and enhance the taste of nutritious ingredients.[29]

However, as noted in chapter 7, nutrition experts and institutions, as
well as popular food writers, often attempt to reduce and generalize the
essential foods or food components in these diets in a way that reflects
their own nutritional recommendations or preferences.[30] The 2010 *Dietary Guidelines for Americans*, for example, highlights the benefits of the
Mediterranean, the Japanese, and the Okinawan diets.[31] Yet other food
and dietary movements draw contrary lessons from traditional dietary
patterns. The paleo movement focuses on the claimed dietary habits of
our hunter-gatherer ancestors and on the presumed health benefits of a
diet high in meat but that excludes grains and, in some cases, dairy products. However, a common feature of all of these dietary patterns—one
that is much less noted—is the lack of highly processed foods they contain,
rather than the presence of any specific types of whole foods. Whether it
is the "French," the "Japanese," or the "Mediterranean" diet, these dietary
patterns are typically defined by their promoters in terms of the whole
food dishes that are distinctive to these cultures or geographical regions,

rather than the vast range of more highly processed foods that people in these countries actually consume today.

Communities living in particular locations and climates have developed their dietary patterns and cuisines largely based on readily available local and seasonal foods. These cuisines have also evolved in a context where deficiency and infectious diseases, rather than chronic diseases, were common. By contrast, many people now lead very sedentary lifestyles and are threatened by a different constellation of disease patterns. The nutritional characteristics of the foods themselves may also be quite different, given the changes wrought by the industrialization of breeding and farming practices. In this context, some traditional foods and dietary patterns may well be better suited than others to contemporary living and eating patterns and body ideals.

Given that we are unlikely to adopt another culture's dietary and lifestyle patterns in their entirety, there is the question of how today we might incorporate parts of the dietary knowledge and practices of one or more cultures. We could—and most people do—take a cosmopolitan and eclectic approach, selectively appropriating some of the tasty, convenient, and "well-balanced" meals from a number of countries' cuisines. In the course of a day, we can eat Swiss muesli for breakfast, Japanese sushi with fish for lunch, and Mexican beans and tortillas for dinner. In doing so, we may risk losing the distinctive balance of types and quantities of foods that define a particular cuisine and may overconsume some of the richer or feast dishes of these cuisines. But embracing this dietary diversity and eclecticism may compensate for the loss or neglect of some of the traditional techniques of food production and preparation that once enhanced the nutritional quality of these foods. While many peoples' diets were, and still are, largely constrained by the availability of immediately local and seasonal foods, people with sufficient incomes now have access to an extraordinary abundance and diversity of foods all year round. A modern diet consisting of a greater variety of good-quality whole foods—and that draws on food preparation methods, food combinations, and recipes from around the world—should be every bit as healthful, if not more so, as the diets consumed by people limited to local, in-season, and culturally specific foods.

There is a certain ideology of traditional diets that infuses the appreciation and glorification of other cultures' eating patterns. It is important not to exaggerate the benefits of particular cultural cuisines or dietary patterns or to romanticize the diets or the health of these communities. To recognize the wisdom embedded in traditional cuisines is not to suggest that everyone ate well. Many people lacked access to adequate food and were also confined to a narrow range of foods for most of the year. The ingeniousness of these cultures is that they have managed to develop techniques and recipes for preparing extremely healthful and tasty foods and food combinations out of this limited availability. Nevertheless, life expectancy in most countries has increased as they have followed the path of industrialization, no doubt in part due to the more widespread availability and affordability of many foods, including of meat and dairy foods.

In places where indigenous peoples' health is poor due to the consumption of a poor-quality, highly processed diet, a number of studies have demonstrated the benefits of returning to traditional foods and eating patterns. Intervention studies with the Inuit in Greenland, Indigenous Australians, and indigenous Hawaiians have found their health improved when they were for a period placed on their cultures' traditional diets.[32] However, these benefits may have more to do with their adopting what is effectively a whole foods diet, and the reduced consumption of highly processed and poor-quality foods, rather than with the unique benefits of the traditional foods consumed in these studies. There is also a tendency among American experts and popular commentators alike to selectively fetishize the foods and diets of foreign and non-Western cultures, rather than looking to the cuisines of local migrant populations or even to mainstream white traditions. The combination of beans and tortillas eaten by many Mexican Americans, for example, has much to offer. Compared with highly processed diets, even the unfashionable meal of "meat and three veg" that in the mid-twentieth century characterized the dominant diets of whites in the southern United States, the United Kingdom, and Australia now looks like a healthy alternative to a fast-food diet.

It is not only *what* foods are consumed by people in other cultures but also *how* they consume them that is of interest to scholars and food commentators. The food habits of the French have long been held up as exemplary compared with American food cultures. Studies by Paul Rozin and Claude Fischler on dietary habits suggest that the French spend more time and take greater pleasure in consuming their food than Americans do. The French are also reported to have a greater focus on quality, rather than quantity, compared with Americans. At the same time, they suggest that Americans are paradoxically more concerned about their health and eating healthily.[33] These factors may go some way toward explaining the different types and quantities of food consumed between these countries. Yet as significant as these cultural differences may be, French dietary patterns and health outcomes have tracked not too far behind those of Americans. For all their celebration of pleasure and eschewing of healthism, the French too have their weight-loss diet fads, such as the currently popular high-protein, low-carb Dukan Diet.[34]

These cross-cultural comparisons, and efforts to learn the lessons of other cultures, should be approached critically. For example, several food commentators have picked up on the traditional principle of Okinawan eating called *hara hachi bu*, which translates as "eat until you are eight parts full" or "eat until you are 80 percent full."[35] Michael Pollan draws on this principle as the basis for one of his food rules: "Stop eating before you're full."[36] This principle may have served the Okinawans well, and it certainly resonates with the current exhortations from Pollan and most obesity experts to "eat less" or "not too much." However, this advice to stop eating before you are "full" may not work so well in a context where people are surrounded by cheap, highly processed, convenience foods. A recent study of ethnocultural groups in Canada quoted a Punjabi Indian who put forward a contrary approach to eating. He suggested that *not eating enough* at mealtime—rather than eating too much—might be contributing to poor diets and health outcomes, particularly among children: "Here, kids don't fill up on their food. That's why they eat so frequently, they eat bread, banana, candy, I'm hungry, have pop, cookies, chips. Me, I don't eat anything between my meals. I eat roti and I stay full until it's time to eat again."[37] In a context where poor-quality snack foods and sweets are readily available, eating until you are 100 percent full—including filling up on *roti* —could be a more sensible eating strategy for reducing the number of poor-quality snacks between meals.

THE SENSUAL AND PRACTICAL EXPERIENCE OF CONSUMING AND PRODUCING FOOD

The human senses discriminate a wide range of quality of natural foods and can also detect bacterial and other types of natural contamination that might be harmful. The technological food system, by separating palatability from nutritional quality, seriously impairs the ability of the individual to assess nutrition. But having made this separation, the technologic food system provides no surrogate function for the intrinsic human sense of food quality the individual possesses.
—ROSS HUME HALL, *FOOD FOR NOUGHT: THE DECLINE IN NUTRITION*, 1974

In *Food for Nought*, Ross Hume Hall argued that in earlier times the human senses allowed individuals to assess the nutritional quality and safety of food. For example, "rotted food looked and smelled rotten." But he argued that this connection between food and the senses has been severed by the "technologic food system" and the manufacturing of highly processed, fabricated, and imitation foods that fool the senses by simulating the taste and texture of "natural" food.[38] At the same time, Hall suggested food-labeling regulations had failed to provide the public with an adequate surrogate for the senses. In 1971 the U.S. Food and Drug Administration (FDA) removed the requirement that imitation foods be labeled imitations, while the new nutrition facts panel gave no clue as to how a food had been processed and transformed.

Hall was an early critic of the way our taste buds have been overwhelmed and seduced by the combinations of ingredients and additives conjured by food scientists and the food manufacturing and service industries. Some critics of fast food and highly processed food emphasize the way our bodies are wired to like and to respond to the taste and texture of fat, sugar, and salt. In *The End of Overeating*, David Kessler, former commissioner of the FDA, argues that loading foods with the right combination of fat, sugar, and salt not only makes them highly palatable but also activates certain "reward centers" in the brain that override other bodily signals, such as for satiety, thereby causing us to overeat.[39] Whatever the merit of these physiological explanations, Kessler sees these three ingredients as tricking our bodies into eating more calories. Another way in which our sense of taste may let us down is in failing to detect the many other "hidden" ingredients in highly processed foods, including the hidden oils, fats, modified starches, and sugars.

Nutrition experts have at times been complicit with this undermining of the senses as a guide to food quality. The promotion of margarine over butter is an example of expert advice encouraging people to override their taste buds in order to eat more healthily. Another is the suggestion of some glycemic index and low-carb experts that despite what our tongues, bodies, and culinary experience may reveal to us, flour and sugar are essentially the same thing since both are turned into glucose in the body.[40]

There is some scientific research that supports the idea that our senses may be able to detect the nutritional value of foods. Biologists Stephen Goff and Harry Klee, for example, have argued that the many types of volatile organic compounds found in plant foods, such as tomatoes, are often derived from essential nutrients—including antioxidants and omega-3 fats—that may provide health benefits.[41] They suggest that humans and animals can taste these compounds, which is one way they have historically been able to identify healthful foods. In *Good Food Tastes Good*, journalist Carol Hart implores us to rediscover our senses as a guide to identifying healthful foods: "Trust your senses more than the labels. Flavor and aroma are reliable guides to food quality. A tomato that smells and tastes like a real tomato is more nutritious than one that just looks like a tomato."[42]

In response to the capture of our senses by the fast-food and manufactured food industries, some critics of these foods have reclaimed the sensual pleasures of eating as a guide to good-quality food. The international Slow Food movement celebrates the pleasures of eating and conviviality and places them at the center of its food philosophy. Alice Waters, chef and founder of the San Francisco restaurant Chez Paniz, has for many years called for a "delicious revolution."[43] These promoters of the pleasure principle acknowledge that our palates need to be trained or reeducated to appreciate the flavors of the foods they consider to be of good quality, rather than assuming that good taste just comes naturally. As Carlo Petrini, the Italian founder and president of the international Slow Food movement, puts it in Slow Food: The Case for Taste: "The education of taste is the Slow way to resist McDonaldization.... To train the senses, refine perception, restore atrophied dimensions of sensory experience—these are the objectives of Slow Food. By 'voting with their feet,' consumers can actually do a lot to signal to producers that quality matters. But quality... has to be discovered, then learned and codified."[44] For Petrini, as for Waters, the rediscovery of the taste and pleasure of consuming good-quality food is a means of resisting the proliferation of poor-quality foods.[45] There is an assumption here that the cultivation of a fine sense of taste—which is a fairly middle-class preoccupation—can empower citizens to reject poor-quality fast foods. However, as with the limits of nutrition education, we need to ask whether people really need to be educated to appreciate the taste of good-quality food, or does it just come fairly "naturally" when one has more disposable income and time to prepare good foods?

Sensual and practical approaches to food can also include the practices of growing, preparing, and cooking food. These are not only strategies for procuring, and making accessible, good-quality foods but also for promoting a better understanding of food and nutritional quality. School kitchen garden programs that teach children growing and cooking skills can foster a better appreciation and understanding of the qualities and taste of good food. This is the approach celebrated by Alice Waters in her Edible Schoolyard project: "When children grow and prepare good, healthy food themselves, they want to eat it, and what's more, they like this way of learning. We need a revolution, a delicious revolution, that will induce children—in a pleasurable way—to think critically about what they eat."[46] Sociologists JoAnn Jaffe and Michael Gertler have also highlighted the connection between consumer deskilling and the ability to prepare good-quality food at a reasonable cost: "Many if not most American consumers have lost (or never acquired) the skills needed to make use of basic commodities in a manner that allows them to enjoy a high quality diet while simultaneously eating lower on the food (marketing) chain, and for less money."[47] Programs that teach growing and cooking skills to adults as well as children are proliferating and are other ways for us to practically and sensually reconnect with good-quality food.

The sensual-practical approach also includes being guided by—and adapting dietary recommendations to—one's own personal experience, bodily disposition, and individual needs. Dietary guidelines have largely prescribed a uniform and culturally specific diet for the whole population. Yet an individual's tastes, cultural background, biological susceptibilities, allergies, lifestyle practices, activity levels, and existing diseases and health conditions may dispose them to choose particular foods over others to meet their own bodily requirements. For example, the tolerance and response to particular foods, such as wheat or legumes, can vary widely among individuals. Similarly, many people seem to maintain extremely good health on vegetarian diets, but others may be more prone to nutritional deficiencies on such restricted diets.

The embodied experience of feeling healthy, eating well, and being physically active can be valued as a legitimate source of knowledge and can be used to contextualize and to question the scientific interpretation of one's internal biomarkers—such as being told by a doctor that you have high blood cholesterol levels and therefore require cholesterol-lowering medication. This individual experimentation is also distinct from more scientific attempts to personalize dietary recommendations, often based on body size, age, biochemical biomarkers of disease risk, metabolic typing, or genetic markers.

The obsessive and reductive focus on the nutritional and health dimensions of food—and the reductive focus on health in general—has also tended to overwhelm the pleasure of eating and to promote a range of anxieties around food. As Michelle Stacey argues in her 1994 book *Consumed*: "It may be that we will have to redefine fundamentally the concept of 'eating well.' The phrase now, in the hands of the food paranoids, is often used to convey the idea of following a diet scientifically programmed to prevent disease, balanced to the last ounce with beta-carotene and whatever other nutrients the latest studies tout, and almost religiously outlawing certain forbidden food."[48] Recovering or cultivating a sensual approach to food may be an antidote to the obsessive culture of control and the anxieties associated with scientific eating and technologically engineered foods.

While the various alternative food movements have challenged some aspects of the dominant food and dietary discourses, they have tended to take for granted and reinforce others. For example, in *Weighing In: Obesity, Food Justice, and the Limits of Capitalism*, Julie Guthman argues that some food movement activists and commentators have bought into the dominant obesity discourse, in that they reinforce the focus on weight loss as the goal of healthy eating, while also assuming that the promotion of fresh, whole, local and organic food will solve the obesity problem.[49] By contrast, the Health at Every Size and "size acceptance" movements promote a different way of understanding the body and of addressing dietary issues related to obesity.[50] The Health at Every Size movement is critical of the equation of body mass index and health status—or what I have referred to as BMI reductionism. It instead promotes the idea that one can be "fat and fit" and emphasizes the importance of people adopting healthy dietary and exercise behaviors rather than focusing on losing weight as an end in itself.[51] They consider the focus on weight reduction promoted by mainstream nutrition experts and dietary guidelines as not only largely ineffective but also potentially detrimental to the goal of attaining good health.

It is important not to assume that promoting alternative ideas about food quality or other ways of identifying and engaging with food will in itself address poor diets or diet-related health problems, or that a lack of nutrition education is the problem. Most people can probably recognize poor-quality foods as they are defined here, even if they have only a sketchy knowledge of the types of ingredients or processing techniques used in their production. If consumers continue to purchase poor-quality foods, it probably has more to do with cost, accessibility, and convenience—as well as taste—rather than any great illusions regarding their healthfulness.[52] Whether in the form of raw ingredients or prepared foods, good-quality foods often cost more.[53] Eating better-quality food may therefore require spending more money on food, preparing more meals at home from scratch, or growing food at home or sourcing it from the local community or region through alternative supply chains. Good-quality meals can take longer to prepare, raising the question of whether everyone has the extra time—and skills—needed to purchase and cook the meals, especially when the burden continues to fall disproportionately on women. There are in this sense many economic and structural barriers preventing healthier food purchasing and preparation practices that cannot be addressed by reforms within the food system alone.

Instead of providing alternative dietary advice and better food labeling, or expecting people to pay more for better-quality food, there should be more stringent policies that regulate the kinds of food produced. This may include placing limits on the types and quantities of agricultural chemicals applied to crops or on the types and quantities of refined and reconstituted ingredients and additives used in processed and fast foods. Hydrogenated oils, for example, do not belong in the food supply, yet there are still no regulations prohibiting their use in the United States nor in most other countries, and they are most likely to be found in cheap, highly processed or fast foods. The use of added sugars in foods and beverages could similarly be directly regulated.

The food quality paradigm outlined here emphasizes the evaluation of foods in terms of their production and processing quality, an appreciation of the wisdom embedded in traditional and culturally contextualized dietary patterns, and the knowledge of food quality gained from our own sensual and practical engagement with growing, preparing, and consuming food. However, while providing other ways of understanding the relationship between food and bodily health, this knowledge is often general in nature and does not specifically link foods or dietary patterns to particular diseases, bodily functions, or health outcomes. Yet this is the kind of precise knowledge that we look to nutrition science to provide, whether the research is focused on nutrients, foods, or dietary patterns. The food quality paradigm does not reject nutritional or scientific forms of knowledge but provides a framework within which all of these approaches can be integrated and contextualized.

CHAPTER TEN

After Nutritionism

Food, not nutrients, is the fundamental unit of nutrition.
—DAVID JACOBS AND LINDA TAPSELL, 2007

Nutritionism, as I have emphasized throughout this book, is characterized by the reductive scientific focus on and interpretation of nutrients, rather than simply by the study or reference to nutrients per se. In recent years, and particularly since the publication of Michael Pollan's *In Defense of Food* in 2008, commentators in the popular media, blogs, and scientific journals have more openly discussed and debated the limitations of nutricentric scientific research and dietary advice. Now the refrain of many nutrition and public health experts is that we "eat food, not nutrients" and that dietary guidelines should therefore be food-based rather than nutrient-based.[1] Nutrition scientists have also directed much more of their research at the level of foods and dietary patterns over the past decade.

The food quality paradigm introduced in chapter 9 places the production and processing quality of food at the center of our understanding of food and health. Traditional and cultural knowledge of food and food combinations and the sensual and practical experience of producing and consuming food provide other ways of understanding and contextualizing the relationship between food and the body. These approaches provide alternatives to the scientific and nutricentric analysis of food and health and may to a certain extent displace our reliance on nutritional knowledge. Yet while these approaches offer valuable insights and criteria for assessing foods and dietary patterns, they do not always provide the kinds of specific knowledge and understanding of foods and bodily health that

we look for from nutrition science. In some situations we may require—
and many people will continue to demand—this more specific form of
scientific knowledge of nutrients, foods, and dietary patterns to inform
our dietary practices and to address diet-related health problems. This is
particularly true for people facing serious diet-related health problems,
such as type 2 diabetes, as well as those people on restricted diets who may
want to ensure that they are not missing out on any important nutrients,
such as vegetarians and vegans. With so many highly processed and novel
food ingredients and products on the market, we also need dedicated scientific research to guide our understanding—and, more important, the
regulation—of these types of food products.

The challenge for nutrition experts is to carry out and interpret scientific research into nutrients, foods, and dietary patterns in a manner that
avoids the decontextualization, oversimpliflication, exaggeration, and hubris that have characterized the nutritionism paradigm. This chapter out-
lines some of these alternative approaches to nutrition research, dietary
guidelines, and food labeling and also suggests how individuals might
navigate the contemporary nutriscape.

Throwing the Baby Out with the Bathwater

A common interpretation of Pollan's critique of nutritionism in his book
In Defense of Food is that he is asking us to stop using nutrition science and
nutritional knowledge altogether as a way of understanding good food. In
Real Food for Mother and Baby, for example, "real food" advocate Nina Planck
begins by acknowledging some of the limitations of nutritionism identified by Pollan: "Nutritionism hasn't served us well, and like the sensible
Michael Pollan, I'm against it." Yet she also admits that her book is filled
with nutritional facts and arguments: "Far better I confess now. I'll talk
about the nutrients you need in order to have a healthy baby and where to
get them. I don't know a better way."[2] Planck calls this a "paradox," having
interpreted Pollan's account of nutritionism as implying we should not
need to refer to nutrients at all to understand what makes a healthy diet.
Similarly, British food policy expert Tim Lang and his colleagues argue
that Pollan "calls on policy-makers and consumers to follow simple or
common-sensical dietary behaviour, rooted in culture and tradition. This
requires no-one to be a nutritionist. 'Don't eat anything your grand-
mother wouldn't recognize as food,' suggested Pollan."[3] They, too, interpret Pollan as rejecting the need for nutrition science, and they respond by

defending the contribution of nutrition science to the understanding of nutrient deficiencies and chronic diseases and to the development of public health policies.

While *In Defense of Food* can certainly be read as a dismissal of nutrition science and nutrient-level knowledge, it is rather ambiguous—and ultimately contradictory—on this key point. Pollan begins by criticizing not just the ideology of nutritionism, but arguing that the whole of nutrition science and dietary advice has done more harm than good to the nation's health. By the end of the book, however, Pollan is selectively, though uncritically, drawing upon nutrition science to explain the benefits of eating some foods rather than others. He provides definitive explanations for the health effects of omega-3 fats, antioxidants, *trans*-fats, and calorie restriction and of the dietary causes of particular diseases and bodily conditions such as diabetes and obesity. Ironically, like those he criticizes, he attributes to single nutrients great explanatory power. His nutritional explanations are also orthodox, rather than offering an alternative interpretation of this nutritional knowledge. His discussion of omega-3, omega-6, and *trans*-fats, for example, falls neatly into the "good-and-bad nutrient" discourse, which he acknowledges yet cannot help but reproduce.

Pollan does not attempt to explain how the nutrient-level science he dismisses differs from the one that he uncritically draws on. For example, why is the science on omega-3 fats any more accurate and reliable than the science on saturated fats which he derides? He apparently cannot imagine any way of doing nutrition research other than in a reductive manner. In drawing upon standard nutritional knowledge to support his own dietary advice, he writes,

> Much of the nutrition science I've presented here qualifies as reductionist science, focusing as it does on individual nutrients (such as certain fats or carbohydrates or antioxidants) rather than on whole foods or dietary patterns. Guilty. But using this sort of science to try to figure out what's wrong with the Western diet is probably unavoidable. However imperfect, it's the sharpest experimental and explanatory tool we have.[4]

Pollan largely defers to the latest knowledge and theories of nutrition as the basis for deciding what's right and wrong in nutrition science, while belittling older and now discredited nutritional theories. In this respect, his criticisms tend to be mounted from within the terms of mainstream nutrition science rather than proposing some other way of evaluating or contextualizing these nutritional theories. He even promotes the taking of multivitamin and mineral supplements for those older than fifty, as well as a fish oil supplement, in much the same terms as many nutrition experts—that is, as a kind of insurance policy against the risk of nutrient deficiencies as the result of an inadequate diet.[5]

Pollan also accepts and repeats nutritionists' definitive statements regarding the relationship between particular foods or dietary patterns and health outcomes, including making definitive declarations on the health impacts of the so-called Western diet. For example, he notes that several studies point to the conclusion that the more meat there is in your diet— especially red meat—the greater your risk of heart disease and cancer.[6] While these studies may have used meat rather than saturated fat as their basic unit of analysis, Pollan does not make clear why we should accept scientists' definitive conclusions in these food-based studies any more than those in nutrient-based studies.

INTEGRATED NUTRITION RESEARCH

If nutrition science is to avoid the pitfalls of nutritionism, then nutrition experts need to design, interpret, and apply the results of nutrient-level research in ways that avoid the kinds of premature, decontextualized, deterministic, oversimplified, and exaggerated interpretations of these relationships that have so often characterized the history of nutrition research and dietary guidelines. This may mean refraining from coming to definitive conclusions on the role of nutrients and foods and resisting the urge to rapidly translate research findings into dietary advice for the lay public. Another problem with generating decontextualized nutritional knowledge—the kind that attributes definitive health effects to single, isolated food components outside of any food or dietary context—is that it is easily appropriated by food companies to market their products.

An alternative approach to scientific research is to more strongly contextualize nutrient-level studies in terms of the types of foods and dietary patterns in which nutrients are embedded and to integrate these various levels of engagement with food. Some researchers have referred to the need for "top-down" approaches to food—that is, starting at the level of dietary patterns and working down to the nutrient level—rather than the currently dominant "bottom-up" approaches that begin with nutrients and work their way up to dietary patterns. These top-down and bottom-up approaches could also be fruitfully combined.[7]

Nutritional epidemiologist David Jacobs has been interrogating the limitations of nutricentric scientific research over the past decade and is particularly critical of the overwhelming focus of nutrition research on single nutrients and its failure to account for the possible synergies among nutrients found in the "food matrix" of whole foods. Jacobs and his colleagues have begun to map out alternatives to this single-nutrient focus, though largely within the terms of mainstream technoscientific approaches. As the title of one of his papers suggests, "Food, not nutrients, is the fundamental unit of nutrition."[8] Jacobs argues that the interactions among nutrients and other food components in whole foods will have greater effects than any single component alone. Studying whole foods, or whole food extracts, may thereby avoid some of the problems associated with attributing health effects to single components. Jacobs focuses on the synergies that may occur not only among nutrients within single foods but also among foods when eaten in combination. He therefore argues for the need to study food combinations and broader dietary patterns.

Jacobs advocates designing studies that work at a number of "food synergy levels"—the levels of single nutrients, food extracts, single foods, food groups, food combinations, and dietary patterns, respectively. Different types of studies may be more appropriate for each of these levels, with observational and clinical studies more appropriate for food and dietary patterns analysis and in vitro and animal studies for studying food components. He suggests that studies at these various levels be interpreted together to find common patterns, though what this means in practice is somewhat unclear, and few studies seem to be explicitly designed to integrate these levels of studying foods.[9] Some of the insights offered from studying foods at these various levels are illustrated by the history of scientists' attempts to explain the relationship between diet and heart disease. Since the 1960s, researchers have focused primarily on fats and their effects on blood cholesterol. Jacobs notes that recent studies on some plant foods and food combinations have also been shown to achieve reductions in blood cholesterol levels. Biochemical markers of heart disease other than blood cholesterol levels have also emerged. These more recent studies and findings, discussed in chapter 4, have thereby contextualized and decentered the earlier theories regarding dietary fats and painted a more complex picture of the various factors that may contribute to cardiovascular diseases.

Jacobs illustrates the importance of food synergy by comparing the results of single-nutrient studies with studies that have examined food extracts, single foods, and dietary patterns. Whole foods and food extracts have been shown to deliver more beneficial outcomes—at least in terms of their effects on particular biomarkers—when compared with the particular nutrients or components within these foods that had been assumed to be the main source of their health benefits. For example, Jacobs cites research comparing pomegranate juice with some of its isolated polyphenol constituents, which showed that the juice produced higher antioxidant activity and greater protection against tumor proliferation. These studies provide a way of contextualizing the study of individual food components in terms of their food source.[10] However, such findings are not particularly surprising, even from a nutricentric perspective, because most scientists would expect that whole foods contain a greater variety and quantity of beneficial nutrients than refined/extracted foods have. The health benefits of these whole foods may also simply be due to the cumulative benefits of each individual nutrient, rather than to synergies among them.[11]

Jacobs's own research group has examined the health effects of whole grains versus refined grains. One study compared two groups of women eating the same amount of fiber in their overall dietary patterns. One group obtained this fiber primarily from whole grain foods—such as whole grain bread, rice, and breakfast cereals—while the other group obtained most of their fiber intake from refined grain foods, such as white bread, pasta, muffins, and desserts. Jacobs found that the whole grain group had a significantly lower mortality from all causes than the refined grain group. He concludes from this that the better health of the whole grain group cannot be attributed to the fiber in the whole grain alone but perhaps to other bioactive components present in the whole grains, such as the antioxidants. He therefore suggests that the differences in outcomes cannot be reduced to the presence or absence of single food components. Perhaps it is the combined effects of these various single nutrients, or the interactions among nutrients, that bring about these beneficial health effects.

It is worth noting that women in the whole grain group also ate more red meat, fish, fruits, and vegetables and were less likely to smoke, which makes attributing the benefits to the whole grains highly questionable. Other studies have found that those who consume more whole grains also tend to eat better-quality diets overall and have healthier lifestyles, including exercising more and being less likely to smoke.[12] Studies examining the relationship between whole grain intake and cardiovascular disease risk have delivered mixed results.[13] What these various trials highlight is the difficulty of conducting and interpreting dietary studies to test even single foods or food components, and the danger of drawing definitive conclusions from epidemiological studies regarding their specific health effects.

Many researchers now advocate dietary pattern analysis as a way to move beyond the limitations of both single-nutrient and single-food research. Jacobs characterizes dietary pattern research as the "highest level in the food synergy approach."[14] He refers to studies reporting the benefits of the Mediterranean diet and the "prudent" diet compared with the so-called Western pattern, while acknowledging the uncertainties associated with attempts to identify the role of particular foods within these dietary patterns. Some of these limitations of dietary pattern research are discussed in chapter 7. Dietary pattern analysis is often a highly statistical enterprise that attempts to evaluate the health of people whose diets approximate particular dietary patterns, rather than actually following the precise dietary pattern under investigation. Researchers also often measure the health effects of these dietary patterns in terms of their impacts on disease biomarkers, rather than directly on disease or health outcomes; they therefore rely on the dominant scientific understanding of these biomarkers. At the same time, particular dietary patterns may be correlated with other socioeconomic and lifestyle patterns, thereby confounding the relationship between dietary patterns and health outcomes.

The beneficial dietary patterns commonly identified by researchers—such as the Mediterranean, prudent, and DASH diets—almost exclusively comprise minimally processed, good-quality foods. These good-quality diets are in turn invariably contrasted with diets high in poor-quality, highly refined and processed foods, usually referred to as the Western dietary pattern or the standard American diet. These studies certainly suggest that any whole food dietary pattern may be healthful when compared with highly processed food diets. But they reveal little about whether particular types of whole foods are more healthful than others. The inclusion of red meat in the Western dietary pattern is particularly problematic. The close association of meat with highly processed food consumption within the standard American/Western dietary pattern potentially confounds the health effects of meat. It also suggests that dietary pattern analysis remains tied to the dominant nutritional understandings of fat and saturated fat, rather than departing from these nutrient-level assumptions.

From the perspective of the food quality paradigm, more research should focus directly on the evaluation of ingredients, foods, and dietary patterns in terms of the levels of processing, and particularly the many synthetic chemicals and technologically transformed and degraded ingredients in the food supply. This would include measuring and comparing foods consumed in observational or controlled studies according to whether they are minimally or highly processed. Until recently, there has been a surprising lack of studies on highly processed foods. Some exceptions are the many studies that have been conducted on *trans*-fats and sugary sodas since the 1990s. Some cancer studies have distinguished between unprocessed and processed meats in their dietary surveys. The studies by Jacobs and others that I referred to earlier comparing whole grains and refined grains do distinguish between levels of processing of grain; however, refined grain and refined flour are used in a range of food products that differ widely in terms of their quality. For example, a loaf of white sourdough bread should not be placed in the same category as a sugary breakfast cereal or a highly sweetened and adulterated muffin, even though they are all high in refined grains or "refined carbs." So it is important to ask about the quality of the foods in which the refined flour is contained. Nutrient-level studies should also more accurately identify and distinguish among the categories of processed foods being consumed or tested. For example, does saturated fat have the same health effects in steaks and sausages?[15] Similarly, the combination of particular nutrients or ingredients in highly processed foods may be important to study, such as the high levels of added fats and sugars that tend to be concentrated in these foods.

Where nutrient-level, food-level, and dietary-level evidence is found to be in conflict rather than in agreement, an alternative to nutritionism is to place our faith in food and dietary pattern evidence. This includes not only the scientific analysis of foods and dietary patterns—in the form of epidemiological, clinical, and lab studies—but also with reference to the food production and processing quality and the cultural-traditional knowledge of food and dietary patterns. For example, the dietary recommendations to reduce total fat intake to less than 30 percent of calories is contradicted by the apparent good health of Mediterranean populations consuming up to 40 percent of calories from fat.[16] Given the uncertainties in the science of fats and blood cholesterol beginning in the 1960s, scientists could have erred on the side of butter rather than margarine, on the basis of both food quality (butter is minimally processed) and traditional-cultural knowledge (butter has a history of safe use and is an integral part of many healthy cuisines).

While food- and dietary-level scientific studies provide a way of contextualizing and decentering nutrient-level knowledge, this research is equally subject to some of the limitations and pitfalls associated with nutricentric research. Identifying the role of single foods or food groups within a given dietary pattern can be as difficult and complex a process as isolating and attributing these effects to a specific nutrient. There are just as many dietary, lifestyle, and environmental factors that can confound the results of food and dietary pattern studies as there are for nutrient-level studies. The measure of a food's or dietary pattern's health impacts may also similarly be based on a narrow range of quantifiable biomarkers—rather than disease incidence or other health outcomes—and therefore be similarly subject to the kinds of biomarker reductionism that characterize nutrient-level studies.

ALTERNATIVE DIETARY GUIDELINES

Some of the limitations of dietary guidelines and nutritional advice dispensed under the sway of the nutritionism paradigm have been identified throughout this book. Since the 1970s, government-endorsed dietary guidelines have been framed in terms of nutrients rather than foods and have promoted the dominant message that we should think about and choose foods on the basis of a fairly narrow set of nutrient components and nutritional concepts. These nutritional recommendations have often prematurely translated nutritional hypotheses into definitive dietary advice, or they have simplified the scientific understanding of the role of these nutrients due to the difficulties of conveying to a general audience any more nuanced, complex, and contextualized advice.

Since the 1980s, government authorities and experts have also issued ample food-level guidance, such as in the form of the *Food Guide Pyramid*. In recent years, many nutrition experts have also called for a substantial shift from nutrient-based to food-based dietary guidelines and food guides.[17] However, there have been two main limitations of food-based dietary guidelines to date. First, food-specific advice has been based primarily on the nutrient composition of foods, rather than on research into specific foods, thereby reinforcing the nutricentric bias. Second, food-level recommendations and food-based guidelines have referred almost exclusively to different categories of whole foods but have made little reference to the level of processing these foods are subjected to.

In 2011 the U.S. Department of Agriculture (USDA) introduced the *MyPlate* food-based guide (figure 10.1) to replace *MyPyramid*, which itself had earlier replaced the original *Food Guide Pyramid*. However, *MyPlate* reproduces many of the limitations of the *Food Guide Pyramid* discussed in chapter 4. *MyPlate* is divided primarily into food groups (fruits, vegetables,

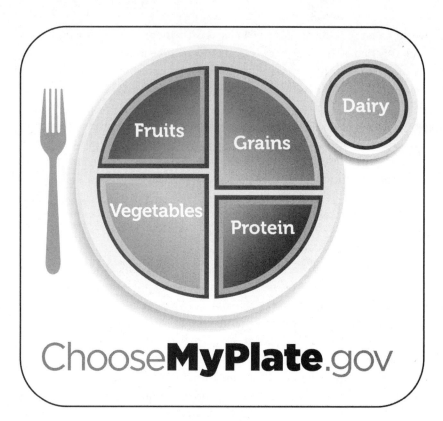

FIGURE 10.1

MyPlate

SOURCE: U.S. Department of Agriculture, *MyPlate* (Washington, D.C.: Center for Nutrition Policy and Promotion, 2011).

grains, and dairy), but it also includes the nutrient group "protein," which refers to protein-rich foods such as meat, seafood, and legumes. The USDA's emphasis on whole food groups reinforces the idea that the primary problem with contemporary American diets is an imbalance between these different whole food groups, rather than the level of processing that each of these types of foods typically undergo. Within the more specific recommendations for the grains food group, a distinction is made between whole grain and refined grain foods, with the recommendation to "Make at least half your grains whole grains."[18] But few such distinctions based on levels of processing are to be found within the other food groups. The fruit and vegetable group, for example, counts 100 percent fruit juice as equivalent to whole fruit.

The kinds of highly processed meals, snacks, and desserts made from combinations of refined-extracted, processed-reconstituted, and deep-fried ingredients are not acknowledged by the plate itself. One has to dig deeper into the *MyPlate* guidelines, to the section on "Empty Calories," to find the advice to cut back on foods high in solid fats, added sugars, and salt.[19] The USDA's message is that these specific nutrients and ingredients need to be avoided, rather than the highly processed foods in which they are often contained. The USDA's definition of empty-calorie foods are those that contain "solid fats" (i.e., saturated and *trans*-fats) and added sugars, but this nutrient-based definition therefore includes whole foods and beneficially processed foods such as whole milk, butter, and bacon. Nevertheless, the 2010 version of the *Dietary Guidelines for Americans* and the accompanying *MyPlate* are more explicit than ever before about the need to restrict intake of products such as sugary soft drinks.

In a 2010 commentary in the *Journal of the American Medical Association*, two leading nutrition scientists, Dariush Mozaffarian and David Ludwig, make the case for a shift from nutrient-based to food-based dietary guidelines.[20] They begin with a blunt assessment of past dietary guidelines, noting some of the flaws in the dominant nutritional recommendations of recent decades regarding the prevention of chronic disease. These include the advice to reduce total energy from fat, and they admit that saturated fat "has little relation to risk of cardiovascular disease within most prevailing dietary patterns." They suggest that "with few exceptions (e.g., omega-3 fats, *trans* fat, salt), individual compounds in isolation have small effects on chronic diseases." Mozaffarian and Ludwig also note how nutrient categories such as "carbohydrates" and "protein" conflate different types of foods that contain these nutrients, such as whole wheat and white bread, or chicken and beans. Nutrient-based guidelines may also lead to "dietary practices that defy common sense," such as the marketing of highly processed foods that have merely substituted refined carbohydrates for fat. What is slightly odd about their arguments is that these authors continue to promote such nutricentric guidelines and concepts in their work. Mozaffarian advocates the replacement of saturated with polyunsaturated fats and is involved in the formulation of the American Heart Association's nutricentric dietary guidelines, while Ludwig promotes the use of the glycemic index for determining food quality.[21]

While acknowledging some of the limits of nutricentric guidelines, Mozaffarian and Ludwig claim that we already have substantial scientific evidence that "specific foods and dietary patterns substantially affect chronic disease risk, as shown by controlled trials of risk factors and prospective cohorts of disease end points."[22] This is arguably an exaggeration of the current state of the science and ignores the limitations of the food and dietary pattern research noted earlier. They refer to the benefits of fruits, vegetables, whole grains, and fish and the detrimental effects of processed meats, packaged and fast foods, and sugar-sweetened beverages. Yet they also claim that "healthy eating patterns share many characteristics, emphasizing whole or minimally processed foods and vegetable oils, with few highly processed foods or sugary beverages. Such diets are also naturally lower in salt, *trans*-fat, saturated fat, refined carbohydrates, and added sugars; [and] are higher in unsaturated fats, fiber, antioxidants, minerals, and phytochemicals."[23]

Here we can see a reinforcement of the conventional nutrient-level assumptions within the dominant nutritional paradigm, including the replacement of saturated fat with unsaturated fat, the celebration of vegetable oils (presumably over butter), and the promotion of "prudent" dietary patterns that embody these nutrient-level assumptions. It becomes clear that Mozaffarian and Ludwig's primary rationale for providing food-level guidelines is that they are a more effective means of ensuring that the public adheres to existing nutrient-level recommendations. Indeed, they note that "a focus on foods increases the likelihood of [people] consuming more healthy nutrients and fewer calories and decreasing [their] chronic disease risk." In other words, food-based guidelines will continue to reflect conventional nutrient-level scientific research, yet the public need only be advised of the food-level advice. They make no mention of how this food-level advice would be presented, such as whether it would refer to levels and types of food processing. But the authors hope that such food-based guidelines might "remedy widespread misperceptions about what constitutes healthful diets." Once again, members of the public, rather than the nutrition experts themselves, are portrayed as confused and plagued by "misperceptions."[24]

A more thorough revision of dietary guidelines that is consistent with the food quality paradigm would question not only their nutricentric character but also how the specific food-level recommendations are derived and represented. This includes questioning the provision of oversimplified food-level and nutrient-level information. An alternative to telling people precisely "what to eat," or giving them "rules" to eat by, is to provide more detailed nutrient-level and food-level information. For example, dietary guidelines could provide information about how to recognize and categorize these various types of foods. An alternative

Food Quality Pyramid could differentiate among three categories of food based on food processing: whole (minimally, beneficially, traditionally processed) foods, refined-processed foods, and processed-reconstituted foods.

Given the diverse range of healthful dietary patterns, diets, and cultural cuisines being followed across the nation, the provision of specific and uniform food-level advice for the whole population, such as "eat two to three serves of dairy a day," is of questionable value. Another approach would be to document various healthful dietary patterns, cuisines, and food combinations that could be followed and that could inspire healthful dietary changes. When presented in this fashion, both food-level and nutrient-level advice can be contextualized, providing a cultural and cuisine-based framework for incorporating dietary advice while acknowledging the limitations of single-nutrient or single-whole food advice. For example, even though white rice is a refined grain, it can be the basis of a healthful meal when eaten in combination with legumes or whole meat.

Dietary guidelines should also be contextualized in terms of their implications for environmental sustainability and animal welfare. Food production and consumption practices have significant environmental impacts resulting from the growing, processing, packaging, transportation, and retailing of food. Some of the greatest impacts arise from the large scale production of meat and dairy products, fish, soy and vegetable oils, highly processed and packaged foods, and the long-distance transportation of both fresh and processed foods.[25] A narrow and prescriptive set of nutritional and dietary recommendations may contribute to, or lock people into, consumption practices that are more resource-intensive, ecologically unsustainable, and cruel to animals. For example, dietary guidelines that promote more omega-3 fats, or two or three servings of dairy, may promote unsustainable fishing practices and increased dairy production.[26] The promotion of white meat as a supposedly healthier alternative to red meat has fueled the rise in per capita poultry consumption in recent decades, and this demand for affordable chicken has largely been met through cruel factory-farming practices. Over the past decade public health nutritionists have been strong promoters of the idea of integrating socioeconomic and ecological concerns into dietary guidelines and public health policies.[27] An acknowledgment of the adaptability of humans to a wide variety of healthful dietary patterns creates space for more sustainable and humane food production and consumption practices, and that are adapted to locally available and seasonal foods.

Detailed Food Labeling and the End of
Nutritional Marketing

Freed of the distorting influences of the nutritionism paradigm—and of food industry lobbying—food labeling and food marketing regulations should be fundamentally overhauled to provide more detailed nutrient and ingredient information, while also denying companies the ability to make decontextualized and exaggerated nutrient-content and health claims.

The Nutrition Facts label could be replaced with a Food Quality label. The most important labeling innovation would be to enhance and prioritize information required to be listed by food companies regarding the type, quality, quantity, and source of the ingredients in foods. This information should be presented more prominently than nutritional information. A more comprehensive ingredients list would specify the types of processing that each of the ingredients and additives has been subjected to and the percentage or weight of each product. The ingredients list could also include relevant information on the source of some of the ingredients, such as place of origin, organic versus chemically grown, and free range or confined, and the presence of genetically modified ingredients, pesticides, hormones, and antibiotics. From a health and ecological perspective, all of this information is relevant to both consumers and experts. Such information about the ingredients in food would require considerably more space than is allocated at present, particularly for highly processed products containing many ingredients and additives.

The selective nutritional information currently included on the Nutrition Facts label presents an oversimplified and misleading view of the nutritional composition of foods. Nutrient-level information—if it is to be of any real value—should be comprehensive and detailed. The full range of relevant nutrient categories and subcategories could be listed. With respect to fats, for example, the various types of saturated fats (e.g., stearic acid) and polyunsaturated fats (e.g., omega-3, omega-6) could be included, since there is some evidence that they each have distinct roles in bodily functioning and health outcomes. The food and technological sources of these nutrients should also be identified. Has the fat been extracted from animal products or vegetable oil? Has the polyunsaturated fat been hydrogenated, interesterified, or used for deep frying? Are the vitamins naturally occurring in the ingredients, or have they been added during processing? For nutrition experts and the public, such detailed information is relevant to their assessment of the nutritional value of a food. For consumers, this information would immediately convey the complexity of the composition of a food and give them opportunity to make a better informed choice about a food while deterring simplistic interpretations. Admittedly, some people will be overwhelmed by more detailed nutritional information and may instead defer to the ingredients list.

The mandatory, front-of-pack traffic-light labeling systems advocated by many public health institutions and experts in the United States, the United Kingdom, and Europe have the potential to provide consumers with simple, at-a-glance, prejudgments on the healthfulness of a food. However, the four criteria that are typically included in most existing or proposed schemes are total fat, saturates (a conflation of saturated fats and *trans*-fats), sugar, and salt. This heavy emphasis on fats maintains the focus of consumers and health experts on nutrients. Sugar and salt, on the other hand, are ingredients and are fairly reliable indicators of the quality of a food—the higher the levels of sugar and salt, the more highly processed and degraded the food is likely to be. Of these four criteria, high sugar content is arguably of greatest concern regarding detrimental health outcomes. However, if the criteria for communicating food quality remain focused on sugar, salt, and fat, this allows—indeed encourages—food companies to merely reformulate some of their products with lower quantities of these components and replace them with other processed ingredients. An alternative traffic light system could focus entirely on the quality of the ingredients, particularly ingredients considered most harmful to health. In addition, the traffic light label could signal the overall quality of the product: a green light for minimally processed, good-quality foods; an amber light for moderate-quality, refined-processed foods; and a red light for poor-quality foods high in refined-extracted and processed-reconstituted ingredients.[28]

Nutrient-content claims and all forms of health claims should simply be prohibited, since invariably they exaggerate or distort the significance of particular nutrients or ingredients in food products and their associated health effects.[29] Nutrient-content claims exaggerate the importance of single nutrients within the context of the whole food product, regardless of the level of scientific evidence of their benefits. Health claims—whether in the form of structure/function or disease prevention claims—go a step further and make definitive claims regarding an ingredient's health benefits. Consumers could instead draw their own conclusions regarding the quality of a food from the more detailed ingredient and nutrition information.

While waiting for scientific research, dietary guidelines, and food labeling regulations to be based on a less reductive and more integrated understanding of food and nutrients, members of the nutri-skeptic lay public must find their own way through the nutritional maze. While ignoring nutrition science altogether is one option, ultimately we need a framework for negotiating and contextualizing existing forms of nutrient-level dietary information. The food quality paradigm provides such a framework for navigating the nutriscape. This approach involves prioritizing food production and processing quality, drawing upon traditional-cultural and sensual-practical ways of understanding food where appropriate, and using these to contextualize and temper scientific claims relating to nutrients, foods, and dietary patterns.

Nutrition science has been most useful in progressively identifying the nutrient components in whole foods and some of the bodily requirements for these nutrients. It can be helpful to know which nutrients are found in particular foods, and this knowledge can suggest some of the benefits of eating some types of food and food combinations. However, the scientific estimates regarding the precise daily allowances of nutrients that people should consume to prevent nutrient deficiencies or to reduce the risk of chronic disease must be treated with a good dose of skepticism. Such claims presuppose a high level of scientific precision in the understanding of food and the body. Similarly, it pays to be skeptical of claims that we require megadoses of particular nutrients, which will most likely need to be consumed in the form of dietary supplements or fortified foods. Nutrient intake recommendations are also invariably for single nutrients and therefore cannot convey information about nutrient interactions and their possible health implications. We should also resist succumbing to the perceptions of nutrient scarcity that have been promoted by some nutrition experts and by the functional food and supplements industries—the idea that we just cannot get enough of the necessary nutrients from everyday and conventionally grown or prepared foods.

Scientific claims regarding the link between a nutrient and a particular bodily function or process can be useful. For example, the claims that calcium helps build bone density or that refined flour produces steep rises in blood glucose and insulin levels give us some insights into the role of these foods and nutrients. Yet interpreting the significance of this relationship can be difficult and risks oversimplification, exaggeration, and decontextualization. For instance, the action of calcium is also mediated by the presence of vitamin D; similarly, the impact of refined flour on blood glucose levels will depend on the types of foods in which it is contained and eaten in conjunction with. An associated danger here is that of biomarker reductionism and biomarker determinism—the mistake of assuming that fluctuations in particular biomarkers in and of themselves directly increase disease incidence or affect metabolic problems.

The least reliable nutritional claims are those purporting to show a direct relationship between nutrients, foods, or dietary patterns and chronic diseases. There are certainly many interesting hypotheses regarding the dietary causes of heart disease, cancer, and diabetes, many of which point to the overconsumption of refined-extracted and processed-reconstituted foods and ingredients, such as between *trans*-fats or oxidized polyunsaturated fats and heart disease and between "refined carbohydrates" (highly refined grain or sugar) and diabetes. But the scientific knowledge underpinning these links is often highly contested and far from definitive. The simplified focus on any one component in the etiology of these chronic diseases ignores the possible interactions among a number of food components and the combination of foods in dietary patterns. Many dietary patterns have been associated with reduced risk of chronic diseases. Yet I have argued that the distinguishing feature of these dietary patterns is that they are all based on good-quality whole foods rather than any specific configuration of whole foods or macronutrient ratios.

An alternative way of interpreting nutrient-level claims is to contextualize them in terms of food production and processing quality, traditional-cultural knowledge, and sensual-practical experience. For example, is the nutrient in question a key component of good-quality whole foods, and has it been a part of some traditional dietary pattern? It can be useful to know, for example, that omega-3 fats, and many other beneficial nutrients, are found in walnuts, but encouraging people to boost their intake of isolated wonder nutrients fetishizes particular foods and distorts what should be our real goal: simply eating a diet consisting of good-quality foods. The important question is, of course, how to define what we mean by "good quality." Ultimately, we need to become *food quality literate*, rather than just nutritionally literate, and to err on the side of skepticism toward decontextualized nutritional advice.

Constructing alternatives to nutritionism ultimately requires more than carrying out and interpreting nutrition science differently, developing alternative dietary guidelines, or adopting personal strategies for navigating the nutriscape. Given food corporations' central role in perpetuating the ideology of nutritionism, their level of influence over government policies and scientific research, and their ability to nutritionally market their products, the power of these corporations must also be addressed. Limiting or removing the food industry's ability to use nutrient and health claims is an important step, as this is the primary means through which nutritional knowledge is now disseminated to the public, as well as a primary strategy for marketing highly processed foods. Limiting industry influence over the governments' dietary guidelines and food regulations is also essential if those guidelines and regulations are to be in the interests of public health, social equity, and ecological sustainability.

The provision of good quality food for all also requires direct government regulation of food quality and of the types of foods that can be produced and marketed. The best way to limit the consumption of processed-reconstituted foods is not through nutrition education campaigns, nor regressive "fat taxes," but by limiting—through strict food composition regulations—the food industry's ability to produce poor-quality foods. Determining the criteria for such food regulations means drawing on the latest nutrition science, and therefore negotiating the limitations, debates, and uncertainties within nutrition research. But the focus of research and debate also needs to shift from differentiating between the health implications of whole foods or naturally occurring nutrients, to differentiating and identifying the health effects of foods on the basis of food production and processing quality. Nutrition experts can either lead or be led by the burgeoning food-quality movement and can choose to play a key role in developing food-quality literacy and food policies that promote and protect the quality of our food.

ACKNOWLEDGMENTS

I would like to thank those colleagues and reviewers who read through all or sections of the manuscript and provided invaluable suggestions at various stages of its development, especially to Kerin O'Dea, Charlotte Biltekoff, Julie Guthman, Rosemary Stanton, Mark Lawrence, Adel Yousif, David Jacobs, and Kristen Lyons. Thanks to Karen Walker who carefully read the manuscript for scientific accuracy, though any remaining errors are my own. Stephen James did a tremendous job editing and improving the manuscript. Cristina Lochert was very generous with her time and editing skills. My thanks also to Clare Forster for her helpful publishing advice.

At Columbia University Press, I'm very grateful to Jennifer Crewe for her commitment to the book, and to Kathryn Schell, Asya Graf, Justine Evans, Marisa Pagano, and Derek Warker for guiding the book through the publishing labyrinth from beginning to end. At Westchester Book Services, Pamela Nelson did a marvelous job managing the production process, and Trish Watson meticulously copyedited the manuscript and ironed out any inconsistencies.

Finally, thanks to Mathilde, Rafi, and Ruli for giving me the space to write and for their love, support, and patience.

APPENDIX: THE NUTRITIONISM AND FOOD QUALITY LEXICON

This appendix lists terms, concepts, categories, distinctions, and expressions that I have developed to help analyze the forms, characteristics, and alternatives to nutritionism.

Forms of Reductionism

Ideology/paradigm of nutritionism	The dominant paradigm of nutrition science and dietary advice, primarily characterized by a nutritionally reductive approach to food
Nutritional reductionism	Reductive focus on the nutrient-level of engagement with food, and a reductive interpretation of the role of nutrients in bodily health
	Characteristics include decontextualization, simplification, fragmentation, exaggeration, and determinism with respect to the role of nutrients
Nutrient-level reductionism	The reduction of the understanding and practical engagement with food *to the* nutrient level
Single-nutrient reductionism	The further reductive focus on single nutrients *within* the nutrient level
Macronutrient reductionism	The reductive focus on and interpretation of the macronutrient profile of a food or dietary pattern with respect to their implications for health or weight impacts
Caloric reductionism	The reductive focus on and interpretation of the caloric value of a food, particularly with respect to the energy balance equation and weight changes
Nutritionally reductive technological products/practices	Translation of nutritionally reductive scientific knowledge into nutritionally engineered food products and nutritional supplements
Biomarker reductionism	Reductive focus on, and interpretation of, bodily health in terms of particular biomarkers (biological markers)
Food-level reductionism, single-food reductionism	Reductive focus on, and interpretation of, foods with respect to their health implications
Nutritionally reductive sociological explanations	Reductive and exaggerated explanation of how nutritional guidelines influence food consumption choices and dietary patterns

TABLE A.2
Levels of Engagement with Food and the Body

Levels of engagement with food	Nutrient level
	Food level (single foods, food groups, food combinations)
	Dietary level (dietary patterns)
Levels of engagement with the body	Whole body/embodied level
	Biochemical level
	Genetic level

TABLE A.3
Characteristics of Nutritionism

Nutritional gaze	Nutrition experts or the lay public seeing and encountering food primarily as a collection of nutrients
Myth of nutritional precision	The claimed precision of the scientific knowledge of the role of nutrients in food and the body
Nutritional hubris	An excessive confidence or arrogance in the precision and infallibility of current nutritional knowledge
Nutriscape	The nutritional landscape, refers to prevailing scientific knowledge, debates, technologies, institutions, industries, ideologies and identities associated with nutrition in a particular place and time
Nutrient-dense language and nutri-speak	Nutrient-level and nutricentric terms, categories, and concepts that displace food-level terms
Nutritional euphemisms	Nutrient-level terms used as euphemisms for types of foods
Everyday nutritionisms	Everyday nutritional expressions based on the logic of nutritionism
Nutri-quantification	A calculating and quantifying approach to nutrients and the body
Nutritional leveling	The flattening out of qualitative distinctions among types of foods based on the quantities of specific nutrients they contain
Nutrient fetishism	The worship of particular nutrients thought to be exceptionally health enhancing
Perception of nutrient scarcity	The perception that modern foods and modern diets are deficient in nutrients
Vitaminsurance	Vitamin insurance policy: the taking of vitamin supplements as a form of "health insurance" against inadequate vitamin intake

(continued)

Scientific management of nutrition	The use of scientific measurement and management techniques to monitor and control the nutritional intake of individuals and populations
Nutrient treadmill	The imperative to keep up with the latest nutrient-level knowledge, dietary advice, and nutritionally engineered products
Nutrient-level contradictions	Where the nutritional modification of a food, or other nutrient-level practices, conflicts with or affects the availability or absorption of other nutrients
Nutritional determinism	Where a nutrient is interpreted as directly determining a particular health outcome
Nutritional techno-fix	The attempt to address nutritionally inadequate foods or dietary patterns through the nutritional engineering of foods
Logic of nutritional interchangeability	The understanding of foods as interchangeable sources of nutrients, and the technological practice of arbitrarily adding and subtracting nutrients from foods
Genetic nutritionism	The intersection of nutrigenomics and nutritionism
Corporate nutritionism	The corporate capture of nutritionism in the contemporary era, such that corporations have become the primary drivers and promoters of nutritionism
Nutrient marker of food quality	A nutrient that is strongly correlated with good- or poor-quality foods and dietary patterns
Food quality literacy	An understanding of food production and processing quality
Nutricentric person	A person/subject whose understanding of and engagement with food and dietary health is nutricentric

TABLE A.4

Eras and Paradigms of Nutritionism

Era of quantifying nutritionism	Mid-nineteenth to mid-twentieth centuries
	Nutrients represented as protective
	Characterized by the logic of nutri-quantification and a focus on attaining an adequate quantity of protective and growth-promoting nutrients
	Bodies represented in quantified-mechanical terms and as nutrient-deficient
	Primary actors/drivers: nutrition scientists
Era of good-and-bad nutritionism	1960s to mid-1990s
	Nutrients differentiated into "good" and "bad" types
	Focus on bad nutrients and chronic disease risk
	Bodies represented as at-risk and overnourished
	Primary actors/drivers: government agencies and public health institutions
Era of functional nutritionism	Mid-1990s to present
	Nutrients and foods represented as functional and health enhancing
	Focus on the relationship between nutrients and internal bodily functions and biomarkers and on enhancing and optimizing health and specific bodily functioning
	Bodies represented as functional and nutritionally enhanced
	Primary actors/drivers: food industry/food corporations

TABLE A.5
Representations of the Body

Quantified-mechanical body & Nutrient-deficient body	Representation and experience of the body in mechanical and quantifiable terms, and as deficient in particular nutrients
	Associated with the era of quantifying nutritionism
At-risk body & Over-nourished body	Representation and experience of the body as being at-risk of disease and poor health, especially from the overconsumption of "bad" nutrients and calories
	Associated with the era of good-and-bad nutritionism
Functional body & Nutritionally-enhanced body	Representation and experience of the body in terms of a heightened focus on the relationship between nutrients and the body's internal processes and functions, and by the targeting and enhancement of particular bodily functions
	Associated with the era of functional nutritionism

TABLE A.6
Types of Nutritional Engineering and Marketing

Nutritionally engineered foods	Foods that have had their nutrient profile deliberately modified
Trans-nutric foods	Short for "trans-nutritionally engineered foods": nutritionally engineered foods that involve the transfer of nutrients across recognized food categories/boundaries
Nutritionally marketed foods	Foods marketed on the basis of their nutrient profile, i.e., with nutrient-content claims
Functionally marketed foods	Foods marketed with health claims, and as having specific and targeted health or functional benefits
Naturally marketed foods	Foods marketed on the basis of their claimed "natural" or "whole" food character
Nutritional facade	An image of a food's nutritional profile and characteristics constructed for marketing purposes, concealing the underlying ingredients and quality of a food

TABLE A.7
Categories/Levels of Processing of Food Ingredients

Whole food ingredients	Whole, minimally processed, and beneficially processed ingredients; fresh, preserved, or enhanced through fermentation, sprouting, and cooking
Refined-extracted ingredients	Extracted, refined, and concentrated ingredients and foods, often involving the removal of other beneficial food components from a whole food
Processed-reconstituted ingredients	Ingredients and foods that are broken down into their constituent components, and transformed, reconstituted, or significantly degraded during processing, preparation, and cooking

TABLE A.8
Categories/Levels of Processing of Foods and Food Products

Whole foods (minimally and beneficially processed foods)	Foods and meals prepared primarily with good-quality whole and minimally or beneficially processed ingredients; beneficial combinations of ingredients and foods; may also include some quantities of refined-extracted ingredients
Refined-processed foods	Foods produced with a combination of whole and refined-extracted ingredients, and only small quantities of processed-reconstituted ingredients
Processed-reconstituted foods	Highly processed foods that are constructed primarily out of processed-reconstituted and refined-extracted ingredients

TABLE A.9
The Food Quality Paradigm

Food production and processing quality	Evaluating food quality on the basis of types of food processing and primary production practices
Cultural-traditional knowledge	Cultural and traditional knowledge of healthful foods, food combinations, dietary patterns, and forms of food preparation
Sensual-practical experience	Knowledge of food quality derived from the senses and from the practical experience of growing, preparing, and consuming food
Nutritional-scientific analysis	Nutritional-scientific approaches to analyzing nutrients, foods, and dietary patterns

NOTES

1. A Clash of Nutritional Ideologies

1. The epigraph is from Robert Feron, "Technology and Production," in *Margarine: An Economic, Social and Scientific History 1869–1969*, ed. J.H. van Stuyvenberg, (Liverpool: Liverpool University Press, 1969), 83–122, 118.

2. The term *nutriscape* is short for nutritional landscape. It refers to the totality of the prevailing scientific knowledge, debates, technologies, institutions, industries, ideologies, and identities associated with nutrition in a particular place and time or time period. It is similar to the sense in which the term *healthscapes* is used by Adele Clarke with respect to medicine and healthcare, in "Charting (Bio) Medicine and (Bio)Medicalization in the United States, 1890–Present," in *Biomedicalization: Technoscience, Health and Illness in the U.S.*, ed. Adele Clarke et al. (Durham, N.C.: Duke University Press, 2010), 88–146, 105. John Coveney uses the term *nutrition landscape* in a slightly different sense, defining it as "the growing expanse of nutrition knowledge, rationales and understandings about food in terms of scientific and medical concerns" (John Coveney, *Food, Morals and Meanings: The Pleasure and Anxiety of Eating*, 2nd ed. [London: Routledge, 2006], 95).

3. Gyorgy Scrinis, "Sorry Marge," *Meanjin* 61, no. 4 (2002): 108–116; Scrinis, "On the Ideology of Nutritionism," *Gastronomica* 8, no. 1 (2008): 39–48; Scrinis, "Nutritionism and Functional Foods," in *The Philosophy of Food*, ed. David Kaplan (Berkeley: University of California Press, 2012), 269–291.

4. R.P. Mensink and M.K. Katan, "Effect of Dietary Trans Fatty Acids on High-Density and Low-Density Lipoprotein Cholesterol Levels in Healthy Subjects," *New England Journal of Medicine* 323 (1990): 439–445.

5. W.C. Willett et al., "Intake of Trans Fatty Acids and Risk of Coronary Heart Disease Among Women," *Lancet* 341 (1993): 581–585.

6. Kim Severson, "Trans Fat Fight Claims Butter as a Victim," *New York Times*, March 7, 2007.

7. U.S. Food and Drug Administration, "Labeling and Nutrition," www.fda.gov/Food/LabelingNutrition/default.htm (accessed August 12, 2009).

8. See, for e.g., Bijal Trivedi, "The Good, the Fad and the Unhealthy," *New Scientist* 191, no. 2570 (2006): 42–49; David Jacobs and Linda Tapsell, "Food, Not Nutrients, Is the Fundamental Unit in Nutrition," *Nutrition Reviews* 65, no. 10 (2007): 439–450.

9. Jacobs and Tapsell, "Food, Not Nutrients."

10. Kellogg Company, "Our Brands," www2.kelloggs.com/ProductDetail.aspx ?id=555 (accessed October 1, 2011); Paul Pestano et al., *Sugar in Children's Cereals: Popular Brands Pack More Sugar Than Snack Cakes and Cookies* (Washington, D.C.: Environmental Working Group, 2011).

11. On the U.S. counterculture's approach to meat in the 1960s and 1970s, see Warren James Belasco, *Appetite for Change: How the Counterculture Took on the Food Industry*, 2nd ed. (New York: Cornell University Press, 2007), 54–61.

12. See, e.g., Walter Mertz, "Food and Nutrients," *Journal of the American Dietetic Association* 84 (1984): 769–770; T. Colin Campbell, "The Dietary Causes of Degenerative Diseases: Nutrients vs Foods," in *Western Diseases: Their Dietary Prevention and Reversibility*, ed. N.J. Temple and D.P. Burkitt (Totowa, N.J.: Humana Press, 1994), 119–152; Margaret Allman-Farinelli, "Food for Thought or Thought for Food," *Australian Journal of Nutrition and Dietetics* 58, no. 1 (2001): 8–9; Ingrid Hoffman, "Transcending Reductionism in Nutrition Research," *American Journal of Clinical Nutrition* 78 (2003): 514S–516S.

13. This "levels of engagement with nature" framework has drawn upon and adapted the "levels of constitutive abstraction" social theoretical framework developed by Australian social theorist Geoff Sharp. See esp. Geoff Sharp, "Constitutive Abstraction and Social Practice," *Arena* 70 (1985): 48–82.

14. I am arguing here that the *form* (i.e., the nutricentric form) and not just the particular *content* of scientific knowledge has "effects" in terms of shaping forms of knowledge and practice. This is similar to the ways in which technologies or technological forms are able to shape or transform the form of social relations, quite aside from the particular ways in which they are used. An early theorist of this substantive understanding of technology, Marshall McLuhan, expressed this concept with his slogan, "The medium is the message." See Marshall McLuhan, *Understanding Media: The Extension of Man* (London: Sphere, 1967). See also Martin Heidegger, *The Question Concerning Technology and Other Essays* (New York: Harper and Row, 1977); Albert Borgmann, *Technology and the Character of Contemporary Life: A Philosophical Inquiry* (Chicago: University of Chicago Press, 1984).

15. Alan Chalmers, *What Is This Thing Called Science?*, 2nd ed. (St Lucia: University of Queensland Press, 1982), 90. Barbara Santich refers to paradigms in nutrition science in terms of the dominant theories within particular periods of the history of nutrition science in "Paradigm Shifts in the History of Dietary Advice in Australia," *Nutrition and Dietetics* 62, no. 4 (2005): 152–157.

16. The term *nutritional gaze* borrows from the Foucauldian notion of the "clinical gaze" or "medical gaze." See Michel Foucault, *The Birth of the Clinic: An Archaeology of Medical Perception* (London: Tavistock, 1976); David Armstrong,

"The Rise of Surveillance Medicine," *Sociology of Health and Illness* 17, no. 3 (1995): 393–404.

17. British doctor and science journalist Ben Goldacre has independently used the term nutritionism to refer to the way some alternative and unqualified nutrition practitioners and "media nutritionists" claim nutritional expertise to promote vitamin supplements and unorthodox nutritional remedies, in *Bad Science* (London: Fourth Estate, 2008).

18. Ross Hume Hall, *Food for Nought: The Decline in Nutrition* (Hagerstown, Md.: Harper and Row, 1974), 98, 193.

19. Hall, *Food for Nought*, 44, 196.

20. Hall, *Food for Nought*, 44.

21. Ross Hume Hall, *The Unofficial Guide to Smart Nutrition* (Foster City, Calif.: IDG Books, 2000), 8.

22. See, e.g., Joan Dye Gussow and Isobel Contento, "Nutrition Education in a Changing World: A Conceptualization and Selective Review," *World Review of Nutrition and Dietetics* 44 (1984): 1–56; Joan Gussow, "Why You Should Eat Food, and Other Nutritional Heresies" (lecture, University of California, Davis, 2003); Joan Dye Gussow and Sharon Akabas, "Are We Really Fixing Up the Food Supply?," *Journal of the American Dietetic Association* 93, no. 11 (1993).

23. Gussow and Akabas, "Are We Really Fixing Up the Food Supply?"

24. Jacobs and Tapsell, "Food, Not Nutrients," 439.

25. T. Colin Campbell, *The China Study: The Most Comprehensive Study of Nutrition Ever Conducted and the Startling Implications for Diet, Weight Loss and Long-Term Health* (Dallas, Tex.: Bendella, 2005), 132.

26. Marion Nestle, *Food Politics: How the Food Industry Influences Nutrition and Health*, 2nd ed. (Berkeley: University of California Press, 2007).

27. Marion Nestle, *What to Eat* (New York: North Point Press, 2006), 10.

28. See Walter Willett, "The Food Pushers," *Science* 297, no. 12 (July 2002): 198–199.

29. See, e.g., Marion Nestle, "Eating Made Simple," *Scientific American* 297, no. 3 (2007): 60–69; Nestle, *Food Politics*; Nestle, "Saturated Fats: Pervasive Poison or Dietary Scapegoat?," *Atlantic*, August 11, 2011; Nestle, *What to Eat*, 155. See also Michael Gard and Jan Wright, *The Obesity Epidemic: Science, Morality and Ideology* (Abingdon, U.K.: Routledge, 2005), 130; Willett, "The Food Pushers."

30. Harvey Levenstein, *Paradox of Plenty: A Social History of Eating in Modern America*, rev. ed. (Berkeley: University of California Press, 2003); Belasco, *Appetite for Change*; Geoffrey Cannon, *The Fate of Nations: Food and Nutrition Policy in the New World* (St. Austell, U.K.: Caroline Walker Trust, 2003). Jessica Mudry has recently published an interesting critique of U.S. dietary guidelines in terms of their focus on quantification, rather than their nutricentric focus per se, in *Measured Meals: Nutrition in America* (Albany: State University of New York Press, 2009). Australian food scholar Jane Dixon has also referred to the "nutritionalisation" of the food supply, particularly in terms of the promotion of food products on the

basis of their nutrient components, in "From the Imperial to the Empty Calorie: How Nutrition Relations Underpin Food Regime Transitions," *Agriculture and Human Values* 26 (2009): 321–333.

31. Michael Pollan, *In Defense of Food: The Myth of Nutrition and the Pleasures of Eating* (New York: Allen Lane, 2008). This book elaborated on Pollan's earlier essay "Unhappy Meals," *New York Times Magazine*, January 28, 2007.

32. See, e.g., Mark Bittman, *Food Matters: A Guide to Conscious Eating* (New York: Simon and Schuster, 2009); "Beyond Nutritionism: Rescuing Dietetics Through Critical Dialogue," conference held June 12–14, 2009, Ryerson University, Toronto, Ontario (www.ryerson.ca/beyondnutritionism/index.html).

33. Pollan, *In Defense of Food*, 28, 139.

34. Pollan, *In Defense of Food*, 139.

35. Pollan, *In Defense of Food*, 61.

36. Pollan, *In Defense of Food*, 40.

37. Pollan, *In Defense of Food*, 28.

38. Michael Pollan, *Food Rules: An Eater's Manual* (New York: Penguin, 2009), xi.

39. Pollan, *In Defense of Food*, 81.

40. See, e.g., Nestle, *Food Politics*, xiii.

41. Nestle, "Eating Made Simple," 60; Gussow, "Why You Should Eat Food."

42. Harriet Friedmann argues with respect to naming food regimes that "when names catch on, it is a sign that the regime is in crisis" in "From Colonialism to Green Capitalism: Social Movements and the Emergence of Food Regimes," in *New Directions in the Sociology of Global Development*, ed. Frederick Buttel and Philip McMichael (London: Elsevier, 2005), 227–264, 232.

43. See, e.g., Geoffrey Cannon and Claus Leitzmann, "The New Nutrition Science Project," *Public Health Nutrition* 8, no. 6A (2005): 673–694. The New Nutrition Science project is now taken up by the World Public Health Nutrition Association: www.wphna.org/2011_june_hp4_Rio_2012_spirals.htm (accessed October 1, 2012). See also Lisa Schubert et al., "Re-imagining the 'Social' in the Nutrition Sciences," *Public Health Nutrition* 15, no. 2 (2011): 352–359.

2. THE NUTRITIONISM PARADIGM

1. Robert Silverman, qtd. in Gina Kolata, "Diabetics Should Lose Weight, Avoid Diet Fads," *Science* 235, no. 9 (January 1987): 163–164. See also Gary Taubes, *Good Calories, Bad Calories: Challenging the Conventional Wisdom on Diet, Weight Control, and Disease* (New York: Knopf, 2007), 184.

2. U.S. Department of Agriculture and Department of Health and Human Services, *Nutrition and Your Health: Dietary Guidelines for Americans* (Washington, D.C., 1980); U.S. Department of Agriculture, *Food Guide Pyramid* (Washington, D.C.: Center for Nutrition Policy and Promotion, 1992).

3. The difficulties of achieving substantial changes in people's eating habits that they can sustain over a long period of time are highlighted by the experience of the Women's Health Initiative study. This study failed, for instance, to reduce people's fat intake to the target of 20 percent of energy and to increase their intake of fruit and vegetables to five servings a day and grains to six servings a day. See Gina Kolata, "Maybe You're Not What You Eat," *New York Times*, February 14, 2006; Agneta Yngve et al., "The Women's Health Initiative: What Is on Trial: Nutrition and Chronic Disease? Or Misinterpreted Science, Media Havoc and the Sound of Silence from Peers?," *Public Health Nutrition* 9, no. 2 (2006): 269–272.

4. For this "levels of engagement with food" framework, I adapt the social theoretical "levels of constitutive abstraction" framework developed by Geoff Sharp. See Sharp, "Constitutive Abstraction and Social Practice," *Arena* 70 (1985): 48–82; Sharp, "Intellectual Interchange and Social Practice," *Arena* 99/100 (1992): 188–216. Sharp also distinguishes between more "abstract" and more "concrete" levels of social integration and forms of social relations, including forms of scientific knowledge and technological practices. See also Paul James, *Globalism, Nationalism, Tribalism: Bringing Theory Back In* (London: Sage, 2006).

5. Even though many food components that are intrinsic to or added to foods (e.g., fiber or plant sterols) are not strictly "nutrients," I use the nutrient level as shorthand to refer to all of these components of food that are understood to affect bodily health.

6. See note 4.

7. For a discussion of scientific reductionism in the philosophy of science literature, see, e.g., John Dupre, *The Disorder of Things: Metaphysical Foundations of the Disunity of Science* (Cambridge, Mass.: Harvard University Press, 1993); Sandra D. Mitchell, *Unsimple Truths: Science, Complexity, and Policy* (Chicago: Chicago University Press, 2009).

8. See, e.g., Martijn Katan, "In Praise of Nutrients," (lecture, Vrije University, Amsterdam, 2011).

9. Ingrid Hoffman, "Transcending Reductionism in Nutrition Research," *American Journal of Clinical Nutrition* 78 (2003): 514S–516S. See also chap. 1, note 12.

10. Hoffman, "Transcending Reductionism in Nutrition Research," 515S. See also Martha Slattery, "Defining Dietary Consumption: Is the Sum Greater Than Its Parts?" *American Journal of Clinical Nutrition* 88 (2008): 14–15.

11. Nutrient-level reductionism is a form of what I call *inter-level* reductionism, while single-nutrient reductionism is a form of *intra-level* reductionism. Similar forms of reductionism can be observed in other branches of science, such as biology and genetics.

12. John Crace, "Jennie Brand-Miller—GI Jennie," *Guardian*, July 19, 2005; K. Foster-Powell, S.H. Holt, and J.C. Brand-Miller, "International Table of Glycemic Index and Glycemic Load Values," *American Journal of Clinical Nutrition* 76 (2002): 5–56.

13. Ross Hume Hall, *Food for Nought: The Decline in Nutrition* (Hagerstown, Md.: Harper and Row, 1974), 192.

14. Bill Lands, "A Critique of Paradoxes in Current Advice on Dietary Lipids," *Progress in Lipid Research* 47 (2008): 77–106.

15. See, e.g., Gary Taubes, "The Soft Science of Dietary Fat," *Science* 291, no. 5513 (2001): 2536–2545; Lee Hooper et al., "Dietary Fat Intake and Prevention of Cardiovascular Disease: Systematic Review," *British Medical Journal* 322 (2001): 757–763; J. Bruce German and Cora Dillard, "Saturated Fats: What Dietary Intakes?," *American Journal of Clinical Nutrition* 80 (2004): 550–559; Lands, "Critique of Paradoxes."

16. Lands, "Critique of Paradoxes"; H. Robert Superko and Radhika R. Gadesam, "Is It L.D.L. Particle Size or Number That Correlates with Risk for Cardiovascular Disease?," *Current Atherosclerosis Reports* 10 (2008): 377–385; Steven Nissen et al., "Effect of Torcetrapib on the Progression of Coronary Atherosclerosis," *New England Journal of Medicine* 356, no. 13 (2007): 1304–1316.

17. David Jacobs and Linda Tapsell, "Food, Not Nutrients, Is the Fundamental Unit in Nutrition," *Nutrition Reviews* 65, no. 10 (2007): 439–450.

18. Joan Gussow, "Why You Should Eat Food, and Other Nutritional Heresies" (lecture, University of California, Davis, 2003); Jacobs and Tapsell, "Food, Not Nutrients."

19. T. Colin Campbell, *The China Study: The Most Comprehensive Study of Nutrition Ever Conducted and the Startling Implications for Diet, Weight Loss and Long-Term Health* (Dallas, Tex.: Bendella, 2005), 229; Gussow, "Why You Should Eat Food"; Institute of Medicine, *Evaluation of Biomarkers and Surrogate Endpoints in Chronic Disease* (Washington, D.C.: National Academies Press, 2010); Alice Lichtenstein and Robert Russell, "Essential Nutrients: Food or Supplements? Where Should the Emphasis Be?," *Journal of the American Medical Association* 294, no. 3 (2005); M. Martínez et al., "Dietary Supplements and Cancer Prevention: Balancing Potential Benefits Against Proven Harms," *Journal of the National Cancer Institute* 104 (2012): 1–8.

20. K. Dun Gifford, "Dietary Fats, Eating Guides, and Public Policy: History, Critique and Recommendations," *American Journal of Medicine* 113, no. 9B (2002): 89S–106S.

21. For a critique of the reductive character of the Nutrient Facts label, see Geoffrey Cannon, *The Fate of Nations: Food and Nutrition Policy in the New World* (St. Austell, U.K.: Caroline Walker Trust, 2003).

22. Cannon, *Fate of Nations*, 21.

23. Dimitrios Trichopoulos, Pagona Lagiou, and Antonia Trichopoulou, "Evidence-Based Nutrition," *Asia Pacific Journal of Clinical Nutrition* 9, suppl. (2000): S4–S9; Ingrid Hoffman, "Transcending Reductionism in Nutrition Research," *American Journal of Clinical Nutrition* 78 (2003): 514S–516S; Mark Messina et al., "Reductionism and the Narrowing Nutrition Perspective: Time for Reevaluation and Emphasis on Food Synergy," *Journal of the American Dietetic Association* 101,

no. 12 (2001): 1416–1419; Martha Slattery, "Defining Dietary Consumption: Is the Sum Greater Than Its Parts?," *American Journal of Clinical Nutrition* 88 (2008): 14–15.

24. David R. Jacobs and Lyn M. Steffen, "Nutrients, Foods, and Dietary Patterns as Exposures in Research: A Framework for Food Synergy," *American Journal of Clinical Nutrition* 78, suppl. (2003): 508S–513S, 508S.

25. Jacobs and Tapsell, "Food, Not Nutrients," 439.

26. David R. Jacobs, "Challenges in Research in Nutritional Epidemiology," in *Nutritional Health: Strategies for Disease Prevention*, ed. N.J. Temple, T. Wilson, and D.R. Jacobs, 2nd edition (Totowa, N.J.: Humana Press, 2006), 25–35, 32.

27. For example, steak is well known as a good source of iron, but this iron will be better absorbed if red peppers or orange juice is consumed at the same time, because the vitamin C they contain aids iron absorption. Conversely, steak is also a source of zinc, but if plants rich in phytates are eaten at the same meal, less zinc will be absorbed.

28. C. Sempos, "Food and Nutrient Exposures: What to Consider When Evaluating Epidemiologic Evidence," *American Journal of Clinical Nutrition* 69, suppl. (1999): 1330S–1338S; E. Ransall et al., "Patterns in Food Use and Their Associations with Nutrient Intakes," *American Journal of Clinical Nutrition* 52 (1990): 739–745; Frank Hu, "Dietary Pattern Analysis: A New Direction in Nutritional Epidemiology," *Current Opinion in Lipidology* 13 (2002): 3–9; Katherine Tucker, "Commentary: Dietary Patterns in Transition Can Inform Health Risk, But Detailed Assessments Are Needed to Guide Recommendations," *International Journal of Epidemiology* 36 (2007): 610–611.

29. Gary Fraser, "A Search for Truth in Dietary Epidemiology," *American Journal of Clinical Nutrition* 78 (2003): 521S–525S.

30. Hu, "Dietary Pattern Analysis"; Tucker, "Commentary."

31. See Taubes, *Good Calories, Bad Calories*, 114–119; John Yudkin, *This Slimming Business* (Harmondsworth, U.K.: Penguin, 1974).

32. Joanne Celentano, "Where Do Eggs Fit in a Healthy Diet?," *American Journal of Lifestyle Medicine* 3 (2009): 274–278.

33. On nutritional equivalence, see Hall, *Food for Nought*.

34. Hall, *Food for Nought*, 55.

35. Hall, *Food for Nought*, 56. See also Michael Pollan, *In Defense of Food: The Myth of Nutrition and the Pleasures of Eating* (New York: Allen Lane, 2008), 35; Joan Dye Gussow and Isobel Contento, "Nutrition Education in a Changing World: A Conceptualization and Selective Review," *World Review of Nutrition and Dietetics* 44 (1984): 1–56; Gussow, "Can an Organic Twinkie Be Certified?," in *For All Generations: Making World Agriculture More Sustainable*, ed. J. P. Madden (Glendale, Calif.: Om Pub Consultants, 1997), 143–153.

36. American Dietetic Association, "Nutrient Density: Meeting Nutrient Goals Within Calorie Needs: Practice Paper of the American Dietetic Association," *Journal of the American Dietetic Association* 107, no. 5 (2007): 860–869.

37. Barbara Santich also emphasizes the way Australian guidelines—which have largely mimicked American guidelines—have also referred to food components, rather than foods, in her history of Australian dietary guidelines, *What the Doctor Ordered: 150 Years of Dietary Advice in Australia* (Melbourne: Hyland House, 1995), 195.

38. Marion Nestle, *Food Politics: How the Food Industry Influences Nutrition and Health*, 2nd ed. (Berkeley: University of California Press, 2007), 2.

39. "Position of the American Dietetic Association: Total Diet Approach to Communicating Food and Nutrition Information," *Journal of the American Dietetic Association* 102, no. 1 (2002): 100–108.

40. Nestle, *Food Politics*.

41. In this respect, it concretizes Ancel Keys's 1960s conflation of saturated and *trans*-fats on the basis of which he attributed the detrimental health effects of hydrogenated vegetable oils to animal fats.

42. Hall, *Food for Nought*, 181.

43. Jill Reedy and Susan Krebs-Smith, "Dietary Sources of Energy, Solid Fats, and Added Sugars Among Children and Adolescents in the United States," *Journal of the American Dietetic Association* 110 (2010): 1477–1484; USDA, Human Nutrition Information Service, Dietary Guidelines Advisory Committee, "Report of the Dietary Guidelines Advisory Committee on the Dietary Guidelines for Americans 2010" (Washington, D.C.: National Technical Information Service, 2010).

44. For a critical perspective on the inclusion of solid fats in the definition of empty calories, see Richard Perlmutter, "Labeling Solid Fats and Added Sugars as Empty Calories," *Journal of the American Dietetic Association* 111, no. 2 (2011): 222–223.

45. T.L. Cleave, *The Saccharine Disease: The Master Disease of Our Time* (New Canaan, Conn.: Keats, 1975), xiii. Cleave also used the term *refined carbohydrates* in "The Conception of the Saccharine Disease: An Outline," in *Just Consequences*, ed. Robert Waller (London: Charles Knight, 1971), 15–33. See also D.P. Burkitt and H.C. Trowell, eds., *Refined Carbohydrate Foods and Disease* (London: Academic Press, 1975), 23. For a discussion of Cleave's work, see Taubes, *Good Calories, Bad Calories*. However, Taubes also uses the term *refined carbohydrates* uncritically. For the chemical classification of types of carbohydrates based on molecular size, see J.H. Cummings and A.M. Stephen, "Carbohydrate Terminology and Classification," *European Journal of Clinical Nutrition* 61 (2007): S5–S18. For a critique of the term *refined carbohydrate foods* in favor of *fiber-depleted foods*, see Hugh Trowell, "Definitions of Refined Carbohydrates and Dietary Fibre," *Human Nutrition: Clinical Nutrition* 37C, no. 4 (1983): 236.

46. Robert C. Atkins, *Dr. Atkins' Diet Revolution* (New York: Bantam, 1973).

47. See, e.g., Robert Lustig, "Fructose: Metabolic, Hedonic, and Societal Parallels with Ethanol," *Journal of the American Dietetic Association* 110 (2010): 1307–1321.

48. Quoted in Taubes, *Good Calories, Bad Calories*, 119. See also John Yudkin, *Pure, White and Deadly: The Problem of Sugar* (London: Davis-Poynter, 1972), chap. 4; Yudkin, *This Nutrition Business* (London: Davis-Poynter, 1976), chap. 16.

49. See, e.g., Walter Willett, *Eat, Drink, and Be Healthy: The Harvard Medical School Guide to Healthy Eating* (New York: Free Press, 2005). For a critical perspective on nutrition supplements, see David Jacobs, Myron Gross, and Linda Tapsell, "Food Synergy: An Operational Concept for Understanding Nutrition," *American Journal of Clinical Nutrition* 89 (2009): 1543S–1548S.

50. Jacobs and Tapsell, "Food, Not Nutrients"; Lotte Holm, "Food Health Policies and Ethics: Lay Perspectives on Functional Foods," *Journal of Agricultural and Environmental Ethics* 16 (2003): 531–544.

51. The term *trans-nutric foods* is a variation on the term *transgenic organisms*.

52. Jacobs and Tapsell, "Food, Not Nutrients."

53. Even though the term *biomarker* or *nutritional biomarker* is commonly used to refer to biochemical markers of diseases, I use the terms as a shorthand way of referring to a range of bodily processes and indicators of bodily health.

54. See, e.g., Michael Gard and Jan Wright, *The Obesity Epidemic: Science, Morality and Ideology* (Abingdon, U.K.: Routledge, 2005); Paul Campos, *The Obesity Myth* (New York: Gotham, 2004); Eric Oliver, *Fat Politics: The Real Story Behind America's Obesity Epidemic* (New York: Oxford, 2006); Julie Guthman and Melanie DuPuis, "Embodying Neoliberalism: Economy, Culture and the Politics of Fat," *Environment and Planning D: Society and Space* 24, no. 3 (2006): 427–448.

55. K. Flegal et al., "Excess Deaths Associated with Underweight, Overweight, and Obesity," *Journal of the American Medical Association* 293, no. 15 (2005): 1861–1867; Oliver, *Fat Politics*, 25.

56. S. Bryn Austin, "Commodity Knowledge in Consumer Culture: The Role of Nutritional Health Promotion in the Making of the Diet Industry," in *Weighty Issues: Fatness and Thinness as Social Problems*, ed. J. Sobal and D. Maurer (Hawthorne, N.Y.: Aldine de Gruyter, 1999), 159–182; Ivan Illich, "Needs," in *The Development Dictionary: A Guide to Knowledge as Power*, ed. Wolfgang Sachs (London: Zed Books, 1992), 88–101.

57. The nutrient treadmill is a variation on the technological treadmill. On the latter, see William Cochrane, *The Development of American Agriculture: A Historical Analysis* (Minneapolis: University of Minnesota Press, 1979).

58. Claude Fischler, "A Nutritional Cacophony or the Crisis of Food Selection in Affluent Societies," in *For a Better Nutrition in the 21st Century*, ed. P. Leathwood, M. Horisberger, and W. James (New York: Vevey/Raven Press, 1993). For a critique of the "what to eat" literature, see Julie Guthman, "Commentary on Teaching Food: Why I Am Fed Up with Michael Pollan et al.," *Agriculture and Human Values* 24 (2007): 261–264; Aaron Bobrow-Strain, "Kills a Body Twelve Ways: Bread Fear and the Politics of 'What to Eat?'," *Gastronomica* 7, no. 3 (2007): 45–52.

59. Steven Shapin, "Expertise, Common Sense, and the Atkins Diet," in *Public Science in Liberal Democracy*, ed. J.M. Porter and W.B. Phillips (Toronto: University of Toronto Press, 2007), 174–193.

60. Robert Crawford, "Healthism and the Medicalisation of Everyday Life," *International Journal of Health Sciences* 10, no. 3 (1980): 365–388. Robert Crawford, "Health as a Meaningful Social Practice," *Health* 10, no. 4 (2006): 401–420.

61. Julie Guthman, *Weighing In: Obesity, Food Justice and the Limits of Capitalism* (Berkeley: University of California Press, 2011), 52.

62. See Steven Bratman, *Health Food Junkies: Overcoming the Obsession with Healthful Eating* (New York: Broadway Books, 2000), for a discussion of what he calls "orthorexia nervosa," an eating disorder defined by the "fixation on healthy food."

63. For other ways of dividing and characterizing eras of nutrition science, see, e.g., Barbara Santich, "Paradigm Shifts in the History of Dietary Advice in Australia," *Nutrition and Dietetics* 62, no. 4 (2005): 152–157; Cannon, *Fate of Nations*. In some of these accounts, the periods of the calorie and of vitamins are cast as separate eras, rather than combined as one era as I have here. The shift from the first to the second eras I identify is commonly acknowledged in the literature, but not that between the second and third eras. Michael Heasman and Julian Mellentin do identify this latter shift in their distinction between what they call the "healthy eating revolution" and the "functional foods revolution" in *The Functional Foods Revolution: Healthy People, Healthy Profits?* (London: Earthscan, 2001), 55.

64. Cannon, *Fate of Nations*.

65. See Warren James Belasco, *Appetite for Change: How the Counterculture Took On the Food Industry*, 2nd ed. (New York: Cornell University Press, 2007).

66. Stephen Kritchevsky, "A Review of Scientific Research and Recommendations Regarding Eggs," *Journal of the American College of Nutrition* 23, no. 6 (2004): 596S–600S.

67. Luc Djousse and J. Michael Gaziano, "Egg Consumption in Relation to Cardiovascular Disease and Mortality: The Physician's Health Study," *American Journal of Clinical Nutrition* 87 (2008): 964–969; Alice Lichtenstein et al., "Diet and Lifestyle Recommendations Revision 2006: A Scientific Statement from the American Heart Association Nutrition Committee," *Circulation* 114 (2006): 82–96, 87; U.S. Department of Agriculture and Department of Health and Human Services, *Dietary Guidelines for Americans, 2010* (Washington, D.C., 2010), x.

68. P.F. Surai and N.H.C. Sparks, "Designer Eggs: From Improvement of Egg Composition to Functional Food," *Trends in Food Science and Technology* 12 (2001): 7–16; P. Crotty, *Good Nutrition? Fact and Fashion in Dietary Advice* (Sydney: Allen and Unwin, 1995), 36; Ronald Watson, ed., *Eggs and Health Promotion* (Ames: Iowa State Press, 2002).

69. See Harriet Friedmann, "From Colonialism to Green Capitalism: Social Movements and the Emergence of Food Regimes," and Philip McMichael, "Global Development and the Corporate Food Regime," in *New Directions in the*

Sociology of Global Development, ed. Frederick Buttel and Philip McMichael (London: Elsevier, 2005).

70. For another account of some of the parallels between nutrition science and food regimes, see Jane Dixon, "From the Imperial to the Empty Calorie: How Nutrition Relations Underpin Food Regime Transitions," *Agriculture and Human Values* 26 (2009): 321–333.

71. Adele Clarke et al., *Biomedicalization: Technoscience, Health, and Illness in the U.S.* (Durham, N.C.: Duke University Press, 2010), chap. 2.

3. THE ERA OF QUANTIFYING NUTRITIONISM

1. Hillel Schwartz, *Never Satisfied: A Cultural History of Diets, Fantasies and Fat* (New York: Doubleday, 1986), 175.

2. Lulu Hunt Peters, *Diet and Health, with Key to the Calories* (Chicago: Reilley and Lee, 1918), 24.

3. Dennis Roth, "America's Fascination with Nutrition," *Food Review* 23, no. 1 (2000): 32–37; Schwartz, *Never Satisfied*, 134.

4. Schwartz, *Never Satisfied*, 175.

5. Kenneth Carpenter, "A Short History of Nutritional Science: Part 1 (1785–1885)," *Journal of Nutrition* 133, no. 3 (2003): 638–645. For an account of approaches to nutrition in the Renaissance, see Ken Albala, *Eating Right in the Renaissance* (Berkeley: University of California Press, 2002).

6. Qtd. in Barbara Santich, *What the Doctor Ordered: 150 Years of Dietary Advice in Australia* (Melbourne: Hyland House, 1995), 7.

7. Ross Hume Hall, *Food for Nought: The Decline in Nutrition* (Hagerstown, Md.: Harper and Row, 1974), 186, 95.

8. William Prout, "On the Ultimate Composition of Simple Alimentary Substances," *Philosophical Transactions of the Royal Society of London* 117 (1827); Elmer Verner McCollum, *A History of Nutrition: The Sequence of Ideas in Nutrition Investigations* (Boston: Houghton Mifflin, 1957), 88.

9. Carpenter, "Short History: Part 1." Liebig coined the term *metabolism* to refer to the chemical transformations in the body involved in digesting foods. See Lawrence Weaver, "The Emergence of Our Modern Understanding of Infant Nutrition and Feeding 1750–1900," *Current Paediatrics* 16 (2006): 342–347.

10. William H. Brock, *Justus von Liebig: The Chemical Gatekeeper* (Cambridge: Cambridge University Press, 1997), 183; J.C. Drummond and Anne Wilbraham, *The Englishman's Food: A History of Five Centuries of English Diet* (London: Jonathan Cape, 1958), 347.

11. Qtd. in Kenneth J. Carpenter, "Nutritional Studies in Victorian Prisons," *Journal of Nutrition* 136 (2006): 1–8, 2.

12. Kenneth J. Carpenter, *Protein and Energy: A Study of Changing Ideas in Nutrition* (Cambridge: Cambridge University Press, 1994), 50, 57.

13. Santich, *What the Doctor Ordered*, 8; Carpenter, "Short History: Part I"; Mark R. Finlay, "Early Marketing of the Theory of Nutrition: The Science and Culture of Liebig's Extract of Meat," in *The Science and Culture of Nutrition, 1840–1940*, ed. Harmke Kamminga and Andrew Cunningham (Amsterdam: Editions Rodopi, 1995), 48–74, 53.

14. Finlay, "Early Marketing," 53.

15. Finlay, "Early Marketing," 53; Barbara Santich, "Paradigm Shifts in the History of Dietary Advice in Australia," *Nutrition and Dietetics* 62, no. 4 (2005): 13, 152–157.

16. Qtd. in McCollum, *A History of Nutrition*, 95.

17. Finlay, "Early Marketing," 58–59; Carpenter, *Protein and Energy*, 74–75.

18. Barbara Griggs, *The Food Factor* (Harmondsworth, U.K.: Viking, 1986), 15.

19. Finlay, "Early Marketing," 60; Walter Gratzer, *Terrors of the Table: The Curious History of Nutrition* (Oxford: Oxford University Press, 2005).

20. Qtd. in Carpenter, *Protein and Energy*, 75.

21. See, e.g., "Position of the American Dietetic Association: Functional Foods," *Journal of the American Dietetic Association* 109, no. 4 (2009): 735–746.

22. Carpenter, *Protein and Energy*, 74.

23. Brock, *Justus von Liebig*, 245; Weaver, "Emergence."

24. Griggs, *Food Factor*, 35. On the invention of "artificial" infant feeding, see Amy Bentley, "Inventing Baby Food: Gerber and the Discourse of Infancy in the United States," in *Food Nations: Selling Taste in Consumer Societies*, ed. Warren Belasco and Philip Scranton (New York: Routledge, 2002).

25. Brock, *Justus von Liebig*, 247.

26. Carpenter, *Protein and Energy*, 74.

27. Griggs, *Food Factor*, 35.

28. Geoffrey Cannon, *The Fate of Nations: Food and Nutrition Policy in the New World* (St. Austell, U.K.: Caroline Walker Trust, 2003).

29. Rima Apple, "What's for Dinner? Science and the Ideology of Meat in Twentieth-Century U.S. Culture," in *Meat, Medicine and Human Health in the Twentieth Century*, ed. David Cantor et al. (London: Pickering and Chatto, 2010), 127–235; S. Welsh, C. Davis, and A. Shaw, "A Brief History of Food Guides in the United States," *Nutrition Today* 27, no. 6 (1992): 6–11; Betsy Haughton, Joan Dye Gussow, and Janice Dodds, "An Historical Study of the Underlying Assumptions for U.S. Food Guides from 1917 Through the Basic Four Food Group Guide," *Journal of Nutrition Education* 19, no. 4 (1987): 3331–3342.

30. Kenneth Carpenter, "A Short History of Nutritional Science: Part 4 (1945–1985)," *Journal of Nutrition* 133, no. 11 (2003): 3336.

31. Urban Jonsson, "Child Malnutrition: From the Global Protein Crisis to a Violation of Human Rights," in *Sustainable Development in a Globalized World: Studies in Development, Security and Culture*, vol. 1, ed. Bjorn Hettne (Basingstoke: Palgrave Macmillan, 2008).

32. Carpenter, "Short History: Part 4."

33. Jonsson, "Child Malnutrition"; G.P. Webb, "Interpreting Nutritional Science: What Have We Learnt from the Past?," *Nutrition Bulletin* 34 (2009): 309–315.

34. Donald McLaren, "The Great Protein Fiasco," *Lancet*, July 13 (1974); Jonsson, "Child Malnutrition."

35. Naomi Aronson, "Nutrition as a Social Problem: A Case Study of Entrepreneurial Strategy in Science," *Social Problems* 29, no. 5 (1982): 474–487; Hamilton Cravens, "The German-American Science of Racial Nutrition, 1870–1920," in *Technical Knowledge in American Culture: Science, Technology, and Medicine Since the Early 1800s*, ed. Hamilton Cravens, Alan I. Marcus, and David M. Katzman (Tuscaloosa: University of Alabama Press, 1996), 125–148; Carpenter, *Protein and Energy*, 66.

36. Jessica Mudry, *Measured Meals: Nutrition in America* (Albany: State University of New York Press, 2009), 26.

37. Mudry, *Measured Meals*, 34; Anson Rabinach, *The Human Motor: Energy, Fatigue and the Origins of Modernity* (New York: Basic Books, 1990), 126.

38. Carpenter, "Short History: Part 1."

39. Carpenter, "Short History: Part 1."

40. Carpenter, "Short History: Part 1."

41. Roth, "America's Fascination with Nutrition."

42. Rabinach, *Human Motor*.

43. Rabinach, *Human Motor*, 66, 124.

44. Bryan Turner, "The Government of the Body: Medical Regimens and the Rationalization of the Diet," *The British Journal of Sociology* 33, no. 2 (1982): 254–269, 258.

45. Mudry, *Measured Meals*, 33.

46. Mudry, *Measured Meals*, 33.

47. Naomi Aronson, "Social Definitions of Entitlement: Food Needs 1885–1920," *Media, Culture and Society* 4 (1982), 321–333; H. Levenstein, *Revolution at the Table: The Transformation of the American Diet* (Berkeley: University of California Press, 2003), 57. See also Jane Dixon, "From the Imperial to the Empty Calorie: How Nutrition Relations Underpin Food Regime Transitions," *Agriculture and Human Values* 26 (2009).

48. Martijn B. Katan and David Ludwig, "Extra Calories Cause Weight Gain—But How Much?," *Journal of the American Medical Association* 303, no. 1 (2010): 65–66.

49. Nick Cullather, "The Foreign Policy of the Calorie," *American Historical Review* 112, no. 2 (2007): 337–364.

50. Cravens, "German-American Science."

51. Schwartz, *Never Satisfied*, 87.

52. Aronson, "Nutrition as a Social Problem."

53. Qtd. in Schwartz, *Never Satisfied*, 86.

54. Adam Drewnowski, "The Cost of U.S. Foods as Related to Their Nutritive Value," *American Journal of Clinical Nutrition* 92 (2010).

55. Cravens, "German-American Science"; Corinna Treitil, "Food Science/ Food Politics: Max Rubner and 'Rational Nutrition' in Fin-de-Siecle Berlin," in *Food and the City in Europe Since 1800*, ed. P. Atkins, P. Lummel, and D. Oddy (Burlington, Vt.: Ashgate, 2008), 51–62; Dietrich Milles, "Working Capacity and Calorie Consumption: The History of Rational Physical Economy," in *The Science and Culture of Nutrition, 1840–1940*, ed. Harmke Kamminga and Andrew Cunningham (Amsterdam: Editions Rodopi, 1995), 48–74.

56. Rabinach, *The Human Motor*, 239.

57. P. Crotty, *Good Nutrition? Fact and Fashion in Dietary Advice* (Sydney: Allen and Unwin, 1995), 19.

58. Aronson, "Nutrition as a Social Problem."

59. Aronson, "Social Definitions of Entitlement"; Levenstein, *Revolution at the Table*, 57.

60. Qtd. in Schwartz, *Never Satisfied*, 86.

61. Carolyn De La Pena, *Empty Pleasures: The Story of Artificial Sweeteners from Saccharin to Splenda* (Chapel Hill: University of North Carolina Press, 2010), 26; Laura Shapiro, *Perfection Salad: Women and Cooking at the Turn of the Century* (New York: Farrar, Straus and Giroux, 1986), 76.

62. Levenstein, *Revolution at the Table*, 57.

63. Aronson, "Nutrition as a Social Problem."

64. Levenstein, *Revolution at the Table*, 75.

65. Michelle Stacey, *Consumed: Why Americans Love, Hate and Fear Food* (New York: Simon and Schuster, 1994), 32. See also Deanna L. Pucciarelli, "Early History and Evolution of Nutrition Science in the United States of America," *Family and Consumer Sciences Research Journal* 38, no. 2 (2009): 106–222.

66. Shapiro, *Perfection Salad*, 76.

67. Schwartz, *Never Satisfied*, 177.

68. Schwartz, *Never Satisfied*, 177; Laura Fraser, *Losing It: America's Obsession with Weight and the Industry That Feeds on It* (New York: Dutton, 1997), 56.

69. Cullather, "Foreign Policy of the Calorie." See also Nick Cullather, *The Hungry World: America's Cold War Battle Against Poverty in Asia* (London: Harvard University Press, 2010); Dixon, "From the Imperial to the Empty Calorie"; Michael Carolan, *The Real Cost of Cheap Food* (London: Earthscan, 2011), ch. 4.

70. Cullather, "Foreign Policy of the Calorie."

71. Robert Olson, "Evolution of Scientific and Popular Ideas of the Nutritional Role of Vitamins and Minerals," in *For a Better Nutrition in the 21st Century*, ed. P. Leathwood, M. Horisberger, and W. James (New York: Vevey/Raven Press, 1993).

72. Robyn Smith, "The Emergence of Vitamins as Bio-political Objects During World War I," *Studies in History and Philosophy of Biological and Biomedical Sciences* 40 (2009): 179–189; Olson, "Evolution of Scientific and Popular Ideas."

73. Griggs, *Food Factor*, 36.

74. For example, although scientists such as Voit used foods in their feeding experiments with animals, he had assumed that the same results would be obtained if the animals were merely fed purified fats, protein, carbohydrates, and mineral salts. Griggs, *Food Factor*, 36; McCollum, *A History of Nutrition*, 204.

75. Qtd. in Olson, "Evolution of Scientific and Popular Ideas," 43.

76. Smith, "Emergence of Vitamins"; Santich, *What the Doctor Ordered*, 68.

77. Kenneth Carpenter, "A Short History of Nutritional Science: Part 3 (1912–1944)," *Journal of Nutrition* 133, no. 10 (2003): 3023–3032.

78. Carpenter, "Short History: Part 3," 3023.

79. Carpenter, "Short History: Part 3," 3023. McCollum considered the term *vitamines* unsatisfactory, but it prevailed over his preferred terms "fat-soluble A" and "water-soluble B." See E.V. McCollum and W. Pitz, "The 'Vitamine' Hypothesis and Deficiency Diseases," *Journal of Biological Chemistry* 31, no. 1 (1917): 229–250.

80. Carpenter, "Short History: Part 3"; Levenstein, *Revolution at the Table*, 148; Santich, *What the Doctor Ordered*, 68. It's worth noting that McCollum was warned by colleagues that he may be wasting his time pursuing nutrition research, since "the subject was already well worked out, with nothing remaining to be discovered." Qtd. in Carpenter, "Short History: Part 3."

81. Levenstein, *Revolution at the Table*, 148.

82. Carpenter, "Short History: Part 3"; Levenstein, *Revolution at the Table*, 148.

83. Jeffrey Backstrand, "The History and Future of Food Fortification in the United States: A Public Health Perspective," *Nutrition Reviews* 60, no. 1 (2002): 15–26; Mark Lawrence and Aileen Robertson, "Reference Standards and Guidelines," in *Public Health Nutrition: From Principles to Practice*, ed. Mark Lawrence and Tony Worsley (Crows Nest, Australia: Allen and Unwin, 2007), 39–70; Institute of Medicine, *Dietary Reference Intakes: Applications in Dietary Assessment* (Washington, D.C.: Food and Nutrition Board, 2000).

84. Richard Semba, "The Impact of Improved Nutrition on Disease Prevention," in *Silent Victories: The History and Practice of Public Health in Twentieth-Century America*, ed. Jihn Ward and Christian Warren (Oxford: Oxford University Press, 2007); D. Bishai and R. Nalubola, "The History of Food Fortification in the United States: Its Relevance for Current Fortification Efforts in Developing Countries," *Economic Development and Cultural Change* 51, no. 1 (2002): 37–53.

85. Geoffrey P. Webb, *Dietary Supplements and Functional Foods*, 2nd ed. (Oxford, U.K.: Wiley-Blackwell, 2011), 7.

86. Alice Lichtenstein and Robert Russell, "Essential Nutrients: Food or Supplements? Where Should the Emphasis Be?," *Journal of the American Medical Association* 294, no. 3 (2005): 351–358; Alice Lichtenstein, "Nutrient Supplements and Cardiovascular Disease: A Heartbreaking Story," *Journal of Lipid Research* 50 (2009): S429–S433.

87. Kenneth Carpenter, *Beriberi, White Rice, and Vitamin B* (Berkeley: University of California Press, 2000), 194.

88. Aronson, "Social Definitions of Entitlement."

89. Griggs, *Food Factor*, 52.

90. Griggs, *Food Factor*, 54.

91. Qtd. in Levenstein, *Revolution at the Table*, 149.

92. Qtd. in Santich, *What the Doctor Ordered*, 68.

93. Melanie DuPuis, *Nature's Perfect Food: How Milk Became America's Drink* (New York: New York University Press, 2002), 107.

94. Harvey Levenstein, *Fear of Food: A History of Why We Worry About What We Eat* (Chicago: University of Chicago Press, 2012), 88–89.

95. Rima Apple, *Vitamania: Vitamins in American Culture* (New Brunswick, N.J.: Rutgers University Press, 1996), 179.

96. Michael Ackerman, "Science and the Shadow of Ideology in the American Health Foods Movement, 1930s–1960s," in *The Politics of Healing: Histories of Alternative Medicine in Twentieth-Century North America*, ed. Robert Johnston (New York: Routledge, 2004), 52–65.

97. Apple, *Vitamania*, 14. On the development of vitamin-fortified foods in Europe, see Sally Horrocks, "The Business of Vitamins: Nutrition Science and the Food Industry in Inter-war Britain," in *Food, Science, Policy and Regulation in the Twentieth Century: International and Comparative Perspectives*, ed. David Smith and Jim Phillips (London: Routledge, 2000), 235–258.

98. Apple, *Vitamania*, 14.

99. Apple, *Vitamania*, 14.

100. Apple, *Vitamania*, 22.

101. Apple, *Vitamania*, 8.

102. Ackerman, "Science and the Shadow of Ideology."

103. Rima Apple, "The More Things Change: A Historical Perspective on the Debate over Vitamin Advertising in the United States," in *Silent Victories: The History and Practice of Public Health in Twentieth-Century America*, ed. John Ward and Christian Warren (New York: Oxford University Press, 2006), 193–208.

104. Apple, *Vitamania*, 136.

105. Levenstein, *Revolution at the Table*, 149.

106. Apple, "The More Things Change."

107. Apple, *Vitamania*, 183.

108. See, e.g., Walter Willett, *Eat, Drink, and Be Healthy: The Harvard Medical School Guide to Healthy Eating* (New York: Free Press, 2005), 203.

109. Willett, *Eat, Drink, and Be Healthy*, 24.

110. Linus Pauling, *Vitamin C and the Common Cold* (San Francisco: W.H. Freeman, 1970); Apple, *Vitamania*, 78.

111. Apple, *Vitamania*, 74–84.

112. For a recent review of the scientific literature, see R.M. Douglas et al., "Vitamin C for Preventing and Treating the Common Cold," *Cochrane Database of Systematic Reviews* 3 (2007): CD000980.

113. Robert Heaney, "Nutrients, Endpoints and the Problem of Proof," *Journal of Nutrition* 138, no. 9 (2008): 1591–1595.

114. Bonnie Worthington-Roberts and Maryann Breskin, "Supplementation Patterns of Washington State Dieticians," in *The Nutrition Debate: Sorting Out Some Answers*, ed. Joan Dye Gussow and Paul Thomas (Palo Alto, Calif.: Bull Publishing, 1986), 275–277.

115. Joan Dye Gussow and Paul Thomas, "Nutritional Supplements: To Pill or Not to Pill?," *The Nutrition Debate: Sorting Out Some Answers*, ed. J. Gussow and P. Thomas (Palo Alto, Calif.: Bull Publishing,1986), 269–271, 269.

116. Apple, *Vitamania*, 3.

117. Carole Davis and Etta Saltos, "Dietary Recommendations and How They Have Changed over Time," in *America's Eating Habits: Changes and Consequences*, ed. E. Frazao, USDA Agriculture Information Bulletin No. 750 (Washington, D.C.: U.S. Department of Agriculture, 1999), 33–49; Haughton, "Historical Study."

118. Davis and Saltos, "Dietary Recommendations."

119. Hugh Sinclair, "Modern Diet and Degenerative Disease," in *Just Consequences*, ed. R. Waller (London: Charles Knight, 1971), 85–95, qtd. in Hall, *Food for Nought*, 185.

120. One of the earliest uses of the term *vitamania* was in William Bean, "Vitamania, Polypharmacy and Witchcraft," *Archives of Internal Medicine* 96, no. 2 (1955): 137–141.

4. THE ERA OF GOOD-AND-BAD NUTRITIONISM

1. C. Fischler, "A Nutritional Cacophony, or The Crisis of Food Selection in Affluent Societies," in *For a Better Nutrition in the 21st Century*, ed. P. Leathwood, M. Horisberger, and W. James (New York: Vevey/Raven Press, 1993).

2. P. Crotty, *Good Nutrition? Fact and Fashion in Dietary Advice* (Sydney: Allen and Unwin, 1995).

3. Warren James Belasco, *Appetite for Change: How the Counterculture Took on the Food Industry*, 2nd ed. (New York: Cornell University Press, 2007). The term *negative nutrition* was used earlier by Ross Hume Hall in a more technical manner to refer to the harmful nutritional and health effects of high levels of exposure to certain chemicals and minerals in *Food for Nought: The Decline in Nutrition* (Hagerstown, Md.: Harper and Row, 1974), chap. 13.

4. Belasco, *Appetite for Change*.

5. Geoffrey Cannon, *Food and Health: The Experts Agree* (London: Consumer's Association, 1992), 199.

6. U.S. Department of Agriculture and Department of Health and Human Services, *Nutrition and Your Health: Dietary Guidelines for Americans* (Washington, D.C., 1980), 1.

7. D.P. Burkitt and H.C. Trowell, eds., *Refined Carbohydrate Foods and Disease* (London: Academic Press, 1975); Hugh Trowell, Denis Burkitt, and Kenneth Heaton, eds., *Dietary Fibre, Fibre-Depleted Foods and Disease* (London: Academic Press, 1985).

8. J.H. Cummings and A.M. Stephen, "Carbohydrate Terminology and Classification," *European Journal of Clinical Nutrition* 61 (2007): S5–S18. The distinction between complex and simple carbohydrates has since been abandoned.

9. See, e.g., M. Katan, "Are There Good and Bad Carbohydrates for HDL Cholesterol?," *Lancet* 353, no. 9158 (1999): 1029–1030; Barry Sears and Bill Lawren, *The Zone: A Dietary Road Map* (New York: Harper Collins, 1995).

10. Paul Rozin, "Food Is Fundamental, Fun, Frightening and Far-Reaching," *Social Research* 66, no. 1 (1999): 9–29; Deborah Lupton, *Food, the Body and the Self* (London: Sage, 1996), 27.

11. N.J. Temple and D.P. Burkitt, eds., *Western Diseases: Their Dietary Prevention and Reversibility* (Totowa, N.J.: Humana Press, 1994).

12. Raymond Reiser, "Oversimplification of Diet: Coronary Heart Disease Relationships and Exaggerated Diet Recommendations," *American Journal of Clinical Nutrition* 31, no. 5 (1978): 865–875, 866.

13. Carolyn De La Pena, *Empty Pleasures: The Story of Artificial Sweeteners from Saccharin to Splenda* (Chapel Hill: University of North Carolina Press, 2010), 199–205.

14. Qtd. in De La Pena, *Empty Pleasures*, 203.

15. Robert A. Aronowitz, *Making Sense of Illness: Science, Society and Disease* (Cambridge: Cambridge University Press, 1998), 122.

16. Geoffrey Cannon, *The Fate of Nations: Food and Nutrition Policy in the New World* (St. Austell, U.K.: Caroline Walker Trust, 2003).

17. Centers for Disease Control and Prevention, "Decline in Deaths from Heart Disease and Stroke—United States, 1900–1999," *Journal of the American Medical Association* 282, no. 8 (1999): 724–728.

18. William G. Rothstein, *Public Health and the Risk Factor: A History of an Uneven Medical Revolution* (Rochester, N.Y.: University of Rochester Press, 2003), 4.

19. Rothstein, *Public Health and the Risk Factor*, 66–72.

20. Rothstein, *Public Health and the Risk Factor*, 224–225.

21. Aronowitz, *Making Sense of Illness*, 112.

22. Aronowitz, *Making Sense of Illness*, 116. See also Michel Accad and Herbert Fred, "Risk-Factor Medicine: An Industry out of Control?," *Cardiology* 117 (2010): 64–67.

23. Aronowitz, *Making Sense of Illness*, 124.

24. A. Petersen and D. Lupton, *The New Public Health: Health and Self in the Age of Risk* (London: Sage, 1996), 48. Petersen and Lupton also refer to the "risky body" (50). See also John Coveney, *Food, Morals and Meanings: The Pleasure and Anxiety of Eating*, 2nd ed. (London: Routledge, 2006), 100.

25. Petersen and Lupton, *The New Public Health*, 48. Charles Rosenberg refers to the "invention of protodiseases," those health conditions that "occupy a posi-

tion somewhere between warning signal and pathology," in *Our Present Complaint: American Medicine, Then and Now* (Baltimore: Johns Hopkins University Press, 2007), 30.

26. In the 1980s, epidemiologist Geoffrey Rose was a key promoter of this approach. Rose argued directing preventive measures at the whole population to achieve a statistically significant improvement in population-wide health outcomes is a legitimate public health strategy, even if these interventions offered tangible health benefits to only a small section of the population. See Geoffrey Rose, "Sick Individuals and Sick Populations," *International Journal of Epidemiology* 14, no. 1 (1985): 32–38.

27. Gary Taubes, *Good Calories, Bad Calories: Challenging the Conventional Wisdom on Diet, Weight Control, and Disease* (New York: Knopf, 2007), 17.

28. Ancel Keys and Margaret Keys, *Eat Well and Stay Well* (New York: Doubleday, 1959), 15.

29. Daniel Steinberg, "An Interpretive History of the Cholesterol Controversy. Part II: The Early Evidence Linking Hypercholesterolemia to Coronary Disease in Humans," *Journal of Lipid Reseach* 46 (2005): 179–190.

30. Thomas Moore, *Heart Failure: A Critical Inquiry into American Medicine and the Revolution in Heart Care* (New York: Random House, 1989), 37; Taubes, *Good Calories, Bad Calories*, 27.

31. Gary Taubes, "The Soft Science of Dietary Fat," *Science* 291, no. 5513 (2001): 2536–2545; Ann F. La Berge, "How the Ideology of Low Fat Conquered America," *Journal of the History of Medicine and Allied Sciences* 63, no. 2 (2008): 139–177; Rothstein, *Public Health and the Risk Factor*, 307.

32. J. Yerushalmey and H. Hilleboe, "Fat in the Diet and Mortality from Heart Disease. A Methodological Note," *New York State Journal of Medicine* 57 (1957), 2343–2354; Taubes, *Good Calories, Bad Calories*, 32; Rothstein, *Public Health and the Risk Factor*, 307; David Kritchevsky, "History of Recommendations to the Public About Dietary Fat," *Journal of Nutrition* 128, no. 2 (1998): 449S–452S.

33. J. Richard, F. Cambien, and P. Ducimetiere, "Particularités épidémiologiques de la maladie coronarienne en France" ("Epidemiological Characteristics of Coronary Disease in France," *Nouvelle presse médicale* 10 (1981): 1111–1114; J. Richard, "Les facteurs de risque coronarien. Le paradoxe Français" ("Coronary Risk Factors: The French Paradox"), *Archives des maladies du coeur et des vaisseaux* 80 (1987): 17–21; S. Renaud and M. de Lorgeril, "Wine, Alcohol, Platelets and the French Paradox for Coronary Heart Disease," *Lancet* 339 (1992): 1523–1526; Hugh Tunstall-Pedoe, "The French Paradox," *Dialogues in Cardiovascular Medicine* 13, no. 3 (2008): 159–179; Taubes, *Good Calories, Bad Calories*, 32; Sabine Artaud-Wild, "Differences in Coronary Mortality Can Be Explained by Differences in Cholesterol and Saturated Fat Intakes in 40 Countries but Not in France and Finland. A Paradox," *Circulation* 88 (1993): 2771–2779.

34. Kritchevsky, "History of Recommendations"; I.H. Page et al., "Atherosclerosis and the Fat Content of the Diet," *Circulation* 16 (1957): 164–178.

35. Taubes, *Good Calories, Bad Calories*, 20; Central Committee for Medical and Community Program of the American Heart Association, "Dietary Fat and Its Relation to Heart Attacks and Strokes," *Circulation* 23 (1961): 133–135.

36. I.H. Page et al., "Dietary Fat and Its Relation to Heart Attacks and Strokes," *Circulation* 23 (1961): 133–136; Karin Garrety, "Social Worlds, Actor-Networks and Controversy: The Case of Cholesterol, Dietary Fat and Heart Disease," *Social Studies of Science* 27, no. 5 (1997): 727–773; Kritchevsky, "History of Recommendations"; Page et al., "Atherosclerosis."

37. Steinberg, "An Interpretive History"; Taubes, *Good Calories, Bad Calories*, 21.

38. Taubes, *Good Calories, Bad Calories*, 21.

39. For a history, see Daniel Steinberg, "An Interpretive History of the Cholesterol Controversy: Part III: Mechanistically Defining the Role of Hyperlipidemia," *Journal of Lipid Research* 46 (2005): 2037–2051.

40. Fred Mattson and Scott Grundy, "Comparison of Effects of Dietary Saturated, Monounsaturated, and Polyunsaturated Fatty Acids on Plasma Lipids and Lipoproteins in Man," *Journal of Lipid Research* 26 (1985); Martijn Katan, Peter Zock, and Ronald Mensink, "Dietary Oils, Serum Lipoproteins, and Coronary Heart Disease," *American Journal of Clinical Nutrition* 61 (1995): 1368S–1373S.

41. C.M. Skeaff and J. Miller, "Dietary Fat and Coronary Heart Disease: Summary of Evidence from Prospective Cohort and Randomised Controlled Trials," *Annals of Nutrition and Metabolism* 55 (2009): 173–201.

42. Joint FAO/WHO Expert Consultation on Fats and Fatty Acids in Human Nutrition, *Interim Summary of Conclusions on Fats and Fatty Acids* (Geneva: World Health Organization, 2010).

43. Germain Brisson, *Lipids in Human Nutrition* (Englewood, N.J.: Jack K. Burgess, 1981), 85.

44. Brisson, *Lipids in Human Nutrition*, 88.

45. U.S. Senate Select Committee on Nutrition and Human Needs, *Dietary Goals for the United States*, 2nd ed. (Washington, D.C., 1977).

46. Reiser, "Oversimplification of Diet."

47. Reiser, "Oversimplification of Diet."

48. T.L. Cleave, *The Saccharine Disease: The Master Disease of Our Time* (New Canaan, Conn.: Keats, 1975).

49. Cleave, *The Saccharine Disease*, 16.

50. John Yudkin, *This Slimming Business* (Harmondsworth, U.K.: Penguin, 1974).

51. John Yudkin, *This Nutrition Business* (London: Davis-Poynter, 1976), 219; Yudkin, *Pure, White and Deadly: The Problem of Sugar* (London: Davis-Poynter, 1972). See also Taubes, *Good Calories, Bad Calories*, 119; Glen D. Lawrence, *The Fats of Life: Essential Fatty Acids in Health and Disease* (New Brunswick, N.J.: Rutgers University Press, 2010), 189.

52. Ancel Keys, "Sucrose in the Diet and Coronary Heart Disease," *Atherosclerosis* 14 (1971): 193–202; John Yudkin, "Dietary Fat and Dietary Sugar in Rela-

tion to Ischemic Heart-Disease and Diabetes," *Lancet* 2, no. 7349 (1964): 155–162; Yudkin, "Diet and Coronary Thrombosis: Hypothesis and Fact," *Lancet* 270, no. 6987 (1957); Taubes, *Good Calories, Bad Calories*, 119–120.

53. See Barbara Griggs, *The Food Factor* (Harmondsworth, U.K.: Viking, 1986), 277.

54. See Gilbert Thompson, *The Cholesterol Controversy* (London: Royal Society of Medicine Press, 2008); Taubes, *Good Calories, Bad Calories*, 119.

55. Mary Enig, "Dietary Fat and Cancer Trends—A Critique," *Federation Proceedings* 37, no. 9 (1978): 2215–2219.

56. Robert E. Olson, "Are Professionals Jumping the Gun in the Fight Against Chronic Diseases?," *Journal of the American Dietetic Association* 74 (1979): 543–550.

57. M. Pearce and S. Dayton, "Incidence of Cancer in Men on a Diet High in Polyunsaturated Fat," *Lancet* 297, no. 7697 (1971): 464–467; Lawrence, *Fats of Life*, 125.

58. Enig, "Dietary Fat and Cancer Trends"; Enig, "Diet, Serum Cholesterol and Coronary Heart Disease," in *Coronary Heart Disease*, ed. George Mann (London: Janus, 1993); Enig, *Trans Fatty Acids in the Food Supply: A Comprehensive Report Covering 60 Years of Research* (Silver Spring, Md.: Enig Associates, 1995).

59. J.T. Anderson, F. Grande, and A. Keys, "Hydrogenated Fats in the Diet and Lipids in the Serum of Man," *Journal of Nutrition* 75 (1961): 388–394. Keys never pursued this line of research. It is worth noting that he may have received funding for his research in subsequent years from the vegetable oil industry. See Barbara Santich, *What the Doctor Ordered: 150 Years of Dietary Advice in Australia* (Melbourne: Hyland House, 1995), 164.

60. Enig, "Dietary Fat and Cancer Trends," 2216.

61. Enig, "Dietary Fat and Cancer Trends," 2216

62. Kritchevsky, "History of Recommendations"; Taubes, *Good Calories, Bad Calories*, chap. 2.

63. Patty W. Siri-Tarino et al., "Saturated Fat, Carbohydrate, and Cardiovascular Disease," *American Journal of Clinical Nutrition* (2010); Siri-Tarino et al., "Meta-analysis of Prospective Cohort Studies Evaluating the Association of Saturated Fat with Cardiovascular Disease," *American Journal of Clinical Nutrition* 91 (2010): 535–546; Joint FAO/WHO Expert Consultation on Fats and Fatty Acids in Human Nutrition, *Interim Summary*.

64. Siri-Tarino et al., "Saturated Fat"; Dariush Mozaffarian, Eric Rimm, and David Herrington, "Dietary Fats, Carbohydrate, and Progression of Coronary Atherosclerosis in Postmenopausal Women," *American Journal of Clinical Nutrition* 80 (2004): 1175–1184.

65. Ronald Mensink et al., "Effects of Dietary Fatty Acids and Carbohydrates on the Ratio of Serum Total to H.D.L. Cholesterol and on Serum Lipids and Apolipoproteins: A Metaanalysis of 60 Controlled Trials," *American Journal of Clinical Nutrition* 77 (2003): 1146–1155.

66. Frank Hu, "Are Refined Carbohydrates Worse Than Saturated Fat?," *American Journal of Clinical Nutrition* 91 (2010): 1541–1542, 1542.

67. M. De Oliveira et al., "Dietary Intake of Saturated Fat by Food Source and Incident Cardiovascular Disease: The Multi-ethnic Study of Atherosclerosis," *American Journal of Clinical Nutrition* 96 (2012): 397–404.

68. H.K. Berneis and R.M. Krauss, "Metabolic Origins and Clinical Significance of LDL Heterogeneity," *Journal of Lipid Research* 43 (2002): 1363–1379; Taubes, *Good Calories, Bad Calories*, 173. For a contrary position, see S. Ip et al., "Association of Low-Density Lipoprotein Subfractions with Cardiovascular Outcomes," *Annals of Internal Medicine* 150 (2009): 474–484.

69. Ip et al., "Association of Low-Density Lipoprotein."

70. Arne Astrup et al., "The Role of Reducing Intakes of Saturated Fat in the Prevention of Cardiovascular Disease: Where Does the Evidence Stand in 2010?," *American Journal of Clinical Nutrition* 93 (2011): 684–688; Peter Parodi, "Has the Association Between Saturated Fatty Acids, Serum Cholesterol and Coronary Heart Disease Been Over Emphasized?," *International Dairy Journal* 19 (2009): 345–361; Taubes, *Good Calories, Bad Calories*, 173.

71. Daniel Steinberg, "The LDL Modification Hypothesis of Atherogenesis: An Update," *Journal of Lipid Research*, 50 suppl. (2009): S376–S381; Lawrence, *Fats of Life*, 76; Taubes, *Good Calories, Bad Calories*, 172; Fred A. Kummerow, *Cholesterol Won't Kill You, but trans-Fats Could* (Bloomington, Ind.: Trafford, 2008).

72. Lawrence, *Fats of Life*, 79.

73. Christopher Ramsden et al., "N-6 Fatty Acid-Specific and Mixed Polyunsaturate Dietary Interventions Have Different Effects on CHS Risk: A Meta-analysis of Randomised Controlled Trials," *British Journal of Nutrition* 104 (2010): 1586–1600.

74. Lawrence, *Fats of Life*, 192; Taubes, *Good Calories, Bad Calories*, 193.

75. Lawrence, *Fats of Life*, 73.

76. H. Katcher et al., "Atherosclerotic Cardiovascular Disease," in *Present Knowledge in Nutrition*, ed. B.A. Bowman et al. (ILSI Press, 2010); J. Pai et al., "Inflammatory Markers and the Risk of Coronary Heart Disease in Men and Women," *New England Journal of Medicine* 351, no. 25 (2004): 2599–2610; P. Libby, P. Ridker, and A. Maseri, "Inflammation and Atherosclerosis," *Circulation* 105 (2002): 1135–1143.

77. See, e.g., D. Kromhout et al., "The Confusion About Dietary Fatty Acid Recommendations for C.H.D. Prevention," *British Journal of Nutrition* 106 (2011); D. Mozaffarian, R. Micha, and S. Wallace, "Effects on Coronary Heart Disease of Increasing Polyunsaturated Fat in Place of Saturated Fat: A Systematic Review and Meta-analysis of Randomized Controlled Trials," *PLoS Medicine* 7, no. 3 (2010): 1–10.

78. U.S. Department of Agriculture and Department of Health and Human Services, *Dietary Guidelines for Americans, 2010* (Washington, D.C., 2010), 24–25, 24.

79. USDA, *Dietary Guidelines*, 2010, 26.

80. Marion Nestle, *Food Politics: How the Food Industry Influences Nutrition and Health*, 2nd ed. (Berkeley: University of California Press, 2007), chap. 1; Lara S. Sims, *The Politics of Fat: Food and Nutrition Policy in America* (New York: M.E. Sharpe, 1998), 229–231.

81. U.S. Senate Select Committee on Nutrition and Human Needs, *Dietary Goals for the United States*, 1st ed. (Washington, D.C., 1977).

82. Taubes, *Good Calories, Bad Calories*. See, e.g., Letitia Brewster and Michael Jacobson, *The Changing American Diet* (Washington, D.C.: Center for Science in the Public Interest, 1978).

83. A.E. Harper, "Dietary Goals: A Skeptical View," *Journal of the American Dietetic Association* 31 (1978): 310–321, 314.

84. Olson, "Are Professionals Jumping the Gun?"

85. U.S. Senate, *Dietary Goals for the United States*, 1st ed.

86. Mark Hegsted, "Food and Nutrition Policy: Probability and Practicality," *Journal of the American Dietetic Association* 74 (1979): 537.

87. See the debate in L. Barness, "Twenty Commentaries," *Nutrition Today* 12, no. 6 (1977): 10–27. See also Stewart Truswell, "Evolution of Dietary Recommendations, Goals and Guidelines," *American Journal of Clinical Nutrition* 45 (1987): 1060–1072; K. Dun Gifford, "Dietary Fats, Eating Guides, and Public Policy: History, Critique and Recommendations," *American Journal of Medicine* 113, no. 9B (2002): 89S–106S; Olson, "Are Professionals Jumping the Gun?"; Harper, "Dietary Goals"; Taubes, *Good Calories, Bad Calories*, 47. Marion Nestle, on the other hand, tends to downplay the lack of scientific consensus and instead emphasizes the objections of the food industry in *Food Politics*, 41.

88. U.S. Senate, *Dietary Goals for the United States*, 1st ed, 3.

89. Sims, *Politics of Fat*, 231.

90. Karin Garrety, "Dietary Policy, Controversy and Proof: Doing Something Versus Waiting for the Definitive Evidence," in *Silent Victories: The History and Practice of Public Health in Twentieth Century America*, ed. J. Ward and C. Warren (Oxford: Oxford University Press, 2006).

91. U.S. Senate, *Dietary Goals for the United States*, 2nd ed.; Gifford, "Dietary Fats, Eating Guides, and Public Policy"; Nestle, *Food Politics*, 40.

92. Nestle, *Food Politics*, 42.

93. See Mark Hegsted, "Washington—Dietary Guidelines," www.scribd.com/doc/18974320/Mark-Hegsteds-history-of-the-Dietary-Guidelines-for-Americans (accessed September 22, 2012); Marion Nestle, "In Memoriam: Mark Hegsted, 1914–2009" (August 18, 2009), in *Food Politics* [blog], www.foodpolitics.com/tag/mark-hegsted/ (accessed September 22, 2012).

94. Michael Pollan, *In Defense of Food: The Myth of Nutrition and the Pleasures of Eating* (New York: Allen Lane, 2008), 23.

95. Gifford, "Dietary Fats, Eating Guides, and Public Policy."

96. USDA and DHHS, *Dietary Guidelines*, 1.

97. Sims, *Politics of Fat*, 239; Belasco, *Appetite for Change*, 152.

98. Crotty, *Good Nutrition?*, 50.

99. Santich, *What the Doctor Ordered*, 185.

100. Santich, *What the Doctor Ordered*, 183, 93. In her history of Australian dietary guidelines, Barbara Santich similarly emphasizes the way these guidelines—which have largely mimicked American guidelines since the late 1970s—have referred to food components rather than foods. She suggests that, as well as reflecting a depersonalized and scientific attitude to eating, the use of such abstract wording may have been intended to "avoid acknowledging or incriminating the food industry, with whom nutritionists have long had an uneasy relationship" (195).

101. U.S. Department of Agriculture, *Food Guide Pyramid* (Washington, D.C.: Center for Nutrition Policy and Promotion, 1992).

102. Gyorgy Scrinis, "Sorry Marge," *Meanjin* 61, no. 4 (2002): 108–116; Scrinis, "On the Ideology of Nutritionism," *Gastronomica* 8, no. 1 (2008): 39–48.

103. Rose Hume Hall, *The Unofficial Guide to Smart Nutrition* (Foster City, Calif.: IDG Books, 2000), 27.

104. Walter Willett, *Eat, Drink, and Be Healthy: The Harvard Medical School Guide to Healthy Eating* (New York: Free Press, 2005), 12. See also W.C. Willett, "The Dietary Pyramid: Does the Foundation Need Repair?," *American Journal of Clinical Nutrition* 68 (1998): 218–219. For an alternative view, see Marion Nestle, "In Defense of the U.S.D.A. Food Guide Pyramid," *Nutrition Today* 33, no. 5 (1998): 189–196.

105. Qtd. in "Diet Wars," *Frontline* [transcript] (PBS, 2004), www.pbs.org /wgbh/pages/frontime/shows/diet/themes/pyramid.htm (accessed April 23, 2010).

106. W.C. Willett and M.J. Stampfer, "Rebuilding the Food Pyramid," *Scientific American* 16 (2003): 12–21.

107. Nestle, "In Defense of the U.S.D.A. Food Guide Pyramid." See also Luise Light's claims of how the *Pyramid*'s food recommendations were substantially changed by the USDA to win the acceptance of the food industry, including increasing the number of servings of bread and cereals from 2–3 to 6–11 and dropping the reference to whole grains. Luise Light, *What to Eat: The Ten Things You Really Need to Know to Eat Well and Be Healthy* (New York: McGraw-Hill, 2005).

5. THE MACRONUTRIENT DIET WARS

1. U.S. Department of Agriculture, Millennium Lecture Series, Symposium on the Great Nutrition Debate, February 24, 2000 [transcript], www.cnpp.usda .gov/publications/otherprojects/symposiumgreatnutritiondebatetranscript.txt (accessed March 5, 2012).

2. U.S. Department of Agriculture and Department of Health and Human Services, *Nutrition and Your Health: Dietary Guidelines for Americans* (Washington, D.C., 1980); U.S. Department of Agriculture, *Food Guide Pyramid* (Washington, D.C.: Center for Nutrition Policy and Promotion, 1992).

3. USDA, Millennium Lecture Series.

4. U.S. Public Health Service, *The Surgeon General's Report on Nutrition and Health* (Washington, D.C.: U.S. Government Printing Office, 1988). See also K. Dun Gifford, "Dietary Fats, Eating Guides, and Public Policy: History, Critique and Recommendations," *American Journal of Medicine* 113, no. 9B (2002): 89S–106S; Gary Taubes, *Good Calories, Bad Calories: Challenging the Conventional Wisdom on Diet, Weight Control, and Disease* (New York: Alfred A. Knopf, 2007), 60.

5. Taubes, *Good Calories, Bad Calories*, 60; S. Bryn Austin, "Commodity Knowledge in Consumer Culture: The Role of Nutritional Health Promotion in the Making of the Diet Industry," in *Weighty Issues: Fatness and Thinness as Social Problems*, ed. J. Sobal and D. Maurer (Hawthorne, N.Y.: de Gruyter, 1999), 159–182.

6. Lara S. Sims, *The Politics of Fat: Food and Nutrition Policy in America* (New York: M.E. Sharpe, 1998), 239.

7. Marion Nestle, *Food Politics: How the Food Industry Influences Nutrition and Health*, 2nd ed. (Berkeley: University of California Press, 2007), 6.

8. Patricia Hausman, *Jack Sprat's Legacy: The Science and Politics of Fat and Cholesterol* (New York: Richard Marek, 1981).

9. Michael Jacobson, "Preface," in Hausman, *Jack Sprat's Legacy*, 15.

10. Harvey Levenstein, *Paradox of Plenty: A Social History of Eating in Modern America*, rev. ed. (Berkeley: University of California Press, 2003), 208; A.E. Harper, "Firm Recommendations, Infirm Basis," *Nutrition Today* 17, no. 4 (1982): 16–19; Taubes, *Good Calories, Bad Calories*, 42.

11. Lori Beth Dixon and Nancy D. Ernst, "Choose a Diet That Is Low in Saturated Fat and Cholesterol and Moderate in Total Fat: Subtle Changes to a Familiar Message," *Journal of Nutrition* 131, no.2 (2001): 510S–526S.

12. Walter C. Willett, "Nutrition Recommendations for the General Population: Where Is the Science?," in *Nutrition and Health: Nutrition and Metabolism*, ed. C.S. Mantzoros (New York: Humana Press, 2009), 209–220; Austin, "Commodity Knowledge."

13. Ann F. La Berge, "How the Ideology of Low Fat Conquered America," *Journal of the History of Medicine and Allied Sciences* 63, no. 2 (2008): 139–177.

14. Dean Ornish, *Eat More, Weigh Less* (New York: Harper Collins, 1993), 31. Nathan Pritikin, *The Pritikin Program for Diet and Exercise* (New York: Grosset & Dunlap, 1979).

15. Willett, "Nutrition Recommendations."

16. Gifford, "Dietary Fats, Eating Guides, and Public Policy." David Jacobs and Linda Tapsell similarly argue that "the total fat message was felt to be satisfactory because it was easy to understand and implement" in "Food, Not Nutrients, Is the Fundamental Unit in Nutrition," *Nutrition Reviews* 65, no. 10 (2007): 439–450, 446.

17. La Berge, "How the Ideology of Low Fat Conquered America."

18. Martijn B. Katan, "Effect of Low-Fat Diets on Plasma High-Density Lipoprotein Concentrations," *American Journal of Clinical Nutrition* 67 (1998), 573S–576S; Patty W. Siri-Tarino et al., "Saturated Fat, Carbohydrate, and Cardiovascular Disease," *American Journal of Clinical Nutrition* (2010), 1541–1542; Frank Hu, "Are Refined Carbohydrates Worse Than Saturated Fat?," *American Journal of Clinical Nutrition* 91 (2010); Renata Micha and D. Mozaffarian, "Saturated Fat and Cardiometabolic Risk Factors, Coronary Heart Disease, Stroke and Diabetes: A Fresh Look at the Evidence," *Lipids* 45, no. 10 (2010): 893–905.

19. Walter Willett, *Eat, Drink, and Be Healthy: The Harvard Medical School Guide to Healthy Eating* (New York: Free Press, 2005), 69.

20. American Heart Association, "You're Your Fats," www.heart.org /HEARTORG/Conditions/Cholesterol/PreventionTreatmentofHighCholesterol /Know-Your-Fats_UCM_305628_Article.jsp (accessed November 1, 2010).

21. See American Heart Association, *Low-Fat, Low-Cholesterol Cookbook: Delicious Recipes to Help You Lower Your Cholesterol*, 4th ed. (New York: Crown, 2010).

22. National Research Council, *Diet, Nutrition and Cancer* (Washington, D.C., 1982).

23. National Research Council, *Diet, Nutrition and Cancer*; W.C. Willett, "Public Health Benefits of Preventive Nutrition," in *Preventive Nutrition: The Comprehensive Guide for Health Professionals*, ed. A. Bendich, R.J. Deckelbaum, and A. Sommer (New York: Humana Press, 2010).

24. W.C. Willett, "Dietary Fat Intake and Cancer Risk: A Controversial and Instructive Story," *Seminars in Cancer Biology* 8 (1998): 245–253.

25. R. Prentice et al., "Low-Fat Dietary Pattern and the Risk of Invasive Breast Cancer: The Women's Health Initiative Randomized Controlled Dietary Modification Trial," *Journal of the American Medical Association* 295, no. 6 (2006): 629–642; S.A.A. Beresford et al., "Low-Fat Dietary Pattern and the Risk of Colorectal Cancer: The Women's Health Initiative Randomized Controlled Dietary Modification Trial," *Journal of the American Medical Association* 295, no. 6 (2010): 643–654.

26. See, e.g., S. Sieri et al., "Dietary Fat and Breast Cancer Risk in the European Prospective Investigation into Cancer and Nutrition," *American Journal of Clinical Nutrition* 88 (2008): 1304–1312; E. Escrich et al., "Molecular Mechanisms of the Effects of Olive Oil and Other Dietary Lipids on Cancer," *Molecular Nutrition and Food Research* 51 (2007): 1279–1292; Y. Chen et al., "Dietary Fat–Gene Interactions in Cancer," *Cancer Metastasis Review* 26 (2007): 535–551.

27. World Cancer Research Fund/American Institute for Cancer Research, *Food, Nutrition, Physical Activity, and the Prevention of Cancer: A Global Perspective* (London: World Cancer Research Fund International, 2007).

28. Barbara Howard, "Dietary Fat and Diabetes: A Consensus View," *American Journal of Medicine* 113, no. 9B (2002): 385–403; J. Mann, "Diet and Diabetes," *Diabetologia* 18 (1980): 89–95.

29. Mann, "Diet and Diabetes."

30. Taubes, *Good Calories, Bad Calories*, chap. 6; B. Thomas, "Nutritional Advice for People with Diabetes: Past, Present, What Next?," *Practical Diabetes International* 21, no. 2 (2004): 69–72.

31. Taubes, *Good Calories, Bad Calories*, 186; D.J.A Jenkins, R.H. Taylor, and T.M.S. Wolever, "The Diabetic Diet, Dietary Carbohydrate and Differences in Digestibility," *Diabetologia* 23, no. 6 (1982): 477–484.

32. Jenkins et al., "Diabetic Diet."

33. J. Wylie-Rosett and F. Vinicor, "Diabetes Mellitus," in *Present Knowledge in Nutrition*, ed. B.A. Bowman et al. (Washington, D.C.: ILSI Press, 2010).

34. American Diabetes Association, "Standards of Medical Care in Diabetes—2010," *Diabetes Care* 33 (2010): S61–S78; American Diabetes Association, "Nutrition Recommendations and Interventions for Diabetes," *Diabetes Care* 31, no. 1 (2008): S11–S25.

35. American Diabetes Association, "Nutrition Recommendations"; Anthony Accurso et al., "Dietary Carbohydrate Restriction in Type 2 Diabetes Mellitus and Metabolic Syndrome: Time for a Critical Appraisal," *Nutrition and Metabolism* 5, no. 9 (2008).

36. American Diabetes Association, "Sugar and Desserts," www.diabetes.org /food-and-fitness/food/what-can-i-eat/sweeteners-and-desserts.html (accessed March 22, 2011); American Diabetes Association, "Nutrition Recommendations."

37. Barry Groves, *Trick and Treat: How Healthy Eating Is Making Us All Ill* (London: Hammersmith, 2008), 294.

38. George Bray, Sahasporn Paeratakul, and Barry Popkin, "Dietary Fat and Obesity: A Review of Animal, Clinical and Epidemiological Studies," *Physiology and Behavior* 83 (2004): 549–555; Barbara Rolls and Victoria Hammer, "Fat, Carbohydrate and the Regulation of Energy Intake," *American Journal of Clinical Nutrition* 62 (1995): 1086S–1095S; A. Astrup et al., "The Role of Low-Fat Diets and Fat Substitutes in Body Weight Management: What Have We Learned from Clinical Studies?," *Journal of the American Dietetic Association* 97, no. 7 (1997): S82–S87.

39. Austin, "Commodity Knowledge"; La Berge, "How the Ideology of Low Fat Conquered America."

40. Ornish, *Eat More, Weigh Less*, 19, 31.

41. Martijn B. Katan, "Alternatives to Low-Fat Diets," *American Journal of Clinical Nutrition* 83 (2006): 989–990; B.V. Howard et al., "Low-Fat Dietary Pattern and Weight Change over 7 Years: The Women's Health Initiative Dietary Modification Trial," *Journal of the American Medical Association* 295 (2006): 39–49; James Shikany et al., "Is Dietary Fat 'Fattening'? A Comprehensive Research Synthesis," *Critical Reviews in Food Science and Nutrition* 50 (2010): 699–715; T.A.B Sanders, "The Role of Fat in the Diet—Quantity, Quality and Sustainability," *Nutrition Bulletin* 35 (2010): 138–146.

42. Allysia Finley, "The Soda Tax," *Stanford Review* 42, no. 8 (1999).

43. On reduced-fat milk, see Groves, *Trick and Treat*, chap. 15.

44. Qtd. in Michael Fumento, *The Fat of the Land: The Obesity Epidemic and How Overweight Americans Can Help Themselves* (New York: Viking, 1997), 70.

45. Pauline Ippolito and Janis Pappalardo, *Nutrition and Health Advertising: Evidence from Food Advertising 1977–1997* (New York: Novinka, 2003), 26. See also Michael Heasman and Julian Mellentin, *The Functional Foods Revolution: Healthy People, Healthy Profits?* (London: Earthscan, 2001), 61; Nestle, *Food Politics*, 300.

46. Fumento, *Fat of the Land*, 74.

47. Felicity Lawrence, *Not on the Label: What Really Goes into the Food on Your Plate* (London: Penguin, 2004), 195.

48. Astrup et al., "The Role of Low-Fat Diets"; D. Miller et al., "Effect of Fat-Free Potato Chips with and without Nutrition Labels," *American Journal of Clinical Nutrition* 68 (1998): 282–290.

49. Qtd. in William G. Rothstein, *Public Health and the Risk Factor: A History of an Uneven Medical Revolution* (Rochester, N.Y.: University of Rochester Press, 2003), 322.

50. La Berge, "How the Ideology of Low Fat Conquered America"; Brian Wansick, *Mindless Eating: Why We Eat More Than We Think* (New York: Bantam Books, 2006), 189; Fumento, *Fat of the Land*, 70.

51. Brian Wansink and Pierre Chandon, "Can 'Low-Fat' Nutrition Labels Lead to Obesity?," *Journal of Marketing Research* 43 (2006): 605–617. See also Wansick, *Mindless Eating*.

52. Qtd. in Fumento, *Fat of the Land*, 73.

53. John Allred, "Too Much of a Good Thing?," *Journal of the American Dietetic Association* 95, no. 4 (1995): 417–418.

54. Adrian Heini and Roland Weinsier, "Divergent Trends in Obesity and Fat Intake Patterns: The American Paradox," *American Journal of Medicine* 102 (1997): 259–264; Helen La Fontaine et al., "Two Important Exceptions to the Relationship Between Energy Density and Fat Content: Foods with Reduced-Fat Claims and High-Fat Vegetable-Based Dishes," *Public Health Nutrition* 7, no. 4 (2003): 563–568; Berit Heitmann and Lauren Lissner, "Fat in the Diet and Obesity," in *International Textbook of Obesity*, ed. Per Bjorntorp (Chichester: John Wiley, 2001), 137–143.

55. G. Austin, L. Ogden, and J. Hill, "Trends in Carbohydrate, Fat and Protein Intakes and Association with Energy Intake in Normal-Weight, Overweight and Obese Individuals: 1971–2006," *American Journal of Clinical Nutrition* 93 (2011): 836–843.

56. N. Schwartz and S. Borra, "What Do Consumers Really Think About Dietary Fat?," *Journal of the American Dietetic Association* 97, no. 7 (1997): S73–S75.

57. J.D. Wright et al., "Trends in Intake of Energy and Macronutrients—United States, 1971–2000," *MMWR Morbidity and Mortality Weekly Report* 53

(2004): 80–82; Eric Oliver, *Fat Politics: The Real Story Behind America's Obesity Epidemic* (New York: Oxford, 2006), 126; Paul R. Marantz, Elizabeth D. Bird, and Michael H. Alderman, "A Call for Higher Standards of Evidence for Dietary Guidelines," *American Journal of Preventive Medicine* 34, no. 3 (2008), 234–266; Reena Oza-Frank et al., "Trends in Nutrient Intake Among Adults with Diabetes in the United States: 1988–2004," *Journal of the American Dietetic Association* 109, no. 7 (2009), 1173–1178; Austin et al., "Trends in Carbohydrate, Fat and Protein Intakes."

58. Judy Putnam, Jane Allshouse, and Linda Scott Kantor, "U.S. Per Capita Food Supply Trends: More Calories, Refined Carbohydrates and Fats," *Food Review* 25, no. 3 (2002): 2–15.

59. Ronette Briefel and Clifford Johnson, "Secular Trends in Dietary Intake in the United States," *Annual Review of Nutrition* 24 (2004): 401–431.

60. Linda van Horn, "Calories Count: But Can Consumers Count on Them?," *Journal of the American Medical Association* 306, no. 3 (2011): 315–316.

61. Barry Popkin et al., "Where's the Fat? Trends in U.S. Diets 1965–1996," *Preventive Medicine* 32, no. 245–254 (2001); Briefel and Johnson, "Secular Trends in Dietary Intake in the United States."

62. P. Chanmugam et al., "Did Fat Intake in the United States Really Decline Between 1989–1991 and 1994–1996?," *Journal of the American Dietetic Association* 103, no. 7 (2003): 867–872.

63. See "Diet Wars," *Frontline* (PBS, 2004), www.pbs.org/wgbh/pages/front line/shows/diet/ (accessed October 1, 2011).

64. Allred, "Too Much of a Good Thing?"

65. Dietary Guidelines Advisory Committee, *Report of the Dietary Guidelines Advisory Committee on the Dietary Guidelines for Americans, 2000* (Washington, D.C.: National Technical Information Service, 2000), 36–37.

66. Quoted in Gifford, "Dietary Fats, Eating Guides, and Public Policy."

67. Gary Taubes, "What If It's All Been a Big Fat Lie?," *New York Times Magazine*, July 7, 2002.

68. Taubes, "What If It's All Been a Big Fat Lie?" These omissions are also evident in Taubes, *Good Calories, Bad Calories*, xvii.

69. Taubes, "What If It's All Been a Big Fat Lie?," 26

70. Michael Pollan, *In Defense of Food: The Myth of Nutrition and the Pleasures of Eating* (New York: Allen Lane, 2008).

71. Pollan, *In Defense of Food*, 50, 61.

72. Pollan, *In Defense of Food*, 51.

73. Elsewhere Pollan gives a different explanation for the obesity epidemic when, following the argument of journalist Greg Crister, he blames the rise in obesity on the increased consumption of high-fructose corn syrup in *The Omnivore's Dilemma: A Natural History of Four Meals* (New York: Penguin, 2006), 102–104.

74. Martijn B. Katan, "Reply to E Roem," *American Journal of Clinical Nutrition* 90 (2009): 699.

75. George Blackburn, "The Low-Fat Imperative," *Obesity Reviews* 16, no. 1 (2008), 5–6; Bray et al., "Dietary Fat and Obesity."

76. See, e.g., Austin et al., "Trends in Carbohydrate, Fat and Protein Intakes; Boyd Swinburn, Gary Sacks, and Eric Ravussin, "Increased Food Energy Supply Is More Than Sufficient to Explain the U.S. Epidemic of Obesity," *American Journal of Clinical Nutrition* 90 (2009): 1453–1456.

77. Qtd. in Candy Sagon, "Butter Is Back—and Other Ideas That Will Change Your Diet in 2003," *Washington Post*, January 1, 2003.

78. Marion Nestle, "Eating Made Simple," *Scientific American* 297, no. 3 (2007): 60–69, 62.

79. Marion Nestle, *What to Eat* (New York: North Point Press, 2006), 285.

80. Nestle, *What to Eat*, 10.

81. U.S. Department of Agriculture and Department of Health and Human Services, *Dietary Guidelines for Americans, 2010* (Washington, D.C., 2010), 836–843.

82. Janet Adamy, "Food Firms Pledge to Cut Calories in Fight on Obesity," *Wall Street Journal*, May 17, 2010. See Healthy Weight Commitment Foundation, "HWCF Milestones," www.healthyweightcommit.org/about/hwcf_milestones (accessed July 18, 2012).

83. George Bray, "Good Calories, Bad Calories by Gary Taubes—Book Review," *Obesity Reviews* 9, no. 3 (2008): 251–263.

84. Martijn B. Katan and David Ludwig, "Extra Calories Cause Weight Gain—But How Much?," *Journal of the American Medical Association* 303, no. 1 (2010): 65–66.

85. Christina Wood Baker and Kelly Brownell, "Physical Activity and Maintenance of Weight Loss: Physiological and Psychological Mechanisms," in *Physical Activity and Obesity*, ed. Claude Bouchard (Champaign, Ill.: Human Kinetics, 2000), 311–328, 316.

86. James Hill et al., "Obesity and the Environment: Where Do We Go from Here?," *Science* 299, no. 7 (2003): 835–855. Also cited in Taubes, *Good Calories, Bad Calories*, 450. See also Steven B. Heymsfield, "How Large Is the Energy Gap That Accounts for the Obesity Epidemic?," *American Journal of Clinical Nutrition* 89 (2009): 1717–1718.

87. Human Nutrition Information Service USDA, Dietary Guidelines Advisory Committee, "Dietary Guidelines for Americans" (2005), qtd. in Taubes, *Good Calories, Bad Calories*, 297.

88. Katan and Ludwig, "Extra Calories Cause Weight Gain"; Heymsfield, "How Large Is the Energy Gap?"

89. Qtd. in Taubes, *Good Calories, Bad Calories*, 339.

90. Marion Nestle and Malden Nesheim, *Why Calories Count: From Science to Politics* (Berkeley: University of California Press, 2012), 187.

91. Nestle and Nesheim, *Why Calories Count*, 144.

92. This may be a case of what philosopher Ivan Illich referred to as "misplaced concreteness." See Barbara Duden, "The Quest for Past Somatics," in *The Challenges of Ivan Illich: A Collective Reflection*, ed. Lee Hoinacki and Carl Mitcham (Albany: State University of New York Press, 2002), 219–230.

93. See, e.g., A. Astrup et al., "Can Bioactive Foods Affect Obesity?," *Annals of the New York Academy of Science* 1190 (2010): 25–41.

94. Nestle and Nesheim, *Why Calories Count*, 35.

95. See, e.g., R. Feinman and E. Fine, "'A Calorie Is a Calorie' Violates the Second Law of Thermodynamics," *Nutrition Journal* 3, no. 9 (2004).

96. M. Zou et al., "Accuracy of Atwater Factors and Related Food Energy Conversion Factors with Low-Fat, High-Fiber Diets When Energy Intake Is Reduced Spontaneously," *American Journal of Clinical Nutrition* 86 (2007): 1649–1656; Bijal Trivedi, "The Calorie Delusion: Why Food Labels Are Wrong," *New Scientist*, July 15, 2009.

97. Nestle and Nesheim, *Why Calories Count*, 67.

98. See, e.g., J. Wells and M. Siervo, "Obesity and Energy Balance: Is the Tail Wagging the Dog?," *European Journal of Clinical Nutrition* 65 (2011): 1173–1189.

99. Jonathan Wells, "Obesity as Malnutrition: The Role of Capitalism in the Obesity Global Epidemic," *American Journal of Human Biology* 24 (2012): 261–276.

100. J.P. Chaput and A. Sharma, "Is Physical Activity in Weight Management More About 'Calories In' Than 'Calories Out'?," *British Journal of Nutrition* 106 (2011): 1768–1769.

101. Dale A. Schoeller, "The Energy Balance Equation: Looking Back and Looking Forward Are Two Different Views," *Nutrition Reviews* 67, no. 5 (2009): 249–254.

102. Schoeller, "The Energy Balance Equation."

103. S.N. El and S. Simsek, "Food Technological Applications for Optimal Nutrition: An Overview of Opportunities for the Food Industry," *Comprehensive Reviews in Food Science and Food Safety* 11 (2012): 2–12.

104. C. Gardner et al., "Nonnutritive Sweeteners: Current Use and Health Perspectives. A Scientific Statement from the American Heart Association and the American Diabetes Association," *American Journal of Clinical Nutrition* 35 (2012): 1798–1808.

105. Frank Sacks et al., "Comparison of Weight-Loss Diets with Different Compositions of Fat, Protein and Carbohydrates," *New England Journal of Medicine* 360, no. 9 (2009): 859–873.

106. M. Hession et al., "Systematic Review of Randomized Controlled Trials of Low-Carbohydrate vs. Low-Fat/Low-Calorie Diets in the Management of Obesity and Its Comorbidities," *Obesity Reviews* 10, no. 1 (2008): 36–50; John Foreyt et al., "Weight-Reducing Diets: Are There Any Differences?," *Nutrition Reviews* 67, suppl. 1 (2009): S99–S101; Richard Kones, "Low-Fat Versus Low-Carbohydrate Diets, Weight Loss, Vascular Health, and Prevention of Coronary

Artery Disease: The Evidence, the Reality, the Challenge and the Hope," *Nutrition in Clinical Practice* 25, no. 5 (2010): 528–541; C. Ebbeling et al., "Effects of Dietary Composition on Energy Expenditure During Weight-Loss Maintenance," *Journal of the American Medical Association* 307, no. 24 (2012): 2627–2634.

107. See, e.g., David J.A. Jenkins et al., "Macronutrients, Weight Control and Cardiovascular Health: A Systematic Review," *Current Cardiovascular Risk Reports* 4, no. 89–100 (2010).

108. Austin et al., "Trends in Carbohydrate, Fat and Protein Intakes."

109. Herman Taller, *Calories Don't Count* (New York: Simon and Schuster, 1961).

110. Robert C. Atkins, *Dr. Atkins' Diet Revolution* (New York: Bantam, 1973), 5.

111. Taubes, *Good Calories, Bad Calories*, xxiii.

112. Gary Taubes, *Why We Get Fat* (New York: Knopf, 2011), 8. Nestle and Nesheim suggest that "Taubes's reductionist view that obesity—a complex problem resulting from the interaction of genetics and behavior and affected by an exceptionally large number of hormonal and other regulatory factors—is largely due to a single cause: the effects of carbohydrate on insulin" in *Why Calories Count*, 162. But while they are right to take Taubes to task for this reductive focus on carbs, they provide a similarly reductive account regarding calories and the energy-balance equation.

113. Elissa Gootman, "Fruit Lovers, Weight Watchers Has Good News; Oreo Fans, Sorry," *New York Times*, December 4, 2010, 1.

114. Gootman, "Weight Watchers," 1.

115. Weight Watchers, "Points Plus® 2012—What It's All About," www.weight watchers.com/util/art/index_art.aspx?tabnum=1&art_id=105421 (accessed March 22, 2004).

116. Taubes, *Good Calories, Bad Calories*, xv.

117. Atkins, *Dr. Atkins' Diet Revolution*; Robert Atkins, *Dr. Atkins' New Diet Revolution* (New York: Harper Collins, 2002); Robert Atkins, *Atkins for Life: The Complete Controlled-Carb Program for Permanent Weight Loss and Good Health* (New York: St. Martin's Press, 2003). In 1961 Herman Taller's popular dieting book *Calories Don't Count* also promoted carbohydrate restriction.

118. Atkins, *Dr. Atkins' Diet Revolution*, 5, 7.

119. Atkins, *Dr. Atkins' Diet Revolution*, 5.

120. Atkins, *Dr. Atkins' Diet Revolution*, 31.

121. Atkins, *Dr. Atkins' New Diet Revolution*, 74.

122. Joel Stein, "The Low-Carb Diet Craze," *Time Magazine*, November 1, 1999.

123. A. Agatston, *The South Beach Diet* (New York: Rodale Books, 2003); Barry Sears and Bill Lawren; *The Zone: A Dietary Road Map* (New York: Harper Collins, 1995); Leighton Steward, Morrison Bethea, et al., *Sugar Busters: Cut Sugar to Trim Fat* (New York Ballantine Books, 1998).

124. Qtd. in Laura Fraser, *Losing It: America's Obsession with Weight and the Industry That Feeds on It* (New York: Dutton, 1997), 64; American Medical Association, "A Critique of Low-Carbohydrate Ketogenic Weight Reduction Regimens: A Review of Dr. Atkins' Diet Revolution," *Journal of the American Dietetic Association* 224 (1974).

125. Katan, "Reply to E Roem."

126. Arne Astrup, "Atkins and Other Low-Carbohydrate Diets: Hoax or an Effective Tool for Weight Loss?," *Lancet* 364 (2004); I. Shai et al., "Weight Loss with a Low-Carbohydrate, Mediterranean or Low-Fat Diet," *New England Journal of Medicine* 359, no. 3 (2008): 229–241; Christopher Gardner et al., "Comparison of the Atkins, Zone, Ornish, and Learn Diets for Change in Weight and Related Risk Factors Among Overweight Premenopausal Women," *Journal of the American Medical Association* 297, no. 9 (2007): 969–977; Foreyt et al., "Weight-Reducing Diets."

127. Qtd. in Marni Jameson, "A Reversal on Carbs," *Los Angeles Times*, December 20, 2010.

128. USDA and DHHS, *Dietary Guidelines for Americans, 2010*.

129. Taubes, *Good Calories, Bad Calories*, 393.

130. For studies supporting the benefits of low-carb diets, see E. Westman et al., "Low-Carbohydrate Nutrition and Metabolism," *American Journal of Clinical Nutrition* 86 (2007): 276–284; Gardner et al., "Comparison of the Atkins, Zone, Ornish, and Learn Diets." For counterevidence, see L. de Koning et al., "Low-Carbohydrate Diet Scores and Risk of Type 2 Diabetes in Men," *American Journal of Clinical Nutrition* 93 (2011): 844–850; T. Fung et al., "Low-Carbohydrate Diets and All-Cause and Cause-Specific Mortality: Two Cohort Studies," *Annals of Internal Medicine* 153 (2010): 289–298.

131. Sacks et al., "Comparison of Weight-Loss Diets."

132. Richard Feinman and Jeff Volek, "Carbohydrate Restriction as the Default Treatment for Type 2 Diabetes and Metabolic Syndrome," *Scandinavian Cardiovascular Journal* 42 (2008): 256–263; Accurso et al., "Dietary Carbohydrate Restriction."

133. S. Ben-Avraham et al., "Dietary Strategies for Patients with Type 2 Diabetes in the Era of Multi-approaches; Review and Results from the Dietary Intervention Randomized Controlled Trial (Direct)," *Diabetes Research and Clinical Practice* 86 (2009): S41–S48.

134. Taubes, *Good Calories, Bad Calories*, 344, 445.

135. Nicole Darmon and Adam Drewnowski, "Does Social Class Predict Diet Quality?," *American Journal of Clinical Nutrition* 87 (2008): 1107–1117.

136. Food quality is a consistent theme on the popular *Livin' La Vida Low-Carb* podcast show (www.thelivinlowcarbshow.com). See also Jonny Bowden, *Living Low Carb*, rev. ed. (New York: Sterling, 2010).

137. Jenkins et al., "Diabetic Diet."

138. David Ludwig et al., "High Glycemic Foods, Overeating and Obesity," *Pediatrics* 103, no. 3 (1999).

139. Dean Ornish, *The Spectrum: A Scientifically Proven Program to Feel Better, Live Longer, Lose Weight, Gain Health* (New York: Ballantine Books, 2008), 147.

140. Helen Mitchell, "The Glycemic Concept in Action," *American Journal of Clinical Nutrition* 87, suppl. (2008).

141. American Diabetes Association, "Glycemic Index and Diabetes," www .diabetes.org/food-and-fitness/food/planning-meals/glycemic-index-and-diabe tes.html?utm_ source=RightHandRail&utm_medium= SitePromotion4&utm _campaign=Glycemic (accessed May 10, 2010). See also Nancy Sheard et al., "Dietary Carbohydrate (Amount and Type) in the Prevention and Management of Diabetes: A Statement by the American Diabetes Association," *Diabetes Care* 27, no. 9 (2004).

142. Stacey Bell et al., "Appetite, Body Weight, Health Implications of a Low-Glycemic Load Diet," in *Obesity: Epidemiology, Pathophysiology and Prevention*, ed. D. Bagchi and H. Preuss (Hoboken, N.J.: CRC Press, 2007), 245–263.

143. Thomas Wolever, *The Glycaemic Index: A Physiological Classification* (Wallingford, U.K.: CABI, 2006), 165.

144. J.C. Brand-Miller et al., *The Low-GI Handbook: The New Glucose Revolution Guide to the Long-Term Health Benefits of Low GI Eating* (Cambridge, Mass.: Da Capo, 2010), 19.

145. Amin Esfahani et al., "The Glycemic Index: Physiological Significance," *Journal of the American College of Nutrition* 28, no. 4, suppl. 1 (2009): 439S–445S; J.C. Brand-Miller et al., "Dietary Glycemic Index: Health Implications," *Journal of the American College of Nutrition* 28, no. 4 (2009): 446S–449S; J. Bao et al., "Prediction of Postprandial Glycemia and Insulinemia in Lean, Young, Healthy Adults: Glycemic Load Compared with Carbohydrate Content Alone," *American Journal of Clinical Nutrition* 93 (2011): 984–996; T. Larsen et al., "Diets with High or Low Protein Content and Glycemic Index for Weight-Loss Maintenance," *New England Journal of Medicine* 363, no. 22 (2010): 2102–2113.

146. K. Grau et al., "Overall Glycaemic Index and Glycaemic Load of Habitual Diet and Risk of Heart Disease," *Public Health Nutrition* 14, no. 1 (2010): 109–118; M. Similia et al., "Low-, Medium- and High-Glycemic Index Carbohydrates and Risk of Type 2 Diabetes in Men," *British Journal of Nutrition* 105, no. 8 (2010): 1258–1264; F.X. Pi-Sunyer, "Glycemic Index and Disease," *American Journal of Clinical Nutrition* 76, suppl. (2002): 290S–298S; J. Mann et al., "F.A.O./W.H.O. Scientific Update on Carbohydrates in Human Nutrition: Conclusion," *European Journal of Clinical Nutrition* 61 (2007): S132–S137; M. Franz, "The Glycemic Index: Not the Most Effective Nutrition Therapy Intervention," *Diabetes Care* 26, no. 8 (2003): 2466–2468; R. Vrolix and R. Mensink, "Effects of Glycemic Load on Metabolic Risk Markers in Subjects at Increased Risk of Developing Metabolic Syndrome," *American Journal of Clinical Nutrition* 92, no. 2 (2010): 366–374.

147. David Ludwig, *Ending the Food Fight: Guide Your Child to a Healthy Weight in a Fast Food/Fake Food World* (Boston: Houghton-Mifflin, 2007), 61.

148. Ludwig, *Ending the Food Fight*, 49.

149. J.H. Cummings and A.M. Stephen, "Carbohydrate Terminology and Classification," *European Journal of Clinical Nutrition* 61 (2007): S5–S18.

150. David Ludwig, "The Glycemic Index: Physiological Mechanisms Relating to Obesity, Diabetes and Cardiovascular Disease," *Journal of the American Medical Association* 287 (2002).

151. Marion Franz, "The Glycemic Index of High-Sugar Foods" (letter), *American Journal of Clinical Nutrition* 107, no. 4 (2007): 564.

152. F.S. Atkinson, K. Foster-Powell, and J.C. Brand-Miller, "International Tables of Glycemic Index and Glycemic Load Values," *Diabetes Care* 31, no. 12 (2008).

153. Atkinson et al., "International Tables."

154. B.J. Venn and T.J. Green, "Glycemic Index and Glycemic Load: Measurement Issues and Their Effect on Diet-Disease Relationships," *European Journal of Clinical Nutrition* 61 (2007): S122–S131.

155. Glen D. Lawrence, *The Fats of Life: Essential Fatty Acids in Health and Disease* (New Brunswick, N.J.: Rutgers University Press, 2010), 189; Robert Lustig, "Fructose: Metabolic, Hedonic, and Societal Parallels with Ethanol," *Journal of the American Dietetic Association* 110 (2010): 1307–1321.

156. Brand-Miller et al., *The Low-GI Handbook*, 170.

157. Anon., "CSR LoGiCane LowGI Sugar", www.csrsugar.com.au/Better-For-You-Products/CSR-LoGiCane-LowGI-Sugar.aspx (accessed October 1, 2011).

158. Venn and Green, "Glycemic Index and Glycemic Load."

159. Mann et al., "F.A.O./W.H.O. Scientific Update"; S. Williams et al., "Another Approach to Estimating the Reliability of Glycaemic Index," *British Journal of Nutrition* 100 (2008): 364–372; R. Vrolix and R. Mensink, "Variability of the Glycemic Index Response to Single Food Products in Healthy Subjects," *Contemporary Clinical Trials* 31 (2010): 5–11.

160. Anne Flint et al., "The Use of Glycaemic Index Tables to Predict Glycaemic Index of Composite Breakfast Meals," *British Journal of Nutrition* 91 (2004): 979–989. For a contrary view, see T. Wolever et al., "Food Glycemic Index, as Given in Glycemic Index Tables, Is a Significant Determinant of Glycemic Responses Elicited by Composite Break Fast Cereals," *American Journal of Clinical Nutrition* 83 (2006): 1306–1312.

161. Vrolix and Mensink, "Effects of Glycemic Load"; Williams et al., "Another Approach to Estimating the Reliability of Glycaemic Index."

162. Manny Noakes and Peter Clifton, *The CSIRO Total Wellbeing Diet* (Camberwell: Penguin, 2005); Gyorgy Scrinis and Rosemary Stanton, "Total Wellbeing or Too Much Meat?," *Australasian Science* 26, no. 9 (2005): 37–38.

1. Gussow's words are quoted in Bryan Miller, "Prescriptions for Dining Out," *New York Times*, April 16, 1986, C1. There are also other, earlier versions of this now-famous quotation, such as, "I trust cows more than I do chemists, and when I want to spread something on my bread, I use butter," in Mimi Sheraton, "Nutrition: Balance May Be the Key," *New York Times*, Feb. 13, 1980, C1.

2. W.G. Hoffman, "100 Years of the Margarine Industry," in *Margarine: An Economic, Social and Scientific History 1869–1969*, ed. J.H. van Stuyvenberg (Liverpool: Liverpool University Press, 1969), 9–36, 13.

3. Richard A. Ball and J. Robert Lilly, "The Menace of Margarine: The Rise and Fall of a Social Problem," *Social Problems* 29, no. 5 (1982): 488–498.

4. Ross Hume Hall, *Food for Nought: The Decline in Nutrition* (Hagerstown, Md.: Harper and Row, 1974), 238; Hoffman, "100 Years of the Margarine Industry."

5. R.D. Tousley, "Marketing," in *Margarine: An Economic, Social and Scientific History 1869–1969*, ed. J.H. van Stuyvenberg (Liverpool: Liverpool University Press, 1969), 227–280.

6. Ball and Lilly, "The Menace of Margarine"; Ruth Dupre, "'If It's Yellow, It Must Be Butter': Margarine Regulation in North America since 1886," *Journal of Economic History* 59, no. 2 (1999): 353–371.

7. Dupre, "'If It's Yellow, It Must Be Butter'"; Charlene Elliot, "Canada's Great Butter Caper," *Food, Culture and Society* 12, no. 3 (2009): 379–396.

8. S.F. Riepma, *The Story of Margarine* (Washington, D.C.: Public Affairs Press, 1970), 69.

9. Mika Pantzar, "Public Dialogue Between Butter and Margarine in Finland 1923–1992," *Journal of Consumer Studies and Home Economics* 19 (1995): 11–24.

10. Paul Clark, "The Marketing of Margarine," *European Journal of Marketing* 20, no. 5 (1986): 52–65; Alastair Frazer, "Nutritional and Dietetic Aspects," in *Margarine: An Economic, Social and Scientific History 1869–1969*, ed. J.H. van Stuyvenberg (Liverpool: Liverpool University Press, 1969), 123–162; Sally Horrocks, "The Business of Vitamins: Nutrition Science and the Food Industry in Inter-war Britain," in *Food, Science, Policy and Regulation in the Twentieth Century: International and Comparative Perspectives*, ed. David Smith and Jim Phillips (London: Routledge, 2000), 235–258.

11. Riepma, *The Story of Margarine*, 69.

12. See Mary Enig and Sally Fallon, *Nourishing Traditions: The Cookbook That Challenges Politically Correct Nutrition and the Diet Dictocrats* (Washington, D.C.: New Trends, 1999); Hall, *Food for Nought*.

13. J. Edward Hunter, "Dietary Trans Fatty Acids: Review of Recent Human Studies and Food Industry Responses," *Lipids* 41, no. 11 (2006): 967–992.

14. Susan Allport, *The Queen of Fats: Why Omega-3s Were Removed from the Western Diet and What We Can Do to Replace Them* (Berkeley: University of California Press, 2006), 118.

15. European Food Safety Authority, "Opinion of the Scientific Panel on Dietetic Products, Nutrition and Allergies on a Request from the Commission Related to the Presence of Trans Fatty Acids in Foods and the Effect on Human Health of the Consumption of Trans Fatty Acids," *EFSA Journal* 81 (2004): 1–49; FSANZ, *Trans Fatty Acids in the New Zealand and Australian Food Supply: Review Report* (Canberra: Food Standards Australia and New Zealand, 2007).

16. G. van Duijn, E.E. Dumelin, and E.A. Trautwein, "Virtually *Trans* Free Oils and Modified Fats," in *Improving the Fat Content of Foods*, ed. Christine Williams and Judith Buttriss (New York: CRC Press, 2006), 490–507; P. Lambelet et al., "Formation of Modified Fatty Acids and Oxyphytosterols During Refining of Low Erucic Acid Rapeseed Oil," *Journal of Agricultural and Food Chemistry* 51 (2003): 4284–4290.

17. Susan Pendleton, "'Man's Most Important Food Is Fat': The Use of Persuasive Techniques in Procter & Gamble's Public Relations Campaign to Introduce Crisco, 1911–1913," *Public Relations Quarterly* 44, no. 1 (1999): 6–14.

18. Steve Ettlinger, *Twinkie, Deconstructed* (New York: Hudson Street Press, 2007), 99.

19. G.R. List and T. Pelloso, "Zero/Low Trans Margarine, Spreads and Shortening," in *Trans Fats in Foods*, ed. Gary R. List, D. Kritchevsky, and N. Ratnayke (Urbana, Ill.: AOCS Press, 2007), 155–176, 156.

20. Mary Enig, *Trans Fatty Acids in the Food Supply: A Comprehensive Report Covering 60 Years of Research* (Silver Spring, Md.: Enig Associates, 1995), 3.

21. B. Bronte-Stewart et al., "Effects of Feeding Different Fats on Serum Cholesterol Level," *Lancet* 1 (1956); E.H. Ahrens, "The Influence of Dietary Fats on Serum Levels in Man," *Lancet* 1 (1957); Don McOsker et al., "The Influence of Partially Hydrogenated Dietary Fats on Serum Cholesterol Levels," *Journal of the American Medical Association* 180, no. 5 (1962): 120–125; J.T. Anderson, F. Grande, and A. Keys, "Hydrogenated Fats in the Diet and Lipids in the Serum of Man," *Journal of Nutrition* 75 (1961): 388–394; Onno Korver and Martijn B. Katan, "The Elimination of Trans Fats from Spreads: How Science Helped to Turn an Industry Around," *Nutrition Reviews* 64, no. 6 (2006): 275–279; Hall, *Food for Nought*, 242; Udo Erasmus, *Fats That Heal, Fats That Kill* (Burnaby, Canada: Alive Books, 1987); Germain Brisson, *Lipids in Human Nutrition* (Englewood, N.J.: Jack K. Burgess, 1981).

22. Anderson et al., "Hydrogenated Fats in the Diet." See also Mary Enig, *Know Your Fats: The Complete Primer for Understanding the Nutrition of Fats, Oils, and Cholesterol* (Bethesda, Md.: Bethesda Press, 2010), 85; and Barbara Santich, *What the Doctor Ordered: 150 Years of Dietary Advice in Australia* (Melbourne: Hyland House, 1995), 164. Jane Brody noted the cholesterol raising effects of *trans*-fats in *Jane Brody's Nutrition Book* (New York: W.W. Norton, 1981), 73.

23. I.H. Page et al., "Atherosclerosis and the Fat Content of the Diet," *Circulation* 16 (1957): 163–178; American Heart Association, Central Committee for Medical and Community Program, "Dietary Fat and Its Relation to Heart Attacks

and Strokes," *Circulation* 23 (1961): 133–136; Santich, *What the Doctor Ordered*, 165; Marion Nestle, *What to Eat* (New York: North Point Press, 2006), 115.

24. Fred A. Kummerow, "Viewpoint on the Report of the National Cholesterol Education Program Expert Panel on Detection, Evaluation and Treatment of High Blood Cholesterol in Adults," *Journal of the American College of Nutrition* 12, no. 1 (1993): 2–13; Kummerow, *Cholesterol Won't Kill You, but Trans-Fats Might* (Bloomington, Ind.: Trafford, 2008), 45.

25. Hall, *Food for Nought*, 243. For an example of this expert advocacy for margarines with lower levels of saturated fats, see A. Gattereau and H. Delisle, "The Unsettled Question: Butter or Margarine?," *Canadian Medical Association Journal* 103 (1970): 268–271.

26. Hall, *Food for Nought*, 239. Some margarines at the time were reported by Hall as containing about 40 percent *trans*-fats.

27. Hall, *Food for Nought*, 242.

28. Mary Enig, "Dietary Fat and Cancer Trends—a Critique," *Federation Proceedings* 37, no. 9 (1978): 2215–2219. See also Brisson, *Lipids in Human Nutrition*; Brody, *Jane Brody's Nutrition Book*, 72; George Mann's entry in Lewis Barness et al., "Twenty Commentaries on the *Dietary Goals for the United States*," *Nutrition Today* (November/December 1977): 10–32.

29. While butter has been more or less equated with saturated fats, and margarine equated with unsaturated fats, both spreads consist of different ratios of saturated, polyunsaturated, and monounsaturated fats. Unilever's Flora Original margarine, for example, currently contains by weight 17 percent saturated, 27 percent polyunsaturated, and 16 percent monounsaturated fats, whereas butter contains around 51 percent saturated, 3 percent polyunsaturated, and 21 percent monounsaturated. See Flora, "Flora Original," www.au-flora.com/Flora/Flora -Spreads-Product-Range/Flora-Original.aspx (accessed September 1, 2012).

30. R.P. Mensink and M.K. Katan, "Effect of Dietary Trans Fatty Acids on High-Density and Low-Density Lipoprotein Cholesterol Levels in Healthy Subjects," *New England Journal of Medicine* 323 (1990): 439–445; Korver and Katan, "Elimination of Trans Fats from Spreads."

31. W.C. Willett et al., "Intake of Trans Fatty Acids and Risk of Coronary Heart Disease Among Women," *Lancet* 341 (1993): 581–585.

32. See, e.g., Willett et al., "Intake of Trans Fatty Acids"; M.B. Katan, P.L. Zock, and R.P. Mensink, "Trans Fatty Acids and Their Effects on Lipoproteins in Humans," *Annual Review of Nutrition* 15 (1995): 473–493; R.P. Mensink et al., "Effects of Dietary Fatty Acids and Carbohydrates on the Ratio of Serum Total to H.D.L. Cholesterol and on Serum Lipids and Apolipoproteins: A Meta-analysis of 60 Controlled Trials," *American Journal of Clinical Nutrition* 77 (2003): 1146–1155; D. Mozaffarian, A. Aro, and W.C. Willett, "Health Effects of Trans-Fatty Acids: Experimental and Observational Evidence," *European Journal of Clinical Nutrition* 63 (2009): S5–S21; Dariush Mozaffarian et al., "Trans Fatty Acids and Cardiovascular Disease," *New England Journal of Medicine* 354, no. 15 (2006):

1601–1613; J.T. Judd et al., "Dietary Trans Fatty Acids: Effects on Plasma Lipids and Lipoproteins of Healthy Men and Women," *American Journal of Clinical Nutrition* 59 (1994): 861–868.

33. Mozaffarian et al., "Health Effects of Trans-Fatty Acids: Experimental and Observational Evidence"; Mozaffarian et al., "Trans Fatty Acids and Cardiovascular Disease."

34. Valentina Remig, "Trans Fats in America: A Review of Their Use, Consumption, Health Implications, and Regulation," *Journal of the American Dietetic Association* 110 (2010): 585–592; Mary Enig, *Know Your Fats: The Complete Primer for Understanding the Nutrition of Fats, Oils, and Cholesterol* (Bethesda, Md.: Bethesda Press, 2010).

35. Samuel Shapiro, "Do Trans Fatty Acids Increase the Risk of Coronary Artery Disease? A Critique of the Epidemiologic Evidence," *American Journal of Clinical Nutrition* 66, suppl. (1997): 1011S–1017S.

36. Shapiro, "Do Trans Fatty Acids Increase the Risk of Coronary Artery Disease?"

37. Gary Taubes, *Good Calories, Bad Calories: Challenging the Conventional Wisdom on Diet, Weight Control, and Disease* (New York: Knopf, 2007), 44.

38. William G. Rothstein, *Public Health and the Risk Factor: A History of an Uneven Medical Revolution* (Rochester, N.Y.: University of Rochester Press, 2003), 320.

39. Karin Garrety, "Social Worlds, Actor-Networks and Controversy: The Case of Cholesterol, Dietary Fat and Heart Disease," *Social Studies of Science* 27, no. 5 (1997): 727–773.

40. Rothstein, *Public Health and the Risk Factor*, 318.

41. "Fat in the Fire," *Time*, December 26, 1960; Garrety, "Social Worlds."

42. Qtd. in Rothstein, *Public Health and the Risk Factor*, 320.

43. Rothstein, *Public Health and the Risk Factor*, 318. See also Janis Kohanski Pappalardo and Debra Jones Ringold, "Regulating Commercial Speech in a Dynamic Environment: Forty Years of Margarine and Oil Advertising Before the NLEA," *Journal of Public Policy and Marketing* 19, no. 1 (2000): 74–92; Harvey Levenstein, *Paradox of Plenty: A Social History of Eating in Modern America*, rev. ed. (Berkeley: University of California Press, 2003), 210. Explicit health claims were disallowed in Australia at this time, and some margarine manufacturers in the 1960s were ordered by food authorities in Australia to stop using misleading claims that margarine reduced the risk of heart disease (Santich, *What the Doctor Ordered*, 165). In the United Kingdom a "high in polyunsaturates" claim was first able to be advertised in 1979. See Felicity Lawrence, *Eat Your Heart Out: Why the Food Business Is Bad for the Planet and Your Health* (Melbourne: Penguin, 2008), 234.

44. In Australia, polyunsaturated margarine replaced butter as the more widely consumed spread in 1977–1978 (Santich, *What the Doctor Ordered*, 203).

45. Gary Taubes, "The Soft Science of Dietary Fat," *Science* 291, no. 5513 (2001): 2536–2545.

46. Center for Science in the Public Interest, *Saturated Fat Attack* (Washington, D.C., 1988), 2.

47. Center for Science in the Public Interest, *Saturated Fat Attack*, 5.

48. Mary Enig, "The Tragic Legacy of Center for Science in the Public Interest," www.westonaprice.org/know-your-fats/tragic-legacy-of-cspi (accessed September 1, 2012).

49. George Inglett, ed., *Fabricated Foods* (Westport, Conn.: AVI Publishing, 1975), 1.

50. Umberto Eco, *Travels in Hyperreality* (London: Picador, 1986), 45. On hyperreality, see also Jean Baudrillard, *Simulations* (New York: Semiotext, 1983).

51. Eco, *Travels in Hyperreality*, 44.

52. Albert Borgmann, *Crossing the Postmodern Divide* (Chicago: University of Chicago Press, 1992), 93.

53. U.S. Department of Agriculture and U.S. Department of Health and Human Services, *Dietary Guidelines for Americans, 2010* (Washington, D.C., 2010).

54. Robert Eckel et al., "Understanding the Complexity of Trans Fatty Acid Reduction in the American Diet: American Heart Association Trans Fat Conference 2006," *Circulation* 115 (2007): 2231–2246. Also qtd. in A. Crawford et al., "Estimated Effect on Fatty Acid Intake of Substituting a Low-Saturated, High-Oleic, Low-Linolenic Soybean Oil for Liquid Oils," *Nutrition Today* 46, no. 4 (2011): 189–196.

55. American Heart Association, "Meet the Fats," www.heart.org/HEARTORG/GettingHealthy/FatsAndOils/MeettheFats/Meet-the-Fats_UCM_304495_Article.jsp (accessed October 20, 2012).

56. American Heart Association, "Know Your Fats," www.heart.org/HEARTORG/GettingHealthy/NutritionCenter/Knowing-Your-Fats_UCM_305976_Article.jsp (accessed October 20, 2012).

57. Phil McKenna, "Out of the Trans-Fat Frying Pan, into the Fire," *New Scientist*, January 6, 2007.

58. W.C. Willett, "The Scientific Basis for T.F.A. Regulations—Is It Sufficient? Comments from the USA," *Atherosclerosis Supplements* 7 (2006): 69–71. See also Mozaffarian et al., "Trans Fatty Acids and Cardiovascular Disease"; Harvard School of Public Health, "The Nutrition Source: Fats and Cholesterol: Out with the Bad, In with the Good," www.hsph.harvard.edu/nutritionsource/what-should-you-eat/fats-full-story (accessed September 23, 2012).

59. Susan Okie, "New York to Trans Fats: You're Out!," *New England Journal of Medicine* 356, no. 20 (2007): 2017–2021.

60. W.C. Willett and Dariush Mozaffarian, "Ruminant or Industrial Sources of Trans Fatty Acids: Public Health Issue or Food Label Skirmish?," *American Journal of Clinical Nutrition* 87 (2008): 515–516. In Europe, on the other hand, only industrially produced *trans*-fats require labeling. See Institute of Food Science and Technology (IFST) (2007) Information Statement: *Trans* fatty acids (TFA), www.iufost.org/iufost-scientific-information-bulletins-sib (accessed September

1, 2012); Mary Enig, "Interesterification," www.westonaprice.org/know-your -fats/interesterification (accessed July 1, 2012).

61. Paul R. Marantz, Elizabeth D. Bird, and Michael H. Alderman, "A Call for Higher Standards of Evidence for Dietary Guidelines," *American Journal of Preventive Medicine* 34, no. 3 (2008): 234–266; Laurian Unnevehr and Evelina Jagmanaite, "Getting Rid of Trans Fats in the US Diet: Policies, Incentives and Progress," *Food Policy* 33 (2008): 497–503.

62. U.S. Food and Drug Administration, "Health Claim Notification for Saturated Fat, Cholesterol, and Trans Fat, and Reduced Risk of Heart Disease," www.fda.gov/Food/LabelingNutrition/LabelClaims/FDAModernizationAct FDAMAClaims/ucm073621.htm (accessed October 1, 2011).

63. Kim Severson, "Trans Fat Fight Claims Butter as a Victim," *New York Times*, March 7, 2007.

64. Walter Willett, *Eat, Drink, and Be Healthy: The Harvard Medical School Guide to Healthy Eating* (New York: Free Press, 2005), 28.

65. Willett, *Eat, Drink, and Be Healthy*, 28.

66. See Mary Enig, "The Tragic Legacy of Center for Science in the Public Interest (CSPI)," *Wise Traditions* (2003). See also Elaine Blume's article in the CSPI newsletter, "The Truth About Trans: Hydrogenated Oils Aren't Guilty as Charged," *Nutrition Action Newsletter*, March 1988.

67. Theodore Frank, "A Taxonomy of Obesity Legislation," *UALR Law Review* 28 (2005): 427–441.

68. Nestle, *What to Eat*, 114–115. See also Marion Nestle, *Food Politics: How the Food Industry Influences Nutrition and Health*, 2nd ed. (Berkeley: University of California Press, 2007), 386.

69. See, e.g., American Heart Association, *Planning Fat Controlled Meals for 1200 and 1800 Calories* (Austin, Tx.: American Heart Association, 1966). See also Hall, *Food for Nought*, 234.

70. Marantz et al., "A Call for Higher Standards of Evidence for Dietary Guidelines," 238.

71. Unnevehr and Jagmanaite, "Getting Rid of Trans Fats."

72. Exceptions to this rule include Mary Enig and the Western Price Foundation (www.westonaprice.org), which have highlighted the potential problems with the interesterification process. British journalist Felicity Lawrence has also highlighted some of these issues related to the interesterification of oils (Lawrence, *Eat Your Heart Out*). See also Julie Jargon, "Out with the Trans Fats, in with a Whole Lot of Others," *Wall Street Journal Online*, November 6, 2007.

73. Annemarie Beers, "Low Trans Hydrogenation of Edible Oils," *Lipid Technology* 19, no. 3 (2007): 56–58.

74. Maria Teresa Tarrago-Trani et al., "New and Existing Oils and Fats Used in Products with Reduced Trans-Fatty Acid Content," *Journal of the American Dietetic Association* 106, no. 6 (2006), 867–880; J.E. Upritchard et al., "Modern Fat

Technology: What Is the Potential for Heart Health?," *Proceedings of the Nutrition Society* 64 (2005): 379–386.

75. Upritchard et al., "Modern Fat Technology."

76. Paul Wassell and Niall Young, "Food Applications of *Trans* Fatty Acid Substitutes," *International Journal of Food Science and Technology* 42 (2007): 503–517.

77. van Duijn et al., "Virtually *Trans* Free Oils and Modified Fats"; J. Edward Hunter, "Applications of Food Science in Implementing Dietary Lipid Recommendations," *Nutrition Today* 46, no. 4 (2011): 182–188.

78. Hunter, "Applications of Food Science."

79. The interesterification process rearranges the order of attachment of constituent fatty acids to the glycerol backbone of triglyceride molecules. In 1974 Ross Hume Hall had already highlighted the way interesterification reorganized the original molecular architecture of vegetable oils in *Food for Nought*, 239.

80. Hall, *Food for Nought*, 239.

81. K.C. Hayes and Pronczuk, "Replacing Trans Fat: The Argument for Palm Oil with a Cautionary Note on Interesterification," *Journal of the American College of Nutrition* 29, no. 3 (2010).

82. van Duijn et al. note that production-scale full hydrogenation itself produces *trans*-fat levels greater than 1 percent in "Virtually *Trans* Free Oils and Modified Fats."

83. Flora, www.florapro-activ.com.au/245_250.htm (accessed September 20, 2008). See also Lawrence, *Eat Your Heart Out*, 241.

84. Upritchard et al., "Modern Fat Technology."

85. Donald Pszczola, "Future Strategies for Fat Replacement," *Food Technology*, no. 6 (2006): 61–84.

86. Tom Tiffany, "Oil Options for Deep Frying," *Food Technology*, no. 7 (2007): 46–56.

87. Tiffany, "Oil Options for Deep Frying"; Hunter, "Applications of Food Science."

88. Unnevehr and Jagmanaite, "Getting Rid of Trans Fats"; Eckel et al., "Understanding the Complexity of Trans Fatty Acid Reduction"; Emily Waltz, "Food Firms Test Fry Pioneer's Trans-Fat Free Soybean Oil," *Nature Biotechnology* 28, no. 8 (2010): 769–770.

89. G.W. Meijer and J.A. Weststrate, "Interesterification of Fats in Margarine: Effect on Blood Lipids, Blood Enzymes, and Hemostasis Parameters," *European Journal of Clinical Nutrition* 51 (1997): 527–534. See also Jan I. Pedersen and Bente Kirkhus, "Fatty Acid Composition of *Post Trans* Margarines and Their Health Implications," *Lipid Technology* 20, no. 6 (2008): 132–135; K. Sundram, T. Karapaiah, and K.C. Hayes, "Stearic Acid-Rich Interesterified Fat and Trans-Rich Fat Raise the LDL/HDL Ratio and Plasma Glucose Relative to Palm Olein in Humans," *Nutrition and Metabolism* 4, no. 3 (2007); Hayes and Pronczuk, "Replacing Trans Fat.

90. Sodeif Azadmard-Damirchi and Paresh Dutta, "Changes in Minor Lipid Components During Interesterification," *Lipid Technology* 20, no. 12 (2008): 273–275.

91. See, e.g., A. Gagliardi et al., "Effects of Margarines and Butter Consumption on Lipid Profiles, Inflammation Markers and Lipid Transfer to H.D.L. Particles in Free-Living Subjects with the Metabolic Syndrome," *European Journal of Clinical Nutrition* 64 (2010): 1141–1149.

92. Hunter, "Applications of Food Science."

93. Pedersen and Kirkhus, "Fatty Acid Composition of *Post Trans* Margarines."

94. Nestle, *Food Politics*, 330; Michael Heasman and Julian Mellentin, *The Functional Foods Revolution: Health People, Healthy Profits?* (London: Earthscan, 2001), 40.

95. Nestle, *Food Politics*, 330.

96. Heasman and Mellentin, *Functional Foods Revolution*, 40.

97. National Heart Foundation of Australia, *Summary of Evidence on Phytosterol/Stanol Enriched Foods* (Canberra: National Heart Foundation of Australia, 2007).

98. Gilbert Thompson, *The Cholesterol Controversy* (London: Royal Society of Medicine Press, 2008), 78.

99. Thompson, *Cholesterol Controversy.*

100. European Food Safety Authority, "Plant Stanol Esters and Blood Cholesterol: Scientific Opinion of the Panel on Dietetics, Nutrition and Allergies," *EFSA Journal* 852 (2008): 1–13; Thompson, *Cholesterol Controversy.*

101. Nestle, *Food Politics*, 331.

102. U.S. Food and Drug Administration, "Labeling and Nutrition," www .fda.gov/Food/LabelingNutrition/default.htm (accessed August 12, 2009).

103. National Heart Foundation of Australia, *Summary of Evidence.*

104. Heidi Fransen et al., "Customary Use of Plant Sterol and Plant Stanol Enriched Margarine Is Associated with Changes in Serum Plant Sterol and Stanol Concentrations in Humans," *Journal of Nutrition* 137 (2007): 1301–1306; Wendy Jessup et al., "Phytosterols in Cardiovascular Disease: Innocuous Dietary Components or Accelerators of Atherosclerosis," *Future Medicine* 3, no. 3 (2008): 301–310; Peter J.H. Jones and Suhad S. AbuMweis, "Phytosterols as Functional Food Ingredients: Linkages to Cardiovascular Disease and Cancer," *Current Opinion in Clinical Nutrition and Metabolic Care* 12 (2009): 147–151; Jorg Kreuzer, "Phytosterols and Phytostanols: Is It Time to Rethink That Supplemented Margarine?," *Cardiovascular Research* 90 (2011): 397–398; Sheila Anne Doggrell, "Lowering LDL Cholesterol with Margarine Containing Plant Stanol/Sterol Esters: Is It Still Relevant in 2011?," *Complementary Therapies in Medicine* 19 (2011); Franca Marangoni and Andrea Poli, "Phytosterols and Cardiovascular Health," *Pharmacological Research* 61 (2010): 193–199.

105. In this sense, margarine has shifted from the world of hyperreality, described earlier, into the more abstract realm of what Jean Baudrillard called "pure simulation." The evolution of margarine somewhat fits Baudrillard's theory of

the successive "orders of simulacra": the first order of the counterfeit, the second order of production, and the third order of simulation governed by the code—in this case, the nutritional code. See Baudrillard, *Symbolic Exchange and Death* (London: Sage, 1976).

106. Gary Genosko, "Better than Butter: Margarine and Simulation," in *Jean Baudrillard: Fatal Theories*, ed. David Clarke (London: Routledge, 2009), 83–90; Pantzar, "Public Dialogue Between Butter and Margarine."

107. A. Fearon and M. Golding, "Butter and Spreads: Manufacture and Quality Assurance," in *Dairy Processing and Quality Assurance*, ed. R. Chandan (Ames, Iowa: Wiley-Blackwell, 2009), 253–272.

108. L. Szente and J. Szejtli, "Cyclodextrins as Food Ingredients," *Trends in Food Science and Technology* 15 (2004); Istvan Siro et al., "Functional Food. Product Development, Marketing and Consumer Acceptance—a Review," *Appetite* 51 (2008): 137–142.

109. William Reed Business Media, "First Cholesterol-Lowering Yogurt Hits US Shelves," February 16, 2005, www.nutraingredients-usa.com/content/view/print/26559 (accessed November 2, 2009); Stephen Daniells, "Tesco Launches Cholesterol-Lowering Milk," William Reed Business Media, March 1, 2006, www.foodanddrinkeurope.com/content/view/print/161094 (accessed November 2, 2009).

7. The Era of Functional Nutritionism

1. Julia Moskin, "Superfood or Monster from the Deep?," *New York Times*, September 17, 2008.

2. American Heart Association, "Beneficial Versus Harmful Fats," www.americanheart.org/presenter.jhtml?identifier=3063259 (accessed December 30, 2010).

3. Robert Lustig, "Fructose: Metabolic, Hedonic, and Societal Parallels with Ethanol," *Journal of the American Dietetic Association* 110 (2010): 1307–1321; Glen D. Lawrence, *The Fats of Life: Essential Fatty Acids in Health and Disease* (New Brunswick, N.J.: Rutgers University Press, 2010), 189; George Bray, "Soft Drink Consumption and Obesity: It Is All About Fructose," *Current Opinion in Lipidology* 21 (2010): 51–57; Kimber Stanhope and Peter Havel, "Fructose Consumption: Recent Results and Their Potential Implications," *Annals of the New York Academy of Sciences* 1190 (2010): 15–24.

4. Lustig, "Fructose."

5. Robert Lustig, Laura Schmidt, and Claire Brindis, "The Toxic Truth About Sugar," *Nature Biotechnology* 482 (2012): 27–29.

6. Jane Dixon, Sarah Hinde, and Cathy Banwell, "Obesity, Convenience and 'Phood,'" *British Food Journal* 108, no. 8 (2006): 634–645.

7. Geoffrey Webb, *Dietary Supplements and Functional Foods* (Oxford: Blackwell Publishing, 2006), 141. See Center for Science in the Public Interest, "Functional Foods Named in the Center for Science in the Public Interest's Complaints to the Food and Drug Administration," www.cspinet.org/reports/func foodcomplaint.htm (accessed October 1, 2011).

8. Robert Heaney, "Nutrients, Endpoints and the Problem of Proof," *Journal of Nutrition* 138, no. 9 (2008): 1591–1595; Susan Whiting et al., "Current Understanding of Vitamin D Metabolism, Nutritional Status and Role in Disease Prevention," in *Nutrition in the Prevention and Treatment of Disease*, ed. Ann Coulston and Carol Boushey (Burlington, Mass.: Elsevier, 2008); Jane Brody, "What Do You Lack? Probably Vitamin D," *New York Times*, July 26, 2010; Michael Holick, *The Vitamin D Solution: A Three-Step Strategy to Cure Our Most Common Health Problem* (New York: Hudson Street Press, 2010).

9. Qtd. in Helene Ragovin, "Vitamin D," *Tufts Nutrition Newsletter* 2008: 13–17.

10. Heaney, "Nutrients."

11. Dannon, Inc., "With Activia®, It's a Feel-Good Day," www.activia.us.com /products/discover/Activia.aspx?l=1 (accessed October 1, 2011).

12. GFA Brands, Inc., "Smart Balance® HeartRight® Fat Free Milk," www .smartbalance.com/products/heartright/heartright-fat-free-milk (accessed October 1, 2011).

13. Clint Carter, "Ditch the Diet, Lose the Weight," *Men's Health*, July/August 2011, 84–86.

14. Susan Allport, *The Queen of Fats: Why Omega-3s Were Removed from the Western Diet and What We Can Do to Replace Them* (Berkeley: University of California Press, 2006).

15. See, e.g., Leif Hallberg, "Bioavailable Nutrient Density: A New Concept Applied in the Interpretation of Food Iron Absorption Data," *American Journal of Clinical Nutrition* 34 (1981): 2242–2247.

16. Gregory Miller et al., "Nutrient Profiling: Global Approaches, Policies and Perspectives," *Nutrition Today* 45, no. 1 (2010): 6–12.

17. U.S. Department of Agriculture and Department of Health and Human Services, *Dietary Guidelines for Americans, 2010* (Washington, D.C., 2010), 94.

18. P. Weber, "Role of Biomarkers in Nutritional Science and Industry—a Comment," *British Journal of Nutrition* 86, suppl. 1 (2001).

19. Institute of Medicine, *Evaluation of Biomarkers and Surrogate Endpoints in Chronic Disease* (Washington, D.C.: National Academies Press, 2010), S93–S95.

20. Jim Kaput, "Nutrigenomics Research for Personalized Nutrition and Medicine," *Current Opinion in Biotechnology* 19 (2008): 110–120.

21. Jennifer Ruth Fosket, "Breast Cancer Risk as Disease," in *Biomedicalization: Technoscience, Health, and Illness in the U.S.*, ed. Adele Clarke et al. (Durham, N.C.: Duke University Press, 2010).

22. Ray Moynihan and Alan Cassels, *Selling Sickness: How the World's Biggest Pharmaceutical Companies Are Turning Us All into Patients* (New York: Nation Books, 2005).

23. Gyorgy Scrinis, "On the Ideology of Nutritionism," *Gastronomica* 8, no. 1 (2008): 39–48.

24. Michel Foucault, *The Birth of the Clinic* (New York: Vintage, 1975), chap. 9.

25. Deborah Lupton, *Food, the Body and the Self* (London: Sage, 1996), 75.

26. Rosalind Coward, *The Whole Truth: The Myth of Alternative Health* (London: Faber and Faber, 1989), 146–147.

27. Lupton, *Food, the Body and the Self.*

28. Qtd. in Alex May, "You Are What You Eat," *The Age—Sunday Life*, March 16, 2008.

29. Byron Richards, *Mastering Leptin: The Key to Energetic Vitality, Youthful Hormonal Balance, Optimum Body Weight, and Disease Prevention!* (Minneapolis, Minn.: Wellness Resources Books, 2002); Natasha Turner, *The Hormone Diet: A 3-Step Program to Help You Lose Weight, Gain Strength, and Live Younger Longer* (New York: Rodale, 2010).

30. Michael Aziz, *The Perfect 10 Diet: 10 Key Hormones That Hold the Secret to Losing Weight and Feeling Great* (Naperville: Ill.: Cumberland House, 2010), back cover.

31. Robert Wildman, *The Nutritionist: Food, Nutrition and Optimal Health*, 2nd ed. (New York: Routledge, 2009), 105.

32. Natalie Riediger et al., "A Systematic Review of the Roles of N-3 Fatty Acids in Health and Disease," *Journal of the American Dietetic Association* 109, no. 4 (2009): 668–679; Alexandra McManus, Margaret Merga, and Wendy Newton, "Omega-3 Fatty Acids: What Consumers Need to Know," *Appetite* 57 (2011): 80–83.

33. Alexander Leaf, "Historical Overview of N-3 Fatty Acids and Coronary Heart Disease," *American Journal of Clinical Nutrition* 87 (2008): 1978S–1980S.

34. Artemis Simopoulos, "The Importance of the Omega-6/Omega-3 Fatty Acid Ratio in Cardiovascular Disease and Other Chronic Diseases," *Experimental Biology and Medicine* 233 (2008): 674–688; Allport, *Queen of Fats*, 8; G. Wardlaw and A. Smith, *Contemporary Nutrition* (New York: McGraw-Hill, 2011), 186; Riediger et al., "Systematic Review."

35. S. Akabas and R. Deckelbaum, "Summary of a Workshop on N-3 Fatty Acids: Current Status of Recommendations and Future Directions," *American Journal of Clinical Nutrition* 83, suppl. (2006): 1536S–1538S.

36. J. Woodside and I. Young, "Fish, N-3 Polyunsaturated Fatty Acids and Cardiovascular Disease," in *Nutritional Health: Strategies for Disease Prevention*, ed. N.J. Temple et al. (Totowa, N.J.: Humana Press, 2006), 133–150; E. Brunner et al., "Fish, Human Health and Marine Ecosystem Health: Policies in Collision," *International Journal of Epidemiology* 38 (2009): 93–100.

37. L. Hooper et al., "Risks and Benefits of Omega 3 Fats for Mortality, Cardiovascular Disease, and Cancer: Systematic Review," *British Medical Journal* 332 (2006): 752–755.

38. G. Danaei et al., "The Preventable Causes of Death in the United States: Comparative Risk Assessment of Dietary, Lifestyle and Metabolic Risk Factors," *PLoS Medicine* 6, no. 4 (2009): 1–23.

39. U.S. Food and Drug Administration, "Omega-3 Fatty Acids and Coronary Heart Disease," www.fda.gov/Food/LabelingNutrition/LabelClaims/Qualified HealthClaims/ucm073992.htm#omega3 (accessed November 1, 2011).

40. For the European Union Register on Nutrition and Health Claims, see European Food Safety Authority, Home Page, www.efsa.europa.eu (accessed May 20, 2012).

41. Allport, *Queen of Fats*, chap. 10.

42. Simopoulos, "Importance of the Omega-6/Omega-3"; Riediger et al., "Systematic Review."

43. J. Hibbeln et al., "Healthy Intakes of N-3 and N-6 Fatty Acids: Estimations Considering Worldwide Diversity," *American Journal of Clinical Nutrition* 83, no. 6 (2006): 1483S–1493S.

44. Jim Mann and Stewart Truswell, *Essentials of Human Nutrition*, 3rd ed. (New York: Oxford University Press, 2007), 51. For contrasting views, see William S. Harris et al., "Omega-6 Fatty Acids and Risk for Cardiovascular Disease," *Circulation* 119 (2009): 902–907; Penny Kris-Etherton, Jennifer Fleming, and William S. Harris, "The Debate About N-6 Polyunsaturated Fatty Acid Recommendations for Cardiovascular Health," *Journal of the American Dietetic Association* 110, no. 2 (2010): 201–204; Simopoulos, "Importance of the Omega-6/Omega-3."

45. Hibbeln et al., "Healthy Intakes of N-3 and N-6 Fatty Acids"; Wardlaw and Smith, *Contemporary Nutrition*, 186.

46. USDA and DHHS, *Dietary Guidelines for Americans, 2010.*

47. R. Deckelbaum and P. Calder, "Dietary N-3 and N-6 Fatty Acids: Are There 'Bad' Polyunsaturated Fatty Acids?," *Current Opinion in Clinical Nutrition and Metabolic Care* 13 (2010): 123–124.

48. Harris et al., "Omega-6 Fatty Acids and Risk for Cardiovascular Disease." For criticisms of the American Heart Association advisory by a number of nutrition scientists, see letters to the editor regarding Harris et al.'s article, at www.americanheart.org/presenter.jhtml?identifier=3070203 (accessed May 10, 2010), and Christopher Ramsden et al., "N-6 Fatty Acid-Specific and Mixed Polyunsaturate Dietary Interventions Have Different Effects on CHD Risk: A Meta-analysis of Randomised Controlled Trials," *British Journal of Nutrition* 104 (2010): 1586–1600; Allport, *Queen of Fats*, 115. Poultry is another major source of omega-6 fats and has otherwise been promoted for its cholesterol-lowering benefits; see Hibbeln et al., "Healthy Intakes of N-3 and N-6 Fatty Acids."

49. D. Mozaffarian et al., "Interplay Between Different Polyunsaturated Fatty Acids and Risk of Coronary Heart Disease in Men," *Circulation* 111 (2005): 157–164.

50. Artemis Simopoulos and Jo Robinson, *The Omega Plan: The Medically Proven Diet That Restores Your Body's Essential Nutritional Balance* (New York: Harper Collins, 1998), 131.

51. S. Gebauer et al., "N-3 Fatty Acid Dietary Recommendations and Food Sources to Achieve Essentiality and Cardiovascular Benefits," *American Journal of Clinical Nutrition* 83, suppl. (2006): 1526S–1535S.

52. I. Graham, T. Larson, and J. Napier, "Rational Metabolic Engineering of Transgenic Plants for Biosynthesis of Omega-3 Polyunsaturates," *Current Opinion in Biotechnology* 18 (2007): 142–147.

53. D.J.A Jenkins, "Are Dietary Recommendations for the Use of Fish Oils Sustainable?," *Canadian Medical Association Journal* 180, no. 6 (2009); B.C. Davis and P.M. Kris-Etheron, "Achieving Optimal Essential Fatty Acid Status in Vegetarians: Current Knowledge and Practical Implications," *American Journal of Clinical Nutrition* 78 (2003): 640S–646S. This omega-3 fetish may increase the already unsustainable levels of global fish catches. See Brunner et al., "Fish, Human Health and Marine Ecosystem Health."

54. L.W. Kinsell et al., "Lipid Peroxidation During N-3 Fatty Acid and Vitamin E Supplementation in Humans," *Lipids* 32, no. 5 (1997): 534–541; L. Frost et al., "Fatty Acids Consumed from Fish and Risk of Atrial Fibrillation or Flutter: The Danish Diet, Cancer and Health Study," *American Journal of Clinical Nutrition* 81 (2005): 50–54.

55. Riediger et al., "Systematic Review."

56. McManus et al., "Omega-3 Fatty Acids."

57. See, e.g., Lynda Gillen et al., "Structured Dietary Advice Incorporating Walnuts Achieves Optimal Fat and Energy Balance in Patients with Type 2 Diabetes Mellitus," *Journal of the American Dietetic Association* 105, no. 7 (2005): 1087–1096; W.C. Willett, "Fruit, Vegetables, and Cancer Prevention: Turmoil in the Produce Section," *Journal of the National Cancer Institute* 102, no. 8 (2010): 510–511.

58. An Pan et al., "Red Meat Consumption and Mortality," *Archives of Internal Medicine* 172, no. 7 (2012): 555–563.

59. Anu Turunen et al., "Fish Consumption in Relation to Other Foods in the Diet," *British Journal of Nutrition* 106 (2011): 1570–1580.

60. Pan et al., "Red Meat Consumption and Mortality."

61. Karen Charlton, "Two Apples and Five Carrots a Day Keep the Doctor Away: Strategies to Increase Fruit and Vegetable Consumption," *Nutrition and Dietetics* 65 (2008): 112–114.

62. Paolo Boffetta, "Fruit and Vegetable Intake and Overall Cancer Risk in the European Prospective Investigation into Cancer and Nutrition," *Journal of the National Cancer Institute* 102, no. 8 (2010): 529–537; Willett, "Fruit, Vegetables, and Cancer Prevention."

63. Willett, "Fruit, Vegetables, and Cancer Prevention."

64. David Jacobs and Nicola McKeown, "In Defence of Phytochemical-Rich Dietary Patterns," *British Journal of Nutrition* 104, no. 1 (2010): 1–3. See also E. Pat-

terson et al., "Dietary Energy Density as a Marker of Dietary Quality in Swedish Children and Adolescents: The European Youth Heart Study," *European Journal of Clinical Nutrition* 64 (2010): 356–363.

65. Jacobs, "In Defence of Phytochemical-Rich Dietary Patterns."

66. Peter Williams, "Evaluation of the Evidence Between Consumption of Refined Grains and Health Outcomes," *Nutrition Reviews* 70, no. 2 (2012).

67. USDA Human Nutrition Information Service, *Report of the Dietary Guidelines Advisory Committee on the Dietary Guidelines for Americans 2010* (Washington, D.C.: National Technical Information Service, 2010), 80–99.

68. David Wolfe, *Superfoods: The Food and Medicine of the Future* (Berkeley, Calif.: North Atlantic Books, 2009); Tonia Reinhard, *Superfoods: The Healthiest Food on the Planet* (London: Apple, 2010); Steven Pratt and Kathy Matthews, *Superfoods Rx: Fourteen Foods That Will Change Your Life* (New York: Morrow, 2004).

69. Mehmet Oz, "The Oz Diet," *Time Magazine*, September 11, 2011.

70. U.S. Food and Drug Administration, "Food Labeling Guide," www.fda .gov/Food/GuidanceComplianceRegulatoryInformation/GuidanceDocuments /FoodLabelingNutrition/FoodLabelingGuide/ucm064919.htm (accessed October 1, 2012).

71. See, e.g., A. Mitchell et al., "Ten-Year Comparison of the Influence of Organic and Conventional Crop Management Practices on the Content of Flavonoids in Tomatoes," *Journal of Agricultural and Food Chemistry* 55 (2007).

72. "Position of the American Dietetic Association: Functional Foods," *Journal of the American Dietetic Association* 109, no. 4 (2009): 6154–6159.

73. M.E. Gershwin et al., "Public Safety and Dietary Supplementation," *Annals of the New York Academy of Sciences* 1190 (2009): 104–117; "Position of the American Dietetic Association: Nutrient Supplementation," *Journal of the American Dietetic Association* 109 (2009): 2073–2085; R. Bailey et al., "Dietary Supplement Use in the United States, 2003–2006," *Journal of Nutrition Education* 141, no. 2 (2011): 735–746.

74. Mark Nichter and Jennifer Thompson, "For My Wellness, Not Just My Illness: North Americans' Use of Dietary Supplements," *Culture, Medicine and Psychiatry* 30 (2006): 175–222.

75. American Dietetic Association, "Position of the American Dietetic Association: Nutrient Supplementation," 2077.

76. American Dietetic Association, "Nutrient Supplementation," 2073. See also Alice Lichtenstein and Robert Russell, "Essential Nutrients: Food or Supplements? Where Should the Emphasis Be?," *Journal of the American Medical Association* 294, no. 3 (2005): 351–358.

77. Robert Fletcher and Kathleen Fairfield, "Vitamins for Chronic Disease Prevention in Adults," *Journal of the American Medical Association* 287, no. 23 (2002): 3127–3129; Walter Willett, *Eat, Drink, and Be Healthy: The Harvard Medical School Guide to Healthy Eating* (New York: Free Press, 2005); Rima Apple, *Vitamania: Vitamins in American Culture* (New Brunswick, N.J.: Rutgers University Press, 1996), 185.

78. Willett, *Eat, Drink, and Be Healthy*, 203.

79. Nicola Napoli et al., "Effects of Dietary Calcium Compared with Calcium Supplements on Estrogen Metabolism and Bone Mineral Density," *American Journal of Clinical Nutrition* 85 (2007): 1428–1433.

80. Lichtenstein and Russell, "Essential Nutrients"; G. Bjelakovic et al., "Mortality in Randomized Trials of Antioxidant Supplements for Primary and Secondary Prevention," *Journal of the American Dietetic Association* 297, no. 8 (2007): 842–857; E.R. Miller et al., "Meta-analysis: High-Dosage Vitamin E Supplementation May Increase All-Cause Mortality," *Nutrition Journal* 6 (2005): 30–41.

81. Gardiner Harris, "Study Finds Supplements Contain Contaminants," *New York Times*, May 25, 2010; Gershwin et al., "Public Safety and Dietary Supplementation"; R.L. Bailey et al., "Examination of Vitamin Intakes among U.S. Adults by Dietary Supplement Use," *Journal of the Academy of Nutrition and Dietetics* 112 (2012): 657–663.

82. Rose Hume Hall, *The Unofficial Guide to Smart Nutrition* (Foster City, Calif.: IDG Books, 2000), 239.

83. Frank Hu, "Dietary Pattern Analysis: A New Direction in Nutritional Epidemiology," *Current Opinion in Lipidology* 13 (2002): 3–9. See also Lawrence Appel, "Dietary Patterns and Longevity: Expanding the Blue Zones," *Circulation* 118 (2008): 214–215; Per Sjogren et al., "Mediterranean and Carbohydrate-Restricted Diets and Mortality among Elderly Men: A Cohort Study in Sweden," *American Journal of Clinical Nutrition* 92 (2010): 967–974.

84. Hu, "Dietary Pattern Analysis," 3–4.

85. S. Moeller et al., "Dietary Patterns: Challenges and Opportunities in Dietary Patterns Research," *Journal of the American Dietetic Association* 107, no. 7 (2007): 1233–1239.

86. Hu, "Dietary Pattern Analysis," 8.

87. Christin Heidemann, "Dietary Patterns and Risk of Mortality from Cardiovascular Disease, Cancer, and All Causes in a Prospective Cohort of Women," *Circulation* 118 (2008): 230–237.

88. Dawn Schwenke, "Dietary Patterns: Designs for Progress and Approaches for Health Impact," *Current Opinion in Lipidology* 21 (2010): 276–279.

89. Katherine Tucker, "Dietary Patterns, Approaches and Multicultural Perspective," *Applied Physiology Nutrition Metabolism* 35 (2010): 211–218.

90. Antonia Trichopoulou, Christina Bamia, and Dimitrios Trichopoulos, "Anatomy of Health Effects of Mediterranean Diet: Greek Epic Prospective Cohort Study," *British Medical Journal* 338 (2009); Antonia Trichopoulou et al., "Adherence to a Mediterranean Diet and Survival in a Greek Population," *New England Journal of Medicine* 348, no. 26 (2003): 2599–2608; L. Serra-Majem et al., "Does the Definition of the Mediterranean Diet Need to Be Updated?," *Public Health Nutrition* 7, no. 7 (2004): 927–929.

91. See, e.g., T. Fung et al., "Mediterranean Diet and Incidence of and Mortality from Coronary Heart Disease and Stroke in Women," *Circulation* 119

(2009): 1093–1100; Trichopoulou et al., "Anatomy of Health Effects of Mediterranean Diet."

92. F. Sofi et al., "Adherence to Mediterranean Diet and Health Status: A Meta-analysis," *British Medical Journal* 337 (2009); Trichopoulou et al., "Anatomy of Health Effects of Mediterranean Diet."

93. M. Slatterry et al., "Eating Patterns and Risk of Colon Cancer," *American Journal of Epidemiology* 148, no. 1 (1998): 4–16.

94. Teresa Fung, "Major Dietary Patterns and the Risk of Colorectal Cancer in Women," *Archives of Internal Medicine* 163 (2003): 309–314. See also Heidemann, "Dietary Patterns and Risk of Mortality."

95. Lin et al., "Food Group Sources of Nutrients in the Dietary Patterns of the DASH-Sodium Trial," *Journal of the American Dietetic Association* 103, no. 4 (2003): 488–496.

96. See, e.g., L.J. Appel et al., "A Clinical Trial of the Effects of Dietary Patterns on Blood Pressure," *New England Journal of Medicine* 336 (1997): 1117–1124.

97. An exception was a recent study comparing the DASH and Mediterranean diets for their effects on the incidence of colorectal cancer: T. Fung et al., "The Mediterranean and Dietary Approaches to Stop Hypertension (DASH) Diets and Colorectal Cancer," *American Journal of Clinical Nutrition* 92 (2010): 1429–1435.

98. A. Anderson et al., "Dietary Patterns and Survival of Older Adults," *Journal of the American Dietetic Association* 111, no. 1 (2011): 84–91; L.R. Harriss et al., "Dietary Patterns and Cardiovascular Mortality in the Melbourne Collaborative Cohort Study," *American Journal of Clinical Nutrition* 86 (2007): 221–229. For a study that shows an association between both unprocessed and processed red meats and higher rates of chronic disease, see Pan et al., "Red Meat Consumption and Mortality."

99. Renata Micha, Sarah Wallace, and D. Mozaffarian, "Red and Processed Meat Consumption and Risk of Incident Coronary Heart Disease, Stroke, and Diabetes Mellitus: A Systematic Review and Meta-analysis," *Circulation* 121 (2010): 2271–2283; S. Larsson, J. Virtamo, and A. Wolk, "Red Meat Consumption and Risk of Stroke in Swedish Men," *American Journal of Clinical Nutrition* 94 (2011): 417–421. Pan et al., in "Red Meat Consumption and Mortality," surprisingly included hamburgers in the unprocessed rather than processed red meat category.

100. Joan Sabate, "The Contribution of Vegetarian Diets to Health and Disease: A Paradigm Shift?," *American Journal of Clinical Nutrition* 78, suppl. (2003).

101. See, e.g., D. Jacobs et al., "Food, Plant Food and Vegetarian Diets in the U.S. Dietary Guidelines: Conclusions of an Expert Panel," *American Journal of Clinical Nutrition* 89 (2009): 1S–4S; Johanna Dwyer, "Convergence of Plant-Rich and Plant-Only Diets," *American Journal of Clinical Nutrition* 70, no. 3 (1999): 620S–622S.

102. "Position of the American Dietetic Association: Vegetarian Diets," *Journal of the American Dietetic Association* 109, no. 7 (2009): 1266–1282.

103. Sabate, "Contribution of Vegetarian Diets."

104. Jacobs et al., "Food, Plant Food and Vegetarian Diets."

105. Timothy Key et al., "Health Effects of Vegetarian and Vegan Diets," *Proceedings of the Nutrition Society* 65 (2006): 35–41; Timothy Key et al., "Mortality in British Vegetarians: Results from the European Prospective Investigation into Cancer and Nutrition (EPIC-Oxford)," *American Journal of Clinical Nutrition* 89 (2009): 1613S–1619S; Claire McEvoy, Norman Temple, and Jayne Woodside, "Vegetarian Diets, Low-Meat Diets and Health: A Review," *Public Health Nutrition*, in press (doi:10.1017/S1368980012000936).

106. Staffan Lindeberg, *Food and Western Disease: Health and Nutrition from an Evolutionary Perspective* (Oxford: Wiley-Blackwell, 2010), 68; W.C. Willett, "Convergence of Philosophy and Science: The Third International Congress on Vegetarian Nutrition," *American Journal of Clinical Nutrition* 70, suppl. (1999): 44S–438S; Key et al., "Health Effects of Vegetarian and Vegan Diets."

107. Dwyer, "Convergence of Plant-Rich and Plant-Only Diets."

108. Gary Fraser, "Vegetarian Diets: What Do We Know of Their Effects on Common Chronic Diseases?," *American Journal of Clinical Nutrition* 89 (2009): 1609S–1612S.

109. Key et al., "Health Effects of Vegetarian and Vegan Diets."

110. T. Colin Campbell, *The China Study: The Most Comprehensive Study of Nutrition Ever Conducted and the Startling Implications for Diet, Weight Loss and Long-Term Health* (Dallas, Tex.: Bendella, 2005).

111. Campbell, *China Study*, 7.

112. Campbell, *China Study*, 132. For a critique of Campbell's statistical analysis in the *China Study*, see Denise Minger's blog: www.rawfoodsos.com.

113. Campbell, *China Study*, 271.

114. Campbell, *China Study*, 281.

115. John Robbins, *Healthy at 100: How to Extend Your Life and Stay Fit* (London: Hodder and Stoughton, 2006).

116. Daphne Miller, *The Jungle Effect: A Doctor Discovers the Healthiest Diets from Around the World, Why They Work and How to Bring Them Home* (New York: Harper Collins, 2010); Bradley Willcox, D. Craig Willcox, and Makoto Suzuki, *The Okinawa Program: How the World's Longest-lived People Achieve Everlasting Health—and How You Can Too* (New York: Three Rivers, 2011).

117. Bradley Willcox et al., "The Okinawan Diet: Health Implications of a Low-Calorie, Nutrient-Dense, Antioxidant-Rich Dietary Pattern Low in Glycemic Load," *Journal of the American College of Nutrition* 28, no. 4 (2009): 500S–516S.

118. Willcox et al., "The Okinawan Diet," 500S.

119. Schwenke, "Dietary Patterns."

120. Weston A. Price, *Nutrition and Physical Degeneration*, 8th ed. (La Mesa, Calif.: Price-Pottenger Nutrition Foundation, 2009). See also Sally Fallon, *Nourishing Traditions: The Cookbook That Challenges Politically Correct Nutrition and the Diet Dicto-*

crats (Washington, D.C.: New Trends, 2001); Ronald Schmid, *Traditional Foods Are Your Best Medicine: Improving Health and Longevity with Native Nutrition* (Rochester, Vt.: Healing Arts Press, 1997); Robbins, *Healthy at 100*; Elizabeth Lipski, "Traditional Non-Western Diets," *Nutrition in Clinical Practice* 25, no. 6 (2010): 585–593.

121. Price, *Nutrition and Physical Degeneration*, 9, 240.

122. Weston A. Price Foundation for Wise Traditions in Food, Farming and the Healing Arts, www.westonaprice.org.

123. Robbins, *Healthy at 100*, 105.

124. C. Daniel et al., "Trends in Meat Consumption in the United States," *Public Health Nutrition* 14, no. 4 (2011): 575–583.

125. Loren Cordain, *The Paleo Diet: Lose Weight and Get Healthy by Eating the Foods You Were Designed to Eat*, rev. ed. (Hoboken, N.J.: Wiley and Sons, 2010); Robb Wolf, *The Paleo Solution: The Original Human Diet* (Las Vegas, Nev.: Victory Belt, 2010); Mark Sisson, *The Primal Blueprint: Reprogram Your Genes for Effortless Weight Loss, Vibrant Health, and Boundless Energy* (Malibu, Calif.: Primal Publishing, 2009).

126. Lindeberg, *Food and Western Disease*, 221.

127. Loren Cordain et al., "Plant-Animal Subsistence Ratios and Macronutrient Energy Estimations in Worldwide Hunter-Gatherer Diets," *American Journal of Clinical Nutrition* 71 (2000): 682–692.

128. Sarah Elton, "Environments, Adaptation and Evolutionary Medicine," in *Medicine and Evolution: Current Applications, Future Proposals*, ed. Sarah Elton and Paul O'Higgins (New York: CRC Press, 2008), 9–34; Marion Nestle, "Paleolithic Diets: A Sceptical View," *British Nutrition Foundation* 25 (2000): 43–47.

129. Cordain, *The Paleo Diet*, 3.

130. Cordain, *The Paleo Diet*, 4.

131. Cordain et al., "Plant-Animal Subsistence Ratios."

132. On parallels between the Mediterranean and paleo diets, see John Mackenback, "The Mediterranean Diet Story Illustrates That 'Why' Questions Are As Important As 'How' Questions in Disease Explanation," *Journal of Clinical Epidemiology* 60 (2007): 105–109; Artemis Simopoulos, "The Mediterranean Diets: What Is So Special About the Diet of Greece? The Scientific Evidence," *Journal of Nutrition* 131 (2001): 3065S–3073S.

133. Not all nutrition experts favor the personalization of dietary advice in *MyPyramid*. Marion Nestle argues that "complexity confuses the public and individualization implies that dietary advice should focus on personal dietary choices, not on how to cope with an 'eat more' food environment" in *Food Politics*, 377.

134. Roger Williams, *Biochemical Individuality: The Basis for the Genetotrophic Concept* (New York: Wiley, 1956).

135. Steven Epstein, *Inclusion: The Politics of Difference in Medical Research* (Chicago: University of Chicago Press, 2007), 135; Adele Clarke, Laura Mamo, Jennifer Ruth Fosket, Jennifer Fishman, and Janet Shim, *Biomedicalization: Technoscience, Health and Illness in the U.S.* (Durham, N.C.: Duke University Press, 2010), 79.

136. Jeffrey Brauer, "Low-Fat or Low-Carb? It Depends," *The Thinker* [blog], jeffreybrauer.blogspot.com/2012/03/low-carb-or-low-fat-it-depends.html (accessed October 1, 2011).

137. Kaput, "Nutrigenomics Research."

138. Qtd. in Helen Wallace, "Your Diet Tailored to Your Genes: Preventing Diseases or Misleading Marketing?" (Buxton, U.K.: GeneWatch, 2006), 14.

139. David Castle, "The Personal and the Public in Nutrigenomics," in *Nutrition and Genomics: Issues of Ethics, Law, Regulation and Communication*, ed. David Castle and Nola Ries (Amsterdam: Elsevier, 2009), 245–262. Bart Penders et al. "From Individuals to Groups: A Review of the Meaning of 'Personalized' in Nutrigenomics," *Trends in Food Science & Technology* 18 (2007): 333–338.

140. Gyorgy Scrinis, "Engineering the Food Chain," *Arena Magazine* 77 (2005): 37–39.

141. Paula Saukko, "Negotiating the Boundary Between Medicine and Consumer Culture: Online Marketing of Nutrigenetic Tests," *Social Science and Medicine* 70 (2010): 744–753.

142. Lynette Ferguson, "Nutrigenomics Approaches to Functional Foods," *Journal of the American Dietetic Association* 109 (2009): 452–458.

8. Functional Foods

1. Linda Milo Ohr, "The Best of Functional Foods 2009," *Food Technology* 63, no. 5 (2009): 93–108; Elizabeth Sloan, "The Top 10 Functional Food Trends," *Food Technology* 62, no. 5 (2008): 25–44; L.M. Ohr, "Functional Sweets," *Food Technology* 60, no. 11 (2006): 57.

2. Mary Sanders, "Overview of Functional Foods: Emphasis on Probiotic Bacteria," *International Dairy Journal* 8 (1998): 341–347; Marion Nestle, *Food Politics: How the Food Industry Influences Nutrition and Health*, 2nd ed. (Berkeley: University of California Press, 2007), 296.

3. Nestle, *Food Politics*, 296.

4. Warren James Belasco, *Appetite for Change: How the Counterculture Took on the Food Industry*, 2nd ed. (New York: Cornell University Press, 2007), 201.

5. Laura Bouwman et al., "I Eat Healthfully But I Am Not a Freak: Consumers' Everyday Life Perspective on Healthful Eating," *Appetite* 53 (2009): 390–398.

6. Michelle Stacey, *Consumed: Why Americans Love, Hate, and Fear Food* (New York: Simon and Schuster, 1994), 58.

7. Red Bull, "Taurine," www.redbull.com/cs/Satellite/en_INT/Red-Bull -Energy-Drink/001242937921959?pcs_cid= 1242937842064&pcs_iid=1242 940968365&pcs_pvt=ingredient (accessed October 1, 2011).

8. Dannon, "What Is Danactive?™," www.danone.ca/en/products/danactive (accessed October 1, 2011).

9. Yakult USA, Inc., "How Does Yakult Work?," www.yakultusa.com/Yakult/HowDoesItWork.php (accessed October 1, 2011).

10. Michael Heasman and Julian Mellentin, *The Functional Foods Revolution: Healthy People, Healthy Profits?* (London: Earthscan, 2001), 4.

11. Martijn B. Katan, "Functional Foods," in *Essentials of Human Nutrition*, ed. Jim Mann and Stewart Truswell (Oxford: Oxford University Press, 2007), 396–404, 397.

12. Nestle, *Food Politics*, 316. See also Ted Wilson and David Jacobs, "Functional Foods: A Critical Appraisal," in *Nutritional Health: Strategies for Disease Prevention*, 2nd ed., ed. Norman Temple, Ted Wilson, and David Jacobs (Totowa, N.J.: Humana Press, 2006), 363–372.

13. Gyorgy Scrinis, "Functional Foods or Functionally Marketed Foods: A Critique of, and Alternatives to, the Category of Functional Foods," *Public Health Nutrition* 11, no. 5 (2008): 541–545.

14. A.T. Diplock et al., "Scientific Concepts of Functional Foods in Europe: Consensus Document," *British Journal of Nutrition* 81, no. 4 (1999): S1–S27.

15. "Position of the American Dietetic Association: Functional Foods," *Journal of the American Dietetic Association* 109, no. 4 (2009): 735–745, 736, my emphasis.

16. J. Lehenraki, "On the Borderline of Food and Drug: Constructing Credibility and Markets for a Functional Food Product," *Science as Culture* 12, no. 4 (2003): 499–525.

17. Mark Lawrence and John Germov, "Functional Foods and Public Health Nutrition Policy," in *A Sociology of Food and Nutrition*, ed. John Germov and Lauren Williams (South Melbourne: Oxford University Press, 2008), 147–175; Heasman and Mellentin, *The Functional Foods Revolution*, xvii.

18. Charlotte Biltekoff, "Functional Foods for Health: Negotiation and Implications," in *Promoting Health by Linking Agriculture, Food, and Nutrition*, NABC Report 22, ed. A. Eaglesham, A. Bennett, and R. Hardy (New York: National Agricultural Biotechnology Council, 2010), 99–108.

19. Qtd. in Bruce Horovitz, "Critics Blast Kellogg's Claim That Cereals Can Boost Immunity," usatoday30.usatoday.com/money/industries/food/2009-11-02-cereal-immunity-claim_N.htm (accessed September 25, 2011).

20. Lotte Holm, "Food Health Policies and Ethics: Lay Perspectives on Functional Foods," *Journal of Agricultural and Environmental Ethics* 16 (2003): 531–544; David Jacobs and Linda Tapsell, "Food, Not Nutrients, Is the Fundamental Unit in Nutrition," *Nutrition Reviews* 65, no. 10 (2007): 439–450.

21. Belasco, *Appetite for Change*, 253.

22. On the logic of interchangeability, see Gyorgy Scrinis and Kristen Lyons, "Nanotechnology and the Techno-Corporate Agri-Food Paradigm," in *Food Security, Nutrition and Sustainability*, ed. Geoffrey Lawrence, Kristen Lyons, and Tabatha Wallington (London: Earthscan, 2010), 252–270.

23. See Joan Dye Gussow and Sharon Akabas, "Are We Really Fixing Up the Food Supply?," *Journal of the American Dietetic Association* 93, no. 11 (1993): 1300–1304; Holm, "Food Health Policies and Ethics."

24. Wilson and Jacobs, "Functional Foods"; Nestle, *Food Politics*, 297; David Kaplan, "What's Wrong with Functional Foods?," in *Readings in the Philosophy of Technology*, ed. David Kaplan (Lanham, Md.: Rowman and Littlefield, 2009), 498–510.

25. Wilson and Jacobs, "Functional Foods."

26. S.N. El and S. Simsek, "Food Technological Applications for Optimal Nutrition: An Overview of Opportunities for the Food Industry," *Comprehensive Reviews in Food Science and Food Safety* 11 (2012): 2–12.

27. National Heart Foundation of Australia, *Summary of Evidence on Phytosterol/Stanol Enriched Foods* (Canberra: National Heart Foundation of Australia, 2007); Peter Jones and Suhad AbuMweis, "Phytosterols as Functional Food Ingredients: Linkages to Cardiovascular Disease and Cancer," *Current Opinion in Clinical Nutrition and Metabolic Care* 12 (2009): 146–151.

28. National Heart Foundation of Australia, *Summary of Evidence on Phytosterol/Stanol Enriched Foods*.

29. Lawrence and Germov, "Functional Foods."

30. On nutrification, see P.A. Lachance and J.C. Bauernfeind, "Concepts and Practices of Nutrifying Foods," in *Nutrient Additions to Food: Nutritional, Technological and Regulatory Aspects*, ed. J.C. Bauernfeind and P.A. Lachance (Trumbull, Conn.: Food and Nutrition Press, 1991).

31. Jacobs and Tapsell, "Food, Not Nutrients."

32. L. Martin et al., "Food Products as Vehicles for N-3 Fatty Acid Supplementation," *Canadian Journal of Dietetic Practice and Research* 69, no. 4 (2008): 203–207.

33. Marion Nestle, *Safe Food: Bacteria, Biotechnology, and Bioterrorism* (Berkeley: University of California Press, 2003); Helena Paul and Ricarda Steinbrecher, *Hungry Corporations: Transnational Companies Colonize the Food Chain* (London: Zed Books, 2003).

34. Ian Graham et al., "Rational Metabolic Engineering of Transgenic Plants for Biosynthesis of Omega-3 Polyunsaturates," *Current Opinion in Biotechnology* 18 (2007): 142–147.

35. Mark Filmer, "New Wheat Promises Dual Benefits," *Farming Ahead* 174 (2006): 50–51.

36. Scrinis and Lyons, "Nanotechnology"; Bhupinder Sekhon, "Food Nanotechnology—An Overview," *Nanotechnology, Science and Applications* 3 (2010): 1–15.

37. Scrinis and Lyons, "Nanotechnology"; Istvan Siro et al., "Functional Food. Product Development, Marketing and Consumer Acceptance—A Review," *Appetite* 51 (2008): 456–467.

38. Meredith Melnick, "Food Is the New Pharma: Nestlé Aims to Enter the Functional Foods Market," *Time*, September 28, 2010.

39. Nestlé, *Nestlé Health Science Launches Next Generation of Boost® Complete Nutritional Drink* (Florham Park, N.J.: Nestlé Health Science, 2011).

40. PepsiCo, "Quaker Launches 'Quaker Oats Center of Excellence,'" June 4, 2012, www.pepsico.com/PressRelease/Quaker-Launches-Quaker-Oats-Center-Of-Excellence06042012.html.

41. Sloan, "Top 10 Functional Food Trends."

42. Sloan, "Top 10 Functional Food Trends."

43. Sarah Colby et al., "Nutritional Marketing on Food Labels," *Journal of Nutrition Education and Behavior* 42, no. 2 (2010): 92–98.

44. Michele Simon, *Appetite for Profit: How the Food Industry Undermines Our Health and How to Fight Back* (New York: Nation Books, 2006).

45. Kellogg Co., "Kellogg's® Froot Loops® Marshmallow Cereal," www.kelloggs.com/en_US/kelloggs-froot-loops-marshmallow-cereal.html#prevpoint (accessed May 10, 2012). See also Paul Pestano et al., *Sugar in Children's Cereals: Popular Brands Pack More Sugar than Snack Cakes and Cookies* (Washington, D.C.: Environmental Working Group, 2011).

46. Marlene Schwartz et al., "Examining the Nutritional Quality of Breakfast Cereals Marketed to Children," *Journal of the American Dietetic Association* 108 (2008): 702–705.

47. Geoffrey Cannon, *The Fate of Nations: Food and Nutrition Policy in the New World* (St. Austell, U.K.: Caroline Walker Trust, 2003), 25.

48. Glacéau, "Vitaminwater," www.vitaminwater.com (accessed August 1, 2012).

49. Nestle, *Food Politics*, 240.

50. Corrina Hawkes, *Nutrition Labels and Health Claims: The Global Regulatory Environment* (Geneva: World Health Organization, 2004).

51. C. Rispin, J. Keenan, and D. Jacobs, "Oat Products and Lipid Lowering: A Meta-analysis," *Journal of the American Medical Association* 267, no. 24 (1992): 3317–3327.

52. Robert Fitzsimmons, "Oh, What Those Oats Can Do. Quaker Oats, the Food and Drug Administration, and the Market Value of Scientific Evidence 1984–2010," *Comprehensive Reviews in Food Science and Food Safety* 11 (2011): 56–99.

53. American Dietetic Association, "Functional Foods"; U.S. Food and Drug Administration, "Labeling and Nutrition," www.fda.gov/Food/LabelingNutrition/default.htm (accessed August 12, 2009).

54. "Position of the American Dietetic Association: Total Diet Approach to Communicating Food and Nutrition Information," *Journal of the American Dietetic Association* 107, no. 7 (2007): 1124–132.

55. Nestle, *Food Politics*, 389; N. Hooker and R. Teratanavat, "Dissecting Qualified Health Claims: Evidence from Experimental Studies," *Critical Reviews in Food Science and Nutrition* 48 (2008): 160–176.

56. General Mills, "Does Cheerios® Cereal Lower Cholesterol?," www.cheerios.com/Answers/Does-Cheerios-lower-cholesterol (accessed September 23, 2012).

57. Martijn B. Katan and Nicole De Roos, "Promises and Problems of Functional Foods," *Critical Reviews in Food Science and Nutrition* 44 (2004): 369–377.

58. On consumers' interpretation of nutrient and health claims, see, e.g., Peter Williams, "Consumer Understanding and Use of Health Claims for Foods," *Nutrition Reviews* 63, no. 7 (2005): 256–264; Clare Hasler, "Health Claims in the United States: An Aid to the Public or a Source of Confusion?," *Journal of Nutrition* 138 (2008): 1216S–1220S.

59. U.S. General Accounting Office, *Food Labeling: FDA Needs to Reassess Its Approach to Protecting Consumers from False or Misleading Claims* (Washington, D.C., 2011), 16. See also American Dietetic Association, "Functional Foods."

60. Gaston Ares, Ana Gimenez, and Adriana Gambaro, "Influence of Nutritional Knowledge on Perceived Healthiness and Willingness to Try Functional Foods," *Appetite* 51 (2008): 663–668.

61. Brian Roe, Alan Levy, and Brenda Derby, "The Impact of Health Claims on Consumer Search and Product Evaluation Outcomes: Results from FDA Experimental Data," *Journal of Public Policy and Marketing* 18, no. 1 (1999): 89–105. See also Brian Wansick, *Mindless Eating: Why We Eat More Than We Think* (New York: Bantam Books, 2006).

62. Roe et al., "Impact of Health Claims."

63. Roe et al., "Impact of Health Claims"; H. van Trijp, "Consumer Understanding and Nutritional Communication: Key Issues in the Context of the New EU Legislation," *European Journal of Nutrition* 48 (2009): S41–S48.

64. Elizabeth Sloan, "Top 10 Functional Food Trends," *Food Technology* 66, no. 4 (2012): 24–41.

65. B. Hornick, C. Dolven, and D. Liska, "The Fiber Deficit, Part II: Consumer Misperceptions About Whole Grains and Fiber," *Nutrition Today* 47, no. 3 (2012): 104–109.

66. Belasco, *Appetite for Change*, 222.

67. Sloan, "Top 10 Functional Food Trends"; IRI Group, *I.R.I. New Product Pacesetters* (Chicago, 2011).

68. Barbara Katz and Lu Anne Williams, "Cleaning Up Processed Foods," *Food Technology* (December 2011): 33–37.

69. Danielle Schor et al., "Nutrition Facts You Can't Miss: The Evolution of Front-of-Pack Labeling," *Nutrition Today* 45, no. 1 (2010): 22–32; Lisa Carlson, "Front-of-the-Pack and On-Shelf Labeling," *Nutrition Today* 45, no. 1 (2010): 15–21.

70. C. Fischler, "A Nutritional Cacophony or the Crisis of Food Selection in Affluent Societies," in *For a Better Nutrition in the 21st Century*, ed. P. Leathwood, M. Horisberger, and W.P. James (New York: Nestlé Nutrition Services, 1993).

71. Joanne Lupton et al., "The Smart Choices Front-of-Package Nutrition Labeling Program: Rationale and Development of the Nutrition Criteria," *American Journal of Clinical Nutrition* 91, suppl. (2010): 1078S–1089S.

72. Bruce Silverglade and Ilene Ringel Heller, *Food Labeling Chaos* (Washington, D.C.: Center for Science in the Public Interest, 2010); C. Roberto et al., "Choosing Front-of-Package Food Labelling Nutritional Criteria: How Smart Were 'Smart Choices'?," *Public Health Nutrition* 15, no. 2 (2011): 262–269.

73. Timothy D. Lytton, "Signs of Change or Clash of Symbols? F.D.A. Regulation of Nutrient Profile Labeling," *Health Matrix* 20, no. 1 (2010): 93–144.

74. Jason Switt, "Labeling Around the Globe: Helping to Direct Food Flow," *Journal of the American Dietetic Association* 107, no. 2 (2007): 199–200.

75. Sophie Hieke and Petra Wilczynski, "Colour Me In—an Empirical Study on Consumer Responses to the Traffic Light Signposting System in Nutrition Labelling," *Public Health Nutrition* 15, no. 5 (2011): 773–782; K.L. Hawley et al., "The Science on Front-of-Package Food Labels," *Public Health Nutrition*, in press (doi:10.1017/S1368980012000754). For a study that showed no changes in consumer purchasing behavior from traffic light labeling, see Gary Sacks et al., "Impact of 'Traffic-Light' Nutrition Information on Online Food Purchases in Australia," *Australia and New Zealand Journal of Public Health* 35, no. 2 (2011): 122–126.

76. "Industry Lobbying Sees EU Reject 'Traffic Light' Food Labelling," *Ecologist,* June 17, 2010, www.theecologist.org/News/news_round_up/511976/industry _lobbying_sees_eu_reject_traffic_light_food_labelling.html.

77. Gregory Miller et al., "Nutrient Profiling: Global Approaches, Policies and Perspectives," *Nutrition Today* 45, no. 1 (2010): 6–12.

78. F. Foltran et al., "Nutritional Profiles in a Public Health Perspective: A Critical Review," *Journal of International Medical Research* 38 (2010): 318–385; Marcella Garsetti, "Nutrient Profiling Schemes: Overview and Comparative Analysis," *European Journal of Nutrition* 46 (2007): 15–28.

79. Adam Drewnowski and Victor Fulgoni, "Nutrient Profiling of Foods: Creating a Nutrient-Rich Food Index," *Nutrition Reviews* 66, no. 1 (2007): 23–29.

80. Nestle, *Food Politics*. See also Jennifer Lisa Falbe and Marion Nestle, "The Politics of Government Dietary Advice," in *A Sociology of Food and Nutrition*, ed. John Germov and Lauren Williams (South Melbourne: Oxford University Press, 2008), 127–146.

81. On the influence of the food industry through involvement in government committees, see G. Jenkin et al., "Nutrition Policy in Whose Interests? A New Zealand Case Study," *Public Health Nutrition* 15 (2011): 1483–1488.

82. Amalia Waxman, "The WHO Global Strategy on Diet, Physical Activity and Health: The Controversy on Sugar," *Development* 47, no. 2 (2004): 75–82; Falbe and Nestle, "Politics of Government Dietary Advice."

83. L. Sharma, S. Teret, and K. Brownell, "The Food Industry and Self-Regulation: Standards to Promote Success and Avoid Public Health Failures," *American Journal of Public Health* 100, no. 2 (2010): 240–246.

84. Nestle, *Food Politics*, 116; Jane Dixon, Colin Sindall, and Cathy Banwell, "Exploring the Intersectoral Partnerships Guiding Australia's Dietary Advice," *Health Promotion International* 19, no. 1 (2004): 5–13; Gyorgy Scrinis and Rosemary Stanton, "Total Wellbeing or Too Much Meat?," *Australasian Science* 26, no. 9 (2005): 37–38; Simon, *Appetite for Profit*; Bart Penders and Annemiek Nelis, "Credibility Engineering in the Food Industry: Linking Science, Regulation, and Marketing in a Corporate Context," *Science in Context* 24, no. 4 (2011): 487–515.

85. L. Lesser et al., "Relationship Between Funding Source and Conclusion Among Nutrition-Related Scientific Articles," *PLoS Medicine* 4, no. 1 (2007): 41–46.

86. Nestle, *Food Politics*, 126; Phil Chamberlain, "Independence of Nutritional Information?," *British Medical Journal* 340 (2010); Dixon et al., "Exploring the Intersectoral Partnerships Guiding Australia's Dietary Advice."

87. Simon, *Appetite for Profit*, 186–191.

88. S. Yanamadala et al., "Food Industry Front Groups and Conflicts of Interest: The Case of Americans Against Food Taxes," *Public Health Nutrition* 15, no. 8 (2012): 1331–1332.

89. See, e.g., Marion Nestle and David Ludwig, "Front-of-Package Food Labels: Public Health or Propaganda?," *Journal of the American Medical Association* 303, no. 8 (2010).

90. Center for Science in the Public Interest, "Biotechnology Project," www.cspinet.org/biotech (accessed July 6, 2012).

9. THE FOOD QUALITY PARADIGM

1. Joan Dye Gussow, "Can an Organic Twinkie Be Certified?," in *For All Generations: Making World Agriculture More Sustainable*, ed. P. Madden (Glendale, Calif.: OM Publications, 1997), 143–153.

2. Claude Fischler, "A Nutritional Cacophony, or the Crisis of Food Selection in Affluent Societies," in *For a Better Nutrition in the 21st Century*, ed. P. Leathwood et al. (New York: Raven Press, 1993), 57–65; Joan Gussow, *Why You Should Eat Food, and Other Nutritional Heresies* (lecture, University of California, Davis, 2003); Michael Pollan, *In Defense of Food: The Myth of Nutrition and the Pleasures of Eating* (New York: Allen Lane, 2008), 1.

3. Rose Hume Hall, *The Unofficial Guide to Smart Nutrition* (Foster City, Calif.: IDG Books, 2000).

4. These categories were introduced in: Gyorgy Scrinis, "From Techno-Corporate Food to Alternative Agri-Food Movements," *Local-Global* 4 (2007): 112–140; Scrinis, "On the Ideology of Nutritionism," *Gastronomica* 8, no. 1 (2008): 39–48.

5. Brazilian public health nutritionist Carlos Monteiro has recently echoed a number of my arguments regarding the need to prioritize degrees of processing. However, he distinguishes between only two categories of ingredients (whole

foods and refined ingredients) and two categories of foods made from those ingredients (minimally processed and "ultraprocessed" foods). See Carlos Monteiro, "Nutrition and Health. The Issue Is Not Food, nor Nutrients, So Much as Processing," *Public Health Nutrition* 12, no. 5 (2009): 729–731.

6. Nina L. Etkin, *Edible Medicines: An Ethnopharmacology of Food* (Tucson: University of Arizona Press, 2006), chap. 4; Sally Fallon, *Nourishing Traditions: The Cookbook That Challenges Politically Correct Nutrition and the Diet Dictocrats* (Washington, D.C.: New Trends, 2001).

7. David Julian McClements et al., "In Defense of Food Science," *Gastronomica* 11, no. 2 (2011): 76–84.

8. Etkin, *Edible Medicines*, 133.

9. Etkin, *Edible Medicines*, 112.

10. Alexandra McManus, Margaret Merga, and Wendy Newton, "Omega-3 Fatty Acids: What Consumers Need to Know," *Appetite* 57 (2011): 80–83.

11. Jill Reedy and Susan Krebs-Smith, "Dietary Sources of Energy, Solid Fats, and Added Sugars Among Children and Adolescents in the United States," *Journal of the American Dietetic Association* 110 (2010): 1477–1484.

12. Alice Lichtenstein, "Nutrient Supplements and Cardiovascular Disease: A Heartbreaking Story," *Journal of Lipid Research* 50 (2009): S429–S433.

13. See Michael Hill, "Pink Slime: Why Is It Now Striking a Chord?," *The Huffington Post*, March 14, 2012, www.huffingtonpost.com/2012/03/14/pinkslime _n_1345310.html?view=print&comm_ref=false (accessed July 20, 2012).

14. Hall, *Unofficial Guide*, 188.

15. Steve Ettlinger, *Twinkie, Deconstructed* (New York: Hudson Street Press, 2007).

16. George Inglett, ed. *Fabricated Foods* (Westport, Conn.: AVI Publishing, 1975), 7.

17. David Kessler, *The End of Overeating: Taking Control of the Insatiable American Appetite* (New York: Rodale, 2009), 94.

18. Felicity Lawrence, *Not on the Label: What Really Goes into the Food on Your Plate* (London: Penguin, 2004), 106.

19. "Position of the American Dietetic Association: Total Diet Approach to Communicating Food and Nutrition Information," *Journal of the American Dietetic Association* 107, no. 7 (2007): 1224–1232.

20. Janet Poppendieck, *Free for All: Fixing School Food in America* (Berkeley: University of California Press, 2010), 279–282.

21. Rachel Laudan, "A Plea for Culinary Modernism: Why We Should Love New, Fast, Processed Food," *Gastronomica* 1 (2001): 36–44.

22. On the possible impacts of environmental toxins on weight regulation, see Julie Guthman, *Weighing In: Obesity, Food Justice and the Limits of Capitalism* (Berkeley: University of California Press, 2011), chap. 5.

23. Walter Willett, *Eat, Drink, and Be Healthy: The Harvard Medical School Guide to Healthy Eating* (New York: Free Press, 2005), 167.

24. A. Mitchell et al., "Ten-Year Comparison of the Influence of Organic and Conventional Crop Management Practices on the Content of Flavonoids in Tomatoes," *Journal of Agricultural and Food Chemistry* 55 (2007): 6154–6159; Alan Dangour, "Nutrition-Related Health Effects of Organic Foods: A Systematic Review," *American Journal of Clinical Nutrition* 92 (2010): 203–210. Crystal Smith-Spangler et al., "Are Organic Foods Safer or Healthier than Conventional Alternatives? A Systematic Review," *Ann Intern Med.* 157, no. 5 (2012): 348–366.

25. Etkin, *Edible Medicines*; Andrea Pieroni and Lisa Leimar Price, eds., *Eating and Healing: Traditional Food as Medicine* (Binghamton, N.Y.: Food Products Press, 2006).

26. For a discussion of some of the contradictory evidence on the health benefits or harmfulness of soy products in research studies, see Marion Nestle, *What to Eat* (New York: North Point Press, 2006), 132–137. See also Kaayla Daniel, *The Whole Soy Story* (Washington, D.C.: New Trends, 2005).

27. John Robbins, *Healthy at 100: How to Extend Your Life and Stay Fit* (London: Hodder and Stoughton, 2006); Daphne Miller, *The Jungle Effect: A Doctor Discovers the Healthiest Diets from Around the World, Why They Work and How to Bring Them Home* (New York: Harper Collins, 2010); Bradley Willcox, Craig Willcox, and Makoto Suzuki, *The Okinawa Diet Plan* (New York: Three Rivers Press, 2005); Dan Buettner, *The Blue Zones: Lessons for Living Longer from the People Who've Lived the Longest* (Washington, D.C.: National Geographic Society, 2008).

28. Jonny Bowden, *Living Low Carb*, rev. ed. (New York: Sterling, 2010), 80; Miller, *The Jungle Effect*.

29. Miller, *The Jungle Effect*. See also Catherine Shanahan and Luke Shanahan, *Deep Nutrition: Why Your Genes Need Traditional Food* (Lawai, Hawaii: Big Box Books, 2009).

30. See, e.g., Robbins, *Healthy at 100*.

31. U.S. Department of Agriculture and Department of Health and Human Services, *Dietary Guidelines for Americans, 2010* (Washington, D.C., 2010), 44.

32. Elizabeth Lipski, "Traditional Non-Western Diets," *Nutrition in Clinical Practice* 25, no. 6 (2010): 585–593. Kerin O'Dea, "The Therapeutic and Preventive Potential of the Hunter-Gatherer Lifestyle," in *Western Diseases: Their Prevention and Reversibility*, ed. N.J. Temple and D.P. Burkitt (Totowa: Humana Press, 1994), 349–380. Kerin O'Dea, "Preventable Chronic Diseases Among Indigenous Australians: The Need for a Comprehensive National Approach," *Heart Lung and Circulation* 14 (2005): 167–171.

33. P. Rozin et al., "Attitudes to Food and the Role of Food in Life in the U.S.A., Japan, Flemish Belgium and France: Possible Implications for Diet-Health Debate," *Appetite* 33 (1999): 163–180.

34. Pierre Dukan, *The Dukan Diet* (London: Hodder and Staughton, 2010).

35. Miller, *The Jungle Effect*, 222; Pollan, *In Defense of Food*, 185.

36. Michael Pollan, *Food Rules: An Eater's Manual* (New York: Penguin, 2009), 103.

37. S. Ristovvski-Slijepcevic, G. Chapman, and B. Beagan, "Engaging with Healthy Eating Discourse(s): Ways of Knowing About Food and Health in Three Ethnocultural Groups in Canada," *Appetite* 50 (2008): 167–178.

38. Ross Hume Hall, *Food for Nought: The Decline in Nutrition* (Hagerstown, Md.: Harper and Row, 1974), 54–55.

39. Kessler, *End of Overeating*, 7.

40. David Ludwig, *Ending the Food Fight: Guide Your Child to a Healthy Weight in a Fast Food/Fake Food World* (Boston: Houghton-Mifflin, 2007), 61.

41. Stephen Goff and Harry Klee, "Plant Volatile Compounds: Sensory Cues for Health and Nutritional Value?," *Science* 311, no. 10 (2006): 815–819.

42. Carol Hart, *Good Food Tastes Good: An Argument for Trusting Your Senses and Ignoring the Nutritionists* (Philadelphia: Spring Street Books, 2007).

43. Alice Waters, "Eating for Credit," *New York Times*, February 24, 2006.

44. Carlo Petrini, *Slow Food: The Case for Taste* (New York: Columbia University Press, 2001), 69.

45. See also Allison Hayes-Conroy and Jessica Hayes-Conroy, "Visceral Difference: Variations in Feeling (Slow) Food," in *Taking Food Public: Redefining Foodways in a Changing World*, ed. P. Williams-Forson and C. Counihan (New York: Routledge, 2012), 515–530.

46. Waters, "Eating for Credit."

47. JoAnn Jaffe and Michael Gertler, "Victual Vicissitudes: Consumer Deskilling and the (Gendered) Transformation of Food Systems," *Agriculture and Human Values* 23 (2006): 143–162. See also M. Caraher et al., "The State of Cooking in England: The Relationship of Cooking Skills to Food Choice," *British Food Journal* 101, no. 8 (1999): 590–609.

48. Michelle Stacey, *Consumed: Why Americans Love, Hate and Fear Food* (New York: Simon and Schuster, 1994), 213.

49. Guthman, *Weighing In*, 144–147.

50. Linda Bacon, *Health at Every Size: The Surprising Truth About Your Weight* (Dallas, Tex.: Benballa Books, 2010). See also the Health at Every Size website, www .haescommunity.org.

51. Linda Bacon and Lucy Aphramor, "Weight Science: Evaluating the Evidence for a Paradigm Shift," *Nutrition Journal* 10, no. 9 (2011). See also Guthman, *Weighing In*, 43.

52. Maria Barton, John Kearney, and Barbara Stewart-Knox, "Knowledge of Food Production Methods Informs Attitudes Toward Food but Not Food Choice in Adults Residing in Socioeconomically Deprived Rural Areas Within the United Kingdom," *Journal of Nutrition Education and Behavior* 43, no. 5 (2011): 374–378.

53. Nicole Darmon and Adam Drewnowski, "Does Social Class Predict Diet Quality?," *American Journal of Clinical Nutrition* 87 (2008): 1107–1117.

10. AFTER NUTRITIONISM

1. E.g., David Jacobs and Linda Tapsell, "Food, Not Nutrients, Is the Fundamental Unit in Nutrition," *Nutrition Reviews* 65, no. 10 (2007): 439–450.

2. Nina Planck, *Real Food for Mother and Baby: The Fertility Diet, Eating for Two, and Baby's First Foods* (New York: Bloomsbury, 2009), 40.

3. Tim Lang, David Barling, and Martin Caraher, *Food Policy: Integrating Health, Environment and Society* (New York: Oxford, 2009).

4. Michael Pollan, *In Defense of Food: The Myth of Nutrition and the Pleasures of Eating* (New York: Allen Lane, 2008), 139.

5. Pollan, *In Defense of Food*, 172.

6. Pollan, *In Defense of Food*, 166.

7. Dimitrios Trichopoulos, Pagona Lagiou, and Antonia Trichopoulou, "Evidence-Based Nutrition," *Asia Pacific Journal of Clinical Nutrition* 9, no. S1 (2000): S4–S9.

8. Jacobs and Tapsell, "Food, Not Nutrients."

9. Jacobs and Tapsell, "Food, Not Nutrients."

10. Another such study in which Jacobs has been involved that differentiates between the food sources of saturated fats is M. De Oliveira et al., "Dietary Intake of Saturated Fat by Food Source and Incident Cardiovascular Disease: The Multi-ethnic Study of Atherosclerosis," *American Journal of Clinical Nutrition* 96, no. 2 (2012): 397–404.

11. It is worth noting that some of these studies have been in vitro and animal studies rather than long-term human studies, so only limited conclusions can be drawn from them.

12. Carol O'Neil et al., "Whole-Grain Consumption Is Associated with Diet Quality and Nutrient Intake in Adults: The National Health and Nutrition Examination Survey, 1999–2004," *Journal of the American Dietetic Association* 110, no. 10 (2010): 1461–1468.

13. Nicola McKeown and David Jacobs, "In Defence of Phytochemical-Rich Dietary Patterns," *British Journal of Nutrition* 104, no. 1 (2010): 1–3.

14. Jacobs and Tapsell, "Food, Not Nutrients."

15. One study has suggested that the fat in cheese and butter has differential effects on LDL cholesterol: P.J. Nestel et al., "Dairy Fat in Cheese Raises LDL Cholesterol Less than That in Butter in Mildly Hypercholesterolaemic Subjects," *European Journal of Clinical Nutrition* 59 (2005): 1059–1063.

16. Trichopoulos et al., "Evidence-Based Nutrition."

17. See, e.g., R. Florentino et al., "Report of a Seminar and Workshop on Food-Based Dietary Guidelines and Nutrition Education: Bridging Science and

Communication," *Asia Pacific Journal of Clinical Nutrition* 8, no. 4 (1999): 291–299; K. Brown et al., "A Review of Consumer Awareness, Understanding and Use of Food-Based Dietary Guidelines," *British Journal of Nutrition* 106, no. 1 (2011): 15–26.

18. U.S. Department of Agriculture, "MyPlate," www.choosemyplate.gov /food-groups/grains.html (accessed July 1, 2012).

19. U.S. Department of Agriculture, "MyPlate," www.choosemyplate.gov /weight-management-calories/calories/empty-calories.html (accessed July 1, 2012).

20. Dariush Mozaffarian and David Ludwig, "Dietary Guidelines in the 21st Century—A Time for Food," *Journal of the American Medical Association* 304, no. 6 (2010): 681–682, 681, 682.

21. D. Mozaffarian, R. Micha, and S. Wallace, "Effects on Coronary Heart Disease of Increasing Polyunsaturated Fat in Place of Saturated Fat: A Systematic Review and Meta-analysis of Randomized Controlled Trials," *PLoS Medicine* 7, no. 3 (2010): 1–10; David Ludwig, *Ending the Food Fight: Guide Your Child to a Healthy Weight in a Fast Food/Fake Food World* (Boston: Houghton-Mifflin, 2007).

22. Mozaffarian and Ludwig, "Dietary Guidelines in the 21st Century," 681.

23. Mozaffarian and Ludwig, "Dietary Guidelines in the 21st Century," 682.

24. Mozaffarian and Ludwig, "Dietary Guidelines in the 21st Century," 682.

25. See, e.g., Joyce D'Silva and John Webster, eds., *The Meat Crisis: Developing More Sustainable Production and Consumption* (London: Earthscan, 2010); David Pimentel et al., "Reducing Energy Inputs in the U.S. Food System," *Human Ecology* 36 (2008): 459–471.

26. E. Brunner et al., "Fish, Human Health and Marine Ecosystem Health: Policies in Collision," *International Journal of Epidemiology* 38 (2009). See also J.L. Wilkins et al., "Increasing Acres to Decrease Inches: Comparing the Agricultural Land Requirements of a Low-Carbohydrate, High-Protein Diet with a MyPyramid Diet," *Journal of Hunger and Environmental Nutrition* 3, no. 1 (2008): 3–16.

27. Joan Dye Gussow and Katherine Clancy, "Dietary Guidelines for Sustainability," *Journal of Nutrition Education* 18, no. 1 (1986): 1–5; Anthony McMichael, "Integrating Nutrition with Ecology: Balancing the Health of Humans and Biosphere," *Public Health Nutrition* 8, no. 6A (2005): 706–715. Tim Lang, David Barling, and Martin Caraher, *Food Policy: Integrating Health, Environment & Society* (New York: Oxford, 2009); Barilla Center for Food and Nutrition, *Double Pyramid: Healthy Food for People, Sustainable Food for the Planet* (Parma, Italy, 2010).

28. For other examples of alternative food labels, see the "Rethink the Food Label" design competition: http://berkeley.news21.com/foodlabel/ (accessed July 12, 2012); and *New York Times* food writer Mark Bittman's proposed food label, with color-coded rankings for nutrition, "foodness," and welfare: Mark Bittman,

"My Dream Food Label," *New York Times*, October 13, 2012, www.nytimes.com /2012/10/14/opinion/sunday/bittman-my-dream-food-label.html (accessed October 20, 2012).

29. Marion Nestle and David Ludwig, "Front-of-Package Food Labels: Public Health or Propaganda?," *Journal of the American Medical Association* 303, no. 8 (2010).

INDEX

Page numbers for figures and tables are in *italics*.

Animal Chemistry or Organic Chemistry in Its Application to Physiology and Pathology (Liebig), 54

animal foods, 2, 11, 16, 19, 28, 35–38, 54, 80, 82, 84, 88, 91, 93, 126, 182, 183, 185, 228; animal fats, 37, 134, 142, 144; on *Food Guide Pyramid* (1992), 95, *95*

antioxidants, 7, 14, 47–49, 85–86, 160, 161, 173, 194

Appetite for Change (Belasco), 17, 208

Appetite for Profit (Simon), 203

Apple, Rima, 63, 66–67, 70

Aronowitz, Robert, 78

artificial fats, 40, 106, 119, 143, 200

artificial sweeteners, 40, 77, 119, 143

at-risk body, 48, 77, 79, 164, 167, *261*, *262*

atherosclerosis: 1957 AHA report on, 81; cholesterol and, 76, 84, 85; diet and, 30; inflammation and, 86; sterol and stanol esters and, 154

Atkins, Robert, 26, 38, 100, 120, 122

Atkins diet, 122, 123, 127

Atkins for Life (Atkins), 122

Atwater, Wilbur, 12, 48, 53, 58, 60, 62, 66, 117, 193

Australia: dietary guidelines, 95, 288n100; health claims on foods, 303n43; and low-GI sugar, 131; and margarine, 303nn43–44; weight-loss diet book, 132

Aziz, Michael, 167

"bad cholesterol." *See* low-density lipoprotein

Bad Fats Brothers (AHA campaign), 145

Baker, Christina, 114

Balade, 155

Bang, Hans Olaf, 168

Basic Four food guide (1956), 56, 95, 212

Basic Seven food guide (1943), 56, 70, 95

Baudrillard, Jean, 307n105

Belasco, Warren, 17, 73, 208

Benecol (margarine), 152–153

beriberi, 63, 64, 65, 68

beta-carotene, 31–32, 33, 177, 200

Bethea, Morrison, 100

biomarker reductionism, 40–42, 164, 189, 245, 253, *258*

biomarkers, 14, 30, 40–42, 46, 73, 76, 83, 86, 146, 164, 172–174, 188, 189, 234, 243, 253, 258, 273n53

biomedicalization, 49–50

Bittman, Mark, 329n28

blood cholesterol levels, 164; biomarker reductionism and, 41; dietary cholesterol and, 82; dietary influences on, 30, 81–82; fiber and, 205; heart disease and, 4, 30–31, 78, 79, 80, 81–82, 84, 85; lowering, 165; saturated fatty acids and, 84; statin drugs and, 78, 165; sterol- and stanol-enriched foods and, 153; *trans*-fats and, 137–140, 144

blood glucose levels: carbohydrates and, 123, 124, 125; glycemic index and, 126, 164; sugars and, 160

The Blue Zones (Buettner), 184, 228

BMI reductionism, 235

body: at-risk, 48, 79, 167, *261*, *262*; characterization of, 47–48; fat storage, insulin, and sugar, 123–124; functional, 43, 48 165–167, *262*; levels of engagement with, *259*; as machine, 58; nutrient-deficient, 48, 68, 167, *261*, *262*; nutritionally enhanced, 48, 166, *262*; and optimal health, 164; overnourished, 48, 74, 79, *262*; quantified-mechanical, 47–48, 58, *262*; summary of types, *262*

body mass index (BMI), 41–42; as biomarker of risk for disease, 164;

DASH diet (Dietary Approaches to Stop Hypertension diet), 178, 179, 243, 315*n*97

De La Pena, Carolyn, 77

De Oliveira, M., 328*n*10

decontextualization, 6, 7, 23, 29, 41, 77, 101, 116, 124, 193, 207, 211, 238, 240, 250

deep-frying oil, 85, 136–137, 142, 147–148, 150, 151

deficiency diseases, 63, 64–65, 77; industrial foods and, 66; nutrient deficiency diseases, 65; single-nutrient deficiency diseases, 5, 30, 31; vitamin deficiency diseases, 64–65

Derby, Brenda, 207

detrimentally processed foods, *219*

detrimentally processed ingredients, *218*

DHA (docosahexanoic acid), 159, 168, 170, 171, 201

diabetes: biomarkers for management of, 164; cause of, 125; chronic inflammation and, 86; dietary guidelines for, 104–105, 238; glycemic index and, 126–127; high-GI foods and, 126–127; insulin resistance and, 124; as leading cause of death, 77; low-fat diets and, 100; management, 165; refined carb consumption and, 160; sugar and, 83; *trans*-fats and, 139; "twin epidemics," 108

Diet and Health: Implications for Reducing Chronic Disease Risk (National Academy of Science, 1989), 101

Diet and Health, with Key to Calories (Peters), 51

Diet Coke Plus, 191–192

diet-heart hypothesis, 30, 79–87, 103, 137, 141, 311*n*48

Diet, Nutrition and Cancer (U.S. National Research Council), 31

Diet Pepsi Max, 192

Dietary Approaches to Stop Hypertension diet. *See* DASH diet

dietary cholesterol, 47, 75, 79; blood cholesterol and, 82; *Dietary Goals* (1977) on, *89*, *92*; *Dietary Guidelines* (1980) on, *94*; dietary guidelines for, 82, 88; heart disease and, 75

Dietary Goals for the United States (1977), 76, 82, 87–93

dietary guidelines: alternative guidelines, 245–249; American, 76; Australian, 95, 288*n*100; *Basic Four* food guide (1956), 56, 95, 212; *Basic Seven* food guide (1943), 56, 70, 95; for diabetes, 104–105; *Dietary Goals for the United States* (1977), 76, 82, 87–93, 102; *Dietary Guidelines for Americans* (1980), 26, 48, 76, 82, 90–94, *94*, 101; *Dietary Guidelines for Americans* (1990), 76, 94, 100, 101; *Dietary Guidelines for Americans* (1995), 94, 100; *Dietary Guidelines for Americans* (2000), 109; *Dietary Guidelines for Americans* (2005), 114; *Dietary Guidelines for Americans* (2010), 37, 38, 47, 86, 113–114, 123, 144, 163, 169, 170, 181, 228, 247; first USDA food guide (1917), 70; *Food Guide Pyramid* (1992), 26, 95–97, *95*, 100, 101, 108, 188, 212, 245, 288*n*107; food-level guidelines, 247–248; good-and-bad nutritionism, 193; individual tastes and, 234; interests of food producers and, 212; low-fat diet, 101–112; Mudry on, 267*n*30; *MyPlate* food guide, 212, 245–247, *246*; *MyPyramid* (2005), 188, 245, 317*n*133; Nestle on, 212; nutricentric focus on, 7, 13, 37; period of reissue, 94; revision of, 248–249; for saturated fats, 86; for vitamin D, 162

Dietary Guidelines Advisory
Committee, 109
dietary healthism, 44–45
dietary pattern analysis, 177–181, 243
diets: Alaskan Eskimo diet, 184;
American Samoan diet, 184;
"ancestral" diet, 185; Atkins diet,
122, 123, 127; Cretan diet, 178;
culturally specific approaches to,
62–63, 227–231; DASH diet, 178,
179, 243, 315n97; Dukan diet, 231;
eclecticism in, 229; French dietary
patterns, 230–231; high-carb diet,
25, 85, 125; high-protein diet, 120;
Japanese diet, 228; low-carb diet,
8, 10, 100, 110, 111, 120–123,
297n130; low-carb/high-fat diet,
26, 100, 110, 122; low-fat diet, 7,
80, 97, 101–112; low-fat/high-carb
diet, 25–26, 96, 102, 104, 105;
low-glycemic-index diets, 100, 110,
126–132; low-glycemic-load diets,
127; Mediterranean diet, 178, 180,
184, 228, 243, 315n97, 316n97,
317n132; Okinawa diet, 178, 184,
228; Ornish diet, 100, 102;
paleolithic diet, 10, 158, 185–187,
228, 317n132; perfect 10 diet, 167;
personalized diets, 21, 44, 187–
188, 189, 190; plant-based diets,
95, 100, 102; of poor and working
class, 66; Pritikin diet, 102;
prudent diet, 179, 184, 243; search
for optimal dietary pattern,
177–181; South Beach diet, 122;
Sugar Busters diet, 122; traditional
diets, 184–185, 227–231; vegan
diets, 181; vegetarian diets,
181–184; weight-loss diet books, 51,
132, 167; The Zone diet, 100. See also
American diet
disease risk: biomarkers as measure of,
173; minimizing, 164; reducing,

176; single foods or food groups
and, 172, 173; whole grain intake
and, 173, 174
disease risk factors: body mass index
(BMI), 164; for chronic diseases,
77–79; epidemiological data and,
78; for heart disease, 102
diseases: lifestyle factors and, 78;
nutrient deficiency diseases, 65;
preventive measures, 283n26;
"protodiseases," 282n25. See also
chronic diseases; deficiency
diseases; and under individual diseases
Dixon, Jane, 267n30
docosahexaenoic acid. See DHA
Dr. Atkins' Diet Revolution (Atkins), 38,
120, 122
Dr. Atkins' New Diet Revolution (Atkins),
122
Dukan diet, 231
Dutch government, regulating
trans-fat content, 146
Dyerberg, Jørn, 168

Eat, Drink, and Be Healthy (Willett), 68,
176
Eat More, Weigh Less (Ornish), 100, 105
Eat Well and Stay Well (Keys), 80
Eat Your Way to Health (Rose), 51–52
"eating smarter," 162
Eaton, Boyd, 187
Eco, Umberto, 143
Edible Schoolyard project, 233–234
eggs: as bad food, 76; changing advice
on, 46–47; Dietary Goals (1977) on,
89, 92; factory-farmed, 170; on Food
Guide Pyramid (1992), 95; as good
food, 47; heart disease risk and,
173; as nutrient-dense food, 174;
nutrient profile of, 226;
stigmatization of, 6, 88, 97
eicosapentaenoic acid. See EPA
Emdee (margarine), 141

Empty Pleasures (De La Pena), 77
The End of Overeating (Kessler), 232
energy-balance equation, 17, 101,
    112–121
energy-dense foods, 8, 36
Enig, Mary, 83, 84, 139, 305n72
Entenmanns, 107
EPA (eicosapentaenoic acid), 168
epidemiology, 78, 178
Epstein, Steven, 188
era of functional nutritionism, *261. See
    also* functional nutritionism
era of good-and-bad nutritionism, *261.
    See also* good-and-bad nutritionism
era of quantifying nutritionism, *261.
    See also* quantifying nutritionism
eras of nutritionism, 12–13, 45–49,
    261, 274n63
Etkin, Nina, 220
Ettlinger, Steve, 223
European Food Safety Authority,
    210
European Prospective Investigation
    into Cancer and Nutrition study,
    173
everyday nutritionisms, 30, 129, 143,
    144, *259*
exaggeration, 5, 23, 29, 31, 41, 82, 132,
    238, 266, *258*
Extract of Meat (Liebig), 55, 56

fabricated foods, 143, 223
Fabricated Foods (1975 text), 143, 223
Facts Up Front (labeling system),
    209
fast food: calories in, 114, 115;
    hydrogenated vegetable oils used in
    preparation of, 142; working off
    calories from, 114
fat substitutes (artificial fats), 40, 106,
    119, 143, 200
fats: American Heart Association on,
    102, 103, 159–160; animal, 37;

artificial, 40, 106, 119, 143; calories
    in, 117; cancer and consumption
    of, 88, 103–104; Center for
    Science in the Public Interest on,
    102; chemically modified, 77;
    cholesterol levels and, 30;
    combination of high-fat and
    high-carb foods, 106; dietary fat,
    75, 76, 82, 84; *Dietary Goals* (1977)
    on, *89,* 92, 102; *Dietary Guidelines*
    (1980) on, 94, *94,* 100, 101; *Dietary
    Guidelines* (1990) on, 101; fat
    reductionism, 7, 80, 97, 101–112;
    on *Food Guide Pyramid* (1992), *95,* 96,
    100, 101, 108; food guides and, 76;
    on food package labeling, 251;
    glycemic index and, 130; good-
    and-bad, 1–3, 7, 26, 75–76, 96,
    103, 133, 144; and heart disease, 2,
    3, 26, 30, 34, 75, 102, 103;
    "hidden," 118; hydrogenated
    vegetable oils, 37, 83, 142, 148;
    hydrogenation of, 3, 134, 135–137,
    142, 306n79; interesterified
    (*i*-fats), 4, 149–152; in the
    low-carb/high-fat diet, 26,
    100, 122; in the low-fat diet,
    7, 80, 97, 101–112; low-fat
    paradox, 107–108; lowering
    consumption of, 101, 103–104;
    macronutrient profile of, 25–26;
    monounsaturated, 80, 141,
    144–145; Pollan on, 19; SoFAS,
    36–37; solid, 36, 37–38, 272n44;
    *Surgeon General's Report on Nutrition
    and Health* (1988) on, 101;
    unsaturated, 77, 83, 88. *See also*
    low-fat diet; oils; omega-3 fats;
    omega-6 fats; polyunsaturated
    fats; saturated fats; *trans*-fats
FDA. *See* Food and Drug
    Administration
fermentation, 218, 220–221, *263*

Marantz, Paul, 148–149

margarine, 133–156, 302nn25–26; advertising, 141; American Heart Association on, 137; Australian regulations of, 303nn43–44; butter vs., 97, 155, 300n1, 302n29; cholesterol-lowering, 4, 8–9, 152–156, 165, 167, 195, 200, 206; fats in, 302nn25–26; hardness of, 150; history, 1–4, 134–135, 140–144; interesterified fats (i-fats) and, 4, 149–152; low-fat, 142; omega-3-fortified, 157; plant sterols and stanols and, 4, 40, 152–153, 165, 167, 200, 206; processing techniques, 150; reduced-fat, 142; restrictions on coloring of, 135; as simulated food, 307n105; spreads, 142; superiority of butter over, 137; United Kingdom regulations of, 303n43; as virtually trans-fat free, 149, 151

marketing. See food marketing; nutritional marketing

Mastering Leptin (Richards), 167

Matthews, Kathy, 174

Mazola Corn Oil, 141

McClennan, Mark, 189

McCollum, Elmer, 12, 53, 64, 66, 279nn79–80

McDonald's, 142, 147–148

McGovern, George, 82, 87, 88, 107

McLuhan, Marshall, 266n14

McMichael, Philip, 49

Measured Meals (Mudry), 58

meat: 19th century view on, 54; in 1960s and 1970s, 266n11; in American diet, 108, 125; as bad food, 76, 172; Basic Four (1956) on, 56, 212; chronic diseases and red meat, 315n98; Dietary Goals (1977) on, 89; Dietary Guidelines (1980) on, 94; factory-farmed, 170; on Food

Guide Pyramid (1992), 95; iron in, 271n27; as nutrient-dense food, 174; nutrient density of, 163; nutrient profile of, 226; in paleo diet, 185, 228; stigmatized, 88

meat extract (Liebig), 55, 56

"Meat Group" (Basic Four), 56

meat ingredients, "pink slime," 222

mechanical metaphor, 68

medical gaze, 266n16

medicalization of food, 49, 197

Mediterranean diet, 178, 180, 184, 228, 243, 316n97, 317n132

"Meet the Fats" (AHA campaign), 145

Mège-Mouriès, Hippolyte, 134

Mellentin, Julian, 274n63

Mensink, Ronald, 139, 144

metabolism, origin of term, 275n9

micronutrients, 53, 64, 66–67

milk: in American diet, 108; Basic Four (1956) on, 56, 212; Dietary Goals (1977) on, 89, 89, 92, 93; fat-soluble vitamins and, 106; low-fat, 40, 112; in paleo diet, 185–186; plant sterol–enriched, 175; as protective food, 66; reduced-fat, 77, 106, 108, 292n43; whole, 76

"Milk Group" (Basic Four), 56

milk products. See dairy products

Miller, Daphne, 228

Miller-Kovach, Karen, 121

minimally processed and beneficially processed foods, 219, 263

minimally processed and beneficially processed ingredients, 218

monounsaturated fats, 80, 141, 144–145

Monsanto, 151

Montanari, Massimo, 227

Monteiro, Carlos, 324n5

Mozaffarian, Dariush, 170, 247–248

Mudry, Jessica, 58, 267n30

nutritional gaze, 13–14, 129, 166, 259, 266n16
nutritional genomics, 188–190
nutritional hubris, 6, 61, 71, 259
nutritional leveling, 35–36, 60, 259
nutritional marketing: budgets of food corporations, 49; Lupton on, 165–166; nutritional facade and, 203; summary, 262; targeting health benefits, 194
nutritional precision, myth of, 6, 31, 71, 146, 259
nutritional quality, 210; deficiency diseases and, 64; eating enough/too much, 231; Hall on, 15; pleasure principle and, 233; processing and, 29, 220; terms used for, 36; of whole foods, 175. See also food quality; nutrient density
nutritional reductionism. See reductionism
nutritional techno-fix, 40, 200, 260
"nutritionalisation," 267n30
nutritionally engineered foods, 8, 9, 13, 36, 43, 106, 140, 149, 155, 158, 183; defined, 39–40, 262; forms of, 175–176, 191–212; history, 56
nutritionally marketed foods, 9, 13, 262
nutritionally reductive scientific knowledge, 4, 7, 39, 199, 258
nutritionally reductive technological explanations, 111, 258
nutritionally reductive technological products/practices, 39, 199, 258
nutritionism: characteristics of, 237, 259–260; corporate, 8–9, 13, 49, 211–214, 260; effect on people, 43; eras, 12–13, 45–49, 261, 274n63; everyday nutritionisms, 30, 143; genetic, 189, 260; Goldacre on, 267n17; ideology, 2, 10, 11, 13; limitations, 21, 238; paradigms, 45,

258, 261; protective, 52; strong and weak critiques of, 14. See also functional nutritionism; good-and-bad nutritionism; quantifying nutritionism
NuVal system, 209–210

oats, 202–203, 213
obesity: American diet and, 128; bariatric surgery, 165; BMI and, 41; calories and, 113–115; cause of, 113, 120, 125; energy-balance equation, 113, 114; fat consumption and, 88, 100, 102, 108; heart disease and, 102–103; high-fructose corn syrup and, 160, 293n73; as leading cause of death, 77; Lichtenstein on, 113; low-fat paradox, 107–108; refined carb consumption and, 160; "size acceptance" movement, 235; sugar and, 117; trans-fats and, 139; "twin epidemics," 108
"obesity epidemic," 132, 160, 293n73
oils: "bad," 144; on Food Guide Pyramid (1992), 95; high-oleic canola oil, 150, 151; stearate-rich, 152; tropical, 142. See also fats; vegetable oils
Okinawa diet, 178, 184, 228
The Okinawa Diet Plan (Willcox), 228
The Okinawa Program (Willcox), 184
Olestra, 40, 106, 107
olive oil, 33, 142, 145, 179
Olson, Robert, 88
omega-3 fats: cancer and, 104; demand for, 170; eggs and, 47; FDA on, 169; foods fortified with, 157; functional nutritionism and, 168–171; hazards of, 85, 171; health effects of, 26, 160, 168–169; high doses of, 69; history, 161–162; insufficient intake of, 30; microcapsules for fortification of

foods, 170; as nutrient marker, 35;
omega-3 enhanced canola seeds,
176, 201; ratio of omega-6 to
omega-3 fats, 85, 169–170;
subtypes, 159, 168
omega-3-fortified orange juice, 157,
175
omega-6 fats: cancer and, 104;
harmful effects of, 85, 170; in
poultry, 311n48; ratio of omega-6
to omega-3 fats, 85, 169–170
"On the Ultimate Composition of
Simple Alimentary Substances"
(Prout), 54
orange juice: calcium-fortified, 191,
199; omega-3-fortified, 157, 175;
vitamin C–fortified, 40, 198
"orders of simulacra," 307–308n105
Oreo cookies, 106
organic foods, 175, 187, 208, 215, 217,
226–227, 235, 250
Ornish, Dean, 99, 100, 102, 105,
107, 127
Ornish diet, 100, 102
"orthorexia nervosa," 274n62
O'Shea, Marianne, 202
Ovaltine, 67
overweight, 42, 75, 91, 107, 113, 114,
122. See also obesity
oxidative stress, 85
Oz, Mehmet, 175

paleo diet, 10, 158, 185–187, 317n132
The Paleo Diet (Cordain), 185, 186
The Paleo Solution (Wolf), 185
palm oil, 142, 144, 150, 151
Paradox of Plenty (Levenstein), 17
partially hydrogenated oils, 136, 142,
150, 151
Pauling, Linus, 69
PepsiCo, 157, 202, 209
perception of nutrient scarcity, 68, 71,
162, 175, 226, 252, 259

Pereira, Jonathan, 54
The Perfect 10 Diet (Aziz), 167
Perfection Salad: Women and Cooking at the
Turn of the Century (Shapiro), 62
personalized diets, 21, 44, 187–188,
189, 190
Peters, Lulu Hunt, 51
Petersen, Alan, 79
Petrini, Carlo, 233
pharmafoods, 197
"pink slime," 222
Pitman-Moore, 141
Planck, Nina, 238
Planeat (documentary), 183
plant-based diet: Food Guide Pyramid
(1992) and, 95; Ornish diet, 100,
102
plant sterols: health benefits of, 158,
160, 161, 165, 167, 206; health
hazards of, 154, 200; margarine
fortified with, 4, 40, 152–153, 165,
206; sterol-fortified milk, 175
Pollan, Michael, 17–20, 110–111, 217,
231, 237, 238–240, 268n31, 293n73
polyunsaturated fats: blood cholesterol
levels and, 80; Dietary Goals (1977)
on, 89, 92; as good fats, 2, 26, 75, 81,
141; hydrogenation of, 137; refined
vegetable oil, 85. See also omega-3
fats
poultry: Dietary Goals (1977) on, 89, 92;
on Food Guide Pyramid (1992), 95;
nutrient density of, 163; omega-6
fats and, 311n48
Pratt, Steven, 174
Price, Weston A., 184
The Primal Blueprint (Sisson), 185
primary production quality, 226
Pritikin diet, 102
Pro Activ (margarine), 153
probiotic ice cream, 191
probiotic yogurt, 9, 158, 167
probiotics, 158, 160, 161

refined vegetable oil, 77, 83, 85, 118, 139, 169, 185, 187, *218*

Reinhard, Tonia, 174

Reiser, Raymond, 77, 82

Revolution at the Table (Levenstein), 17, 61

Richards, Byron, 167

rickets, 63, 64

risk. *See* disease risk; disease risk factors

Robbins, John, 184, 228

Roe, Brian, 207

Rose, Geoffrey, 283*n*26

Rose, Robert, 51–52

Rozin, Paul, 230

Rubner, Max, 57, 58

The Saccharine Disease (Cleave), 38, 82–83

Sacks, Frank, 119

salt: *Dietary Goals* (1977) on, 89, *89, 92*; *Dietary Guidelines* (1980) on, 94, *94*; in food guides, 76, 88; in food package labeling, 251

Santich, Barbara, 266*n*15, 272*n*37, 288*n*100

Saturated Fat Attack (CSPI), 142

saturated fats: in the American diet, 174; American Heart Association and, 3; as bad fats, 2, 26, 76, 144; cancer and, 104; diet-heart hypothesis, 79, 80, 81, 103, 137, 141, 311*n*48; *Dietary Goals* (1977) on, *89*, 92, *92*; dietary guidelines on, 86, 88, *89, 92, 92, 94*; *Dietary Guidelines* (1980) on, *94*; *Dietary Guidelines* (2010) on, 144; food sources of, 328*n*10; heart disease and, 1, 2, 30, 34, 75, 102; Keys on, 2, 26, 34, 75, 272*n*41; red meat and, 35; replacing with carbohydrates, 103

Schwartz, Hillel, 60, 62

scurvy, 63, 64, 68

Sears, Barry, 100

Senate Select Committee on Nutrition and Human Needs (McGovern Committee), 82, 87, 88, 107

sensual-practical experience, 13, 22, 60, 216, 231–235, 236, 237, 252, 253, *263*

Shapin, Steven, 43–44

Shapiro, Laura, 62

Shapiro, Samuel, 140

Sharp, Geoff, 266*n*13, 269*n*4

Silverman, Robert, 25

Simon, Michele, 203

Simopoulos, Artemis, 317*n*132

simplification, 5, 29, 32, 39, 41, 48, 57, 97, 252, 258

simulated foods, 223

Sisson, Mark, 185

"size acceptance" movement, 235

Sloan, Elizabeth, 203

"slow carbs," 129

Slow Food: The Case for Taste (Petrini), 233

Slow Food movement, 215, 233

Smart Balance (margarine), 162

Smart Choices program (promotional logo), 209

Smart Spot (promotional logo), 209

Snackwells phenomenon, 107

Snickers (candy bar), 130

soda, 38, 59, 77, 90, 94, 108, 112, 118, 193, 224

SoFAS (solid fats and added sugars), 36–37

solid fats, 36, 37–38, 144, 163, 247, 272*n*44

South Beach Diet (Agatston), 122

soy products, 227, 326*n*26

soybean oil, 144–145, 151

The Spectrum (Ornish), 127

sports drinks, 194

Stacey, Michelle, 193, 234
stanols, 152–153, 154, 161
Stare, Fred, 115
statin drugs, 78, 165
sterols. *See* plant sterols
Steward, Leighton, 122–123
sugar: artificial sweeteners, 40, 77, 119, 143; as bad carb, 160; chronic diseases and, 77; consumption and metabolic consequences, 7; diabetes and, 83, 104; *Dietary Goals* (1977) on, 89, *89*, 92; *Dietary Guidelines* (1980) on, 94, *94*; *Dietary Guidelines* (1990) on, 94; *Dietary Guidelines* (1995) on, 94; *Dietary Guidelines* (2010), 123; extracted/refined sugars, 38; on *Food Guide Pyramid* (1992), *95*, 96; in food guides, 76, 88; in food package labeling, 251; fructose, 39, 85, 117, 131, 160, *218*; glycemic index and, 131; heart disease and, 34, 82–83; LoGiCane, 131; obesity and, 117; sucrose, 39, 160
Sugar Busters! Cut Sugar to Trim Fat (Steward and Bethea), 100, 122–123
"superfoods," 36, 158, 174–175
Superfoods: The Food and Medicine of the Future (Wolf), 174
Superfoods: The Healthiest Food on the Planet (Reinhard), 174
SuperFoods Rx: Fourteen Foods That Will Change Your Life (Pratt and Matthews), 174
supplements: calcium, 68, 177; multinutrient, 39, 68, 176; vitamin, 39, 53, 65, 68, 69, 70, 176, 177
Surgeon General's Report on Nutrition and Health (1988), 101
sweets, on *Food Guide Pyramid* (1992), *95*, 96
synthetic foods, 223

Take Control (margarine), 153–154
Taller, Herman, 120, 296n117
Tapsell, Linda, 200, 237, 289n16
Taubes, Gary, 19–20, 88, 99, 110, 120, 121–122, 123, 124, 272n45, 296n112
taurine, 194
Taylorism, 61
"techno-foods," 192. *See also* functional foods
Tesco, GI labeling scheme, 127
Thomas, Paul, 69
Thompson, Jennifer, 176
Tickel, John, 166
traditional diets, 22, 184–185, 227–231
traffic light labeling systems, 209, 210, 212, 251
trans-fats: American Heart Association on, 145, 146; as bad fat, 1, 2, 26, 133, 144–149; blood cholesterol levels and, 137–140; consumption, 83; *Dietary Guidelines* (2010) on, 144; early studies of, 137; harmful effects of, 133; heart disease and, 139, 140m, 3; history, 7; Keys on, 272n41; labeling, 146, 304n60; low-*trans*-fat foods, 146–147; in margarine, 97, 133; naturally occurring, 136; production, 136–138; regulation, 146; research, 137–140; sources, 136; *trans*-fat-free foods, 146
trans-nutric foods, 40, 198–199, *262*, 273n51
A Treatise on Food and Diet (Pereira), 54
triglyceride levels, 83, 103, 164
Tropicana Healthy Heart Orange Juice, 157
Turner, Bryan, 58
Turner, Natasha, 167
Twinkie, Deconstructed (Ettlinger), 223
Twinkies, 225
type 2 diabetes. *See* diabetes

weight management: *Dietary Guidelines* (2010) on, 113–114; environmental toxins and, 325*n*22

Weight Watchers point plan, 120–121

Wesson Oil, 141

Western diet, 180–181, 240. *See also* American diet

Weston A. Price Foundation, 184–185, 215, 305*n*72

"What If It's All Been a Big Fat Lie?" (Taubes), 110

What to Eat (Nestle), 148

whole food ingredients, food classification system, *218*, 220, 222, *263*

whole foods: animal-based, 36; condemnation of, 77; in food classification system, 22, *218*, *219*, 220, 222; "health claim" status of, 175; omega-3 fats and, 19; plant-based, 36; promotion of, 20, 175; stigmatized as empty calories, 38

Whole Grain Stamp (Whole Grains Council), 209

whole grains, 38; *Dietary Guidelines* (1980) on, 94; disease risk and, 173, 174; on *Food Guide Pyramid*

(1992), 96; as good food, 76–77; research studies of, 242

Whole Grains Council, 209

whole milk: in American diet, 108; as bad food, 76; *Dietary Goals* (1977) on, 89, *89*, *92*

The Whole Soy Story (Daniel), 326*n*26

Why Calories Count (Nestle and Nesheim), 116, 296*n*112

Why We Get Fat (Taubes), 120

Willcox, Bradley, 184, 228

Willcox, Craig, 184

Willett, Walter, 3, 68, 96–97, 103, 123, 146, 147, 170, 176, 177

Wolf, David, 174

Wolf, Robb, 185

Women's Health Initiative, 103, 269*n*3

Women's Wonder Bar, 191

"wonder nutrients," 160

World Health Organization, 212

"world protein gap," 57

Yakult (yogurt drink), 194

yogurt, probiotic, 9

Yudkin, John, 34, 39, 77, 82, 83

The Zone (Sears), 100